COMPETENCIES FOR ADVANCED NURSING PRACTICE

COMPETENCIES FOR ADVANCED NURSING PRACTICE

Edited by

Sue Hinchliff RGN RNT BA MSc
Consultant in Advanced Nursing Practice to the Nursing and Midwifery
Council, UK
Visiting Professor in Nursing & Nursing Education, London South Bank
University, UK
and Consultant to RCN Accreditation Unit, London, UK

Rosemary Rogers BA RGN
Projects Director (Public Sector), Emap Inform, UK

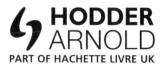

HODDER ARNOLD
PART OF HACHETTE LIVRE UK

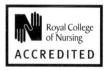
Royal College of Nursing
ACCREDITED

First published in Great Britain in 2008 by
Hodder Arnold, part of Hodder Education and a member of the Hachette Livre UK Group,
338 Euston Road, London NW1 3BH

http://www.hoddereducation.com

Hachette's policy is to use papers that are natural, renewable and recyclable products and made from wood grown in sustainable forests. The logging and manufacturing processes are expected to conform to the environmental regulations of the country of origin.

Whilst the advice and information in this book are believed to be true and accurate at the date of going to press, neither the author[s] nor the publisher can accept any legal responsibility or liability for any errors or omissions that may be made. In particular, (but without limiting the generality of the preceding disclaimer) every effort has been made to check drug dosages; however it is still possible that errors have been missed. Furthermore, dosage schedules are constantly being revised and new side-effects recognized. For these reasons the reader is strongly urged to consult the drug companies' printed instructions before administering any of the drugs recommended in this book.

British Library Cataloguing in Publication Data
A catalogue record for this book is available from the British Library

Library of Congress Cataloging-in-Publication Data
A catalog record for this book is available from the Library of Congress

ISBN   978-0-340-92768-7

1 2 3 4 5 6 7 8 9 10

Commissioning Editor:	Jo Koster
Development Editor:	Naomi Wilkinson
Project Editor:	Clare Patterson
Production Controller:	Andre Sim
Cover Design:	Laura De Grasse
Index:	Laurence Errington

Typeset in 10/12 Minion by Charon Tec Ltd., A Macmillan Company.

Printed and bound in Malta

CONTENTS

CONTRIBUTORS

Thomas D Barton PhD, MPhil, Bed, DipN, RNT, RGN
Chair of the Association of Advanced Nursing
Practice Educators, Council Member of the Welsh
Nursing Academy, Senior Lecturer, Coordinator of
Advanced Clinical Studies, School of Health Science,
Faculty of Health and Human Sciences, University of
Wales Swansea, UK

Audrey M Callum MSc, BSc(Hons), Pg Dip Ed, NP Dip, FETC, RGN
Senior Lecturer, Community Nursing and Nurse
Practitioner Programme, Buckinghamshire New
University, Faculty of Society and Health,
Department of Continuing and Advanced Practice,
Buckinghamshire, UK

Alison Crumbie RGN, Dip App SC N, BSc, MSN, NP, PGCE,
Doctorate NSc
Nurse Practitioner and Nurse Partner, Windermere
and Bowness Health Centre, Cumbria, UK

Heather Griffith MA, BSc (Hons), RGN, RSCN, RNT
Registered Independent Prescriber
Lecturer Practitioner for Advanced Nurse
Practitioner Programmes, School of Health and
Social Care, Bournemouth University, UK;
Committee member of the Association of Advanced
Nursing Practice Educators; Advanced Nurse
Practitioner, Royal Crescent Surgery, Weymouth, UK

Sue Hinchliff RGN, RNT, BA, MSc
Consultant in Advanced Nursing Practice to the
Nursing and Midwifery Council, UK; Visiting
Professor in Nursing & Nursing Education, London
South Bank University, UK; and Consultant to RCN
Accreditation Unit, London, UK

Caroline J Pennels BSc, MSc, MA, RGN, Barrister
Head of Legal Services, Gloucestershire Hospitals
NHS Foundation Trust, UK

Fiona Smart PhD, MEducation (Child Development), BEd (Hons)
Nurse Education, RGN, RSCN, RNT, DipN
Director of Studies for Learning Beyond Initial
Registration, School of Nursing and Midwifery,
University of Cumbria, Carlisle

Renate Thome MSc, BA, RN, HV, PGCE, Dip Couns
Lecturer, Course Director Advanced Clinical
Practice, Faculty of Health and Human Sciences,
Swansea University, UK

Nicola Whiteing PGDip HE, MSc, BSc (Hons), RN, RNT
Lecturer in Adult Nursing, St Bartholomew School
of Nursing and Midwifery, City University,
London, UK

Annaliese Willis MSc, BSc (Hons), NP Dip, Cert Ed, RN
Senior Lecturer and Course Director for MSc
Nurse Practitioner Programme at London
South Bank University, London, UK

HOW TO USE THIS BOOK

In 2002 the Royal College of Nursing Accreditation Unit (RCN AU), working with the course leaders of RCN accredited nurse practitioner programmes, developed a document called *Nurse Practitioners – an RCN guide to the nurse practitioner role, competencies and programme accreditation*. This detailed the domains and competencies for UK nurse practitioner practice.

As explained in the Preface, these domains and competencies later formed the basis for the NMC standards of proficiency for advanced nurse practitioners, that were consulted on in 2005 and signed off by the NMC Nursing Committee in September 2006. The profession is still awaiting (as of May 2008) confirmation by the Privy Council that advanced nursing practice will be registerable within the UK.

During the process of consultation and presentation to lay personnel and focus groups the ordering of the domains was altered and the working of some of the competencies was subtly changed. This text uses the order of domains and wording of competencies used in the NMC consultation document (NMC 2005) – but they differ only very slightly from the original RCN version. The differences are minor and not of substance.

We started to compile this text at a time when the NMC was confident that a level of practice beyond initial registration would be in place within a shorter timeframe than presently appears to be the case. However, the decision has been taken to go ahead with publication. This may mean that some of the wording may alter slightly when (and if) NMC finalise their standards. Essentially, though, this text contains the essence of what practitioners will be required to demonstrate in order to prove that they are competent to practice at an advanced level.

As editors it was our intention that the reader (most frequently we saw him or her as someone who was undertaking a course of preparation for practicing at an advanced level, or someone who was hoping to gain accreditation as an ANP by virtue of being able to produce a portfolio of evidence of practice at this level) would dip in and out of the book, rather than reading it from cover to cover.

It should be seen as a handbook, a guide to putting together credible evidence of advanced nursing practice. The reader might want to start off by studying chapters 1, 2 and 10 for background information on what advanced practice is, how it started in the UK, the legal and regulatory context and frameworks for it – and how to compile a portfolio and collect relevant and compelling evidence.

In chapters 3 to 9 the text explains each of the seven domains and the competencies that they contain. Readers will find that these chapters – each written by a different lecturer in advanced practice – differ in how they approach the various domains and competencies. Some take a micro approach, discussing each competency in turn – others are more broad brush. We hope that each will be of value.

Scenarios are frequently used to illustrate how ANPs might demonstrate their competence within a portfolio. Sometimes the authors offer reflective points where the reader is encouraged to draw on their own practice.

Essentially, each reader will use and apply what they find here in a different way – but we hope that it will become a key tool in the journey towards recognition of practising at an advanced level. We wish you a satisfying journey and a fulfilling outcome!

REFERENCES

Nursing & Midwifery Council (2005) *Consultation on a framework for the standards for post-registration nursing.* London: NMC.

RCN (2002) *Nurse Practitioners – an RCN guide to the nurse practitioner role, competencies and programme accreditation.* London: Royal College of Nursing.

FOREWORD

"If you want to walk fast, walk alone. But if you want to reach farther, look for a companion", Gabbra proverb, Marsabit District, Northern Kenya.

Writing this foreword has been, for me, something of a visit to the past. I was asked some months ago to do this, and I accepted the honor with particular pleasure because two of the authors are colleagues and friends from long ago and another was once a student of mine. And of course, the subject was absolutely compelling for me, having been an early supporter of advanced nursing roles. There is a sense of triumph in reading how far nursing has come in the last decade – arriving at a destination that was not even on the map when I was at the start of this journey. At that time the nurse practitioner programme had begun, but there was no official recognition of the advanced nursing role that it exemplified. We longed for overnight revolution! Yet the stronger way forward has proved to be a steady evolution, building on what was known and being practised and ensuring that there is now a robust, sustainable framework to support and nurture the advanced nursing role.

In Chapter 1 Griffith reminds us that the debate about the nature of advanced practice continues even now. While this may be frustrating to professional development, the ongoing debate does serve to remind us of the complexity of describing what nursing offers to health care. I have been away from the nursing field in the UK for some 15 years now but the impact that exploring the advanced nursing practice role had on my development stays with me still. One reason that those years are so unforgettable is the challenge that was inherent in unraveling those complexities of nursing and describing them to others. I relied heavily on Benner's domains of nursing practice (Benner, 1984), as a map constructed by one who had sought a route to clarity based on observations of practice, and it is heartening now to see these domains brought into this century and into the broader picture of the NHS skills framework. What a great (and rare) example of practice leading to theory which then underpins policy development! In Chapter 7 Crumbie looks in detail at the iteration between policy and practice in the nurse practitioner role, and how nurse practitioners have continued to collect and provide evidence to support their role development – is this unique to nursing? I think so!

So it is inspiring to read this book that articulates so clearly the competencies associated with the components of advanced nursing practice and conveys, through case studies, the ways in which each of the facets of nursing is intricately linked to the others. Just as striking is the way in which the competencies addressed here are relevant to all areas of nursing practice, marking a move towards shared identity in advanced practice across the many specialist areas in nursing. It is this unity that does indeed make it possible to walk further together – and that is one of the observations on this book that prompted me to include the saying from Kenya which begins this foreword. But it is not the only reason that this particular saying came to mind.

I heard this saying from a colleague who is actually from the North Central Province of Kenya. He was telling me that a companion can be a person, but could also be a camel – a common form of transport for the nomadic people in that area. He told me that it is vital to take care of your camel, so that it continues to support you and he said that he thinks of this as a message about supporting partnerships that enable us to continue to make progress. And that caused me to reflect on the many partnerships that advanced nursing practice has nurtured, both within nursing, as I have mentioned already, and outside nursing too.

In the early days of developing advanced nursing practice there were seemingly endless battles about territory – what was medicine and what nursing? What has evolved over time, it seems, is a way of working in partnership with physicians that brings out the best in both practitioners. Nurses are in a network of partnerships and as nursing becomes more expert the quality of these partnerships changes too. The advanced nurse practitioner engages, contributes and consults with others, secure in the boundaries of her knowledge and brave in asking for opinions and in acting as an advocate for patients. As this book reminds us, the willingness to reflect on our roles and relationships with others is characteristic of advanced practice.

More significant is the role that patients are now playing – experts in their own care, supporters of others, partners in their care plans. Thome talks about walking alongside patients in their journeys through illness and health, and this is a vivid image of partnership. And as the saying reminds us when two people walk together, they walk further. It is our privileged partnership with patients that teaches us how far we can walk! Advanced nursing practice has developed in the UK to meet the needs of those who had no other access to care, or to provide care that was previously not available at all (see p148). We can be proud that advanced nursing practice has grown out of our commitment to patients and our partnerships with them.

This is a book worth reading! It will guide you through the exciting world of advanced practice nursing, giving you enough history to show how far we have all come, but also practical information to help us continue to move forward. May you enjoy the journey!

Barbara Stilwell
Chapel Hill, North Carolina, USA

REFERENCE

Benner P. (1984). *From novice to expert: Excellence and power in clinical nursing practice.* Menlo Park, CA: Addison-Wesley.

PREFACE

The road towards the recognition of an advanced level of practice on the UK's register of nurses, midwives and health visitors has been long and tortuous - and is still not over. The latest proposal, at the time of going to press, awaits the outcome of a major consultation on a new nursing careers framework (DH, 2006) and decisions regarding the future regulation of advanced practice arising from the Department of Health's White Paper on the future regulation of health professionals (DH, 2007), before final ratification can be achieved.

The quest for full professional recognition began back in the early 1980s when the development of the first nurse practitioner role by Barbara Stilwell (distinguished author of the Foreword to this book) led to calls for the recognition and regulation of a branch of nurses beginning to extend their practice way beyond traditional roles. Since then its gestation has seen the publication of three different sets of competencies, has absorbed the Knowledge and Skills Framework set out in Agenda for Change (DH 2004) and the introduction of the nurse consultant role and it has emerged into a post-Shipman era determined (rightly) that public protection must be paramount.

In the absence of a recognized and distinct place on the register, however, and the enabling legislation to create one, nursing practice has burgeoned and few now could imagine a UK health service without the existence of nurse practitioners. As nursing practice itself has developed, driven by an impatience to prove that nursing values can successfully and beneficially complement the knowledge and skills traditionally located within a medical model of care, so the pressures of the modern health service have conspired to create conditions in which the development of the advanced nurse practitioner role is not just desirable but inevitable. The working time directive which limited the hours junior hospital doctors were allowed to work, the new General Medical Services contract and the development of nurse prescribing have all made it economically, as well as professionally, desirable that whole swathes of care – for those requiring anticoagulant therapy, those with Parkinson's disease or dementia, those receiving intravenous or oxygen therapy at home, and many others in both primary and secondary care settings – should be not just delivered but directed and managed by nurses operating at an advanced level of practice.

The first set of RCN-accredited nurse practitioner programmes started running in UK universities in 2002, based on competencies anglicized from those developed in the US by the National Organization of Nurse Practitioner Faculties (NONPF). Many nurses have completed these RCN-accredited courses, or sought alternative routes to advanced practice and are practising at that level today. These competencies formed the basis of the current RCN framework for nurse practitioners which was subsequently adopted by the NMC and received Council's approval in December 2005. They are reproduced in full in the Appendix to this book.

Although yet to be formally ratified, such is their currency and importance that the decision was taken not to delay publication further and these competencies or domains therefore form the backbone to this book. It describes each of the domains in turn but begins and ends with chapters which seek to explain the nature and history of advanced practice, its legal base and the academic and accreditation process required to achieve it.

Heather Griffith's chapter charts in some detail the journey towards advanced practice and offers profiles of nurses working at that level. Caroline Pennels then sets out the legal implications of advanced practice – looking at what it means in law to be called an advanced practitioner, the different standards expected in comparison with those required of the 'ordinary' practitioner, and how this relates to the professional backdrop. Subsequent chapters take each individual domain in turn, detailing its theoretical base but explaining what that means in practice. Each one is liberally illustrated with stories, profiles and practical examples of how the theory is put into practice. Finally, Sue Hinchliff examines the accreditation process required of the nurse seeking to be recognized as an advanced practitioner – the evidence and profiling he or she is expected to maintain and the different ways in which an advanced level can be proved.

The book is aimed largely at those nurses seeking to become advanced practitioners – but we hope it will also be used by those already practising at that level as well as by lecturers and by those who manage or work with advanced nurse practitioners (ANPs). It is the first of its kind and is meant to support both their studies and their practice. Similarly, as advanced practice is not a concept that is confined to nursing but also increasingly evident in the practice and education of allied health professionals, this book should also prove a valuable resource in that arena.

In an ideal world the publication of this book would have been timed to coincide with – indeed to celebrate - the final definite creation of a separate place on the register for advanced nurse practitioners. But just as ANPs themselves have decided that the needs and demands of their patients, their health service and their own professional development could not wait, and have developed their practice and their standards accordingly, so we feel that neither could a publication to support that practice be further delayed. By the time of publication we hope the decision is finally ratified – and look forward to a second edition reflecting that fact!

Sue Hinchliff and Rosemary Rogers,
May 2008

REFERENCES

Department of Health (2004). *Agenda for Change: Final Agreement.* London: DH.
Department of Health (2006). *Modernising Nursing careers – setting the direction.* London: DH.
Department of Health (2007). *Trust, Assurance and Safety – The Regulation of Health professionals in the 21st Century.* London: HMSO.

ACKNOWLEDGEMENTS

The editors would like to thank Katrina Maclaine for her help in the early stages of the book's development.

1 WHAT IS ADVANCED NURSING PRACTICE?

HEATHER GRIFFITH

INTRODUCTION

The decision by the Nursing and Midwifery Council (NMC) in 2005 to support the regulation of the advanced nurse practitioner (ANP) role has major implications that will prompt significant debate. For the first time in United Kingdom (UK) history the regulatory council agreed that an advanced part of the nursing register should be opened. For the many nurses who have been leading and developing advanced nursing roles in the past 20 years throughout the UK, this was a welcome verdict. There is compelling evidence to suggest that ANPs contribute significantly to health care delivery (Horrocks et al. 2002, Laurant et al. 2004a) and clarifying the concept of 'advanced nursing practice' will facilitate further innovation. However, despite this decision being centrally relevant, it will have profound repercussions.

The aim of this chapter is to present an overview of the history and development of advanced nursing practice roles in the UK, to outline the definition and competencies agreed by the NMC (2005), and to consider future issues as modernization and reform of the National Health Service (NHS) continues. Personal reflection is included which reveals the perspectives of four nurses, currently engaged in advanced practice roles, for whom the NMC decision has implications.

BACKGROUND

Social trends are increasing demands on health care as the population lives longer and treatments advance with technology. However, there are significant gaps within the workforce in meeting patient needs, and the current pattern of service provision will not be sustainable (Wanless 2002). Nurses play a prominent role in health care provision in the NHS, and advanced nursing roles have been identified in policy documents (NAfW 1999, DoH 2000a, DoH 2002, SEHD 2005, NIPEC 2005) as key to further reform and to cost savings. Policy changes encouraged entrepreneurship and nurses in primary care are now able to run nurse-led primary care practices and become partners in general practices (DoH 2006). In secondary care, pioneering roles have succeeded in demonstrating improved quality of care for patients, as traditional role boundaries are challenged and new ways of working are actively encouraged (DoH 2005a). These changes not only apply to the nursing and medical professions but there is also a focus on innovation and remodelling in all health care occupations. Allied health professionals (AHPs) such as pharmacists, physiotherapists and optometrists are being actively encouraged to advance their scope of practice and work autonomously (DoH 2000b). The *Future Health Worker* report (Kendall and Lissaur 2003) recommended that workforce planning needs to focus on developing existing staff to work in different ways (across traditional boundaries) in addition to creating new roles.

The framework that underpins the current career changes was introduced in *Agenda for Change* (NHSE 1999, DoH 2004a), a strategy that signalled the Government's intention for a more flexible workforce. This established a direct link between pay thresholds and professional competencies with the intention that all NHS employees might have more flexible career opportunities with greater transfer of skills. The Knowledge and Skills Framework (KSF) is a key part of the NHS *Agenda for Change* (DoH 2004b) and is the mechanism through which pay progression operates. It applies to all staff employed in the NHS across the UK (with the exception of doctors, dentists and board-level managers). As the KSF is a broad generic framework it does not describe the exact knowledge and skills that people need to develop. The specific competencies for ANPs, as defined by the NMC, have been mapped against the KSF Framework (Appendix 1) and it is the application of these that must be demonstrated. The British Medical Association (BMA 2002) recognized the workforce challenge that the NHS faces and has acknowledged the vital contribution of ANPs in care delivery.

The development of a national career framework for the NHS (SfH 2005) also has implications for advanced nursing roles. The generic framework offers nine levels through which careers can be progressed (Table 1.1) and is intended to ensure consistency across the entire NHS workforce. It is based on the concept of 'skills escalation' offering staff guidance on career progression through development of their personal skills and competencies. Career frameworks have been published for health care scientists (DoH 2005b) but work is still in progress regarding the alignment of nursing roles with the Careers Framework. It would seem reasonable to presume that the competencies agreed for ANPs (NMC 2005) correspond with level 7, Advanced Practitioner, although this has yet to be confirmed. *Modernising nursing careers* (DoH 2006) was launched to examine strategies for defining and clarifying career pathways for nurses and is a joint project between the four UK countries. Currently, Scotland is leading on initiatives for 'advanced' practice and is piloting a framework to support the development of advanced practice attributes (NES 2007).

The current scrutiny of professional regulation is another important contextual consideration for health care workers. The Bristol Inquiry (BRII 2003) prompted a review of professional self-regulation and in 2003 the Council for Health Care Regulatory Excellence (CHRE) was established by parliament to ensure consistency and good practice across each of the nine regulators (including the NMC). The Government has specifically requested that the CHRE work with regulators on the development of 'common standards and systems' across professional groups with

TABLE 1.1 *NHS career framework for health*

9	More senior staff – Level 9 Staff with the ultimate responsibility for clinical caseload decision-making and full on-call accountability
8	Consultant practitioners – Level 8 Staff working at a very high level of clinical expertise and/or have responsibility for planning services
7	Advanced practitioners – Level 7 Experienced clinical professionals who have developed their skills and theoretical knowledge to a very high standard. They are empowered to make high-level clinical decisions and will often have their own caseload. Non-clinical staff at level 7 will typically be managing a number of service areas
6	Senior practitioners/specialist practitioners – Level 6 Staff who would have a higher level of autonomy and responsibility than 'practitioners' in the clinical environment, or would be managing one or more service areas in the non-clinical environment
5	Practitioners – Level 5 Most frequently registered practitioners in their first or second post-registration/ professional qualification jobs.
4	Assistant practitioners/associate practitioners – Level 4 Probably studying for foundation degree, BTEC (Business & Technician Education Council) Higher or HND. Some of their remit will involve them in delivering protocol-based clinical care that had previously been in the remit of registered professionals, under the supervision of a state registered practitioner.
3	Senior health care assistants/technicians – Level 3 Have a higher level of responsibility than support worker, probably studying for, or have attained NVQ level 3, or Assessment of Prior Experiential Learning (APEL)
2	Support workers – Level 2 Frequently with the title of 'health care assistant' or 'health care technician' – probably studying or has attained NVQ level 2
1	Initial entry level jobs – Level 1 Such as 'domestics' or 'cadets' requiring very little formal education or previous knowledge, skills or experience in delivering or supporting the delivery of health care

http://www.skillsforhealth.org.uk/page/career-frameworks (accessed 04/04/08)

regards to advanced practitioners in nursing and AHPs (DoH 2007). Although it is clear that each individual regulatory body will be in charge of approving standards which registrants will need to meet, it seems likely that coherence will be demanded in defining 'advanced practitioner' across all non-medical professions. In many ways ANPs are at an advantage, in that the NMC has agreed regulatory documentation in support of this specific role (Table 1.2), although legislation has yet to be approved at the time of writing. In order for the NMC to open a further subpart of the nurses' register it has to seek permission from the Privy Council and a response is still awaited (NMC 2007).

TABLE 1.2 *Nursing and Midwifery Council approved definition for advanced nurse practitioners*

Advanced nurse practitioners are highly experienced and educated members of the care team who are able to diagnose and treat your health care needs or refer you to an appropriate specialist if needed.
Advanced nurse practitioners are highly skilled nurses who can:

- take a comprehensive patient history
- carry out physical examinations
- use their expert knowledge and clinical judgement to identify the potential diagnosis
- refer patients for investigations where appropriate
- make a final diagnosis
- decide on and carry out treatment, including the prescribing of medicines, or refer patients to an appropriate specialist
- use their extensive practice experience to plan and provide skilled and competent care to meet patients' health and social care needs, involving other members of the health care team as appropriate
- ensure the provision of continuity of care including follow-up visits
- assess and evaluate, with patients, the effectiveness of the treatment and care provided and make changes as needed
- work independently, although often as part of a health care team
- provide leadership
- make sure that each patient's treatment and care is based on best practice.

Only nurses who have achieved the competencies set by the Nursing and Midwifery Council for a registered advanced nurse practitioner are permitted to use the title advanced nurse practitioner. The title will be protected through a registrable qualification in the Council's register.

NMC 2005.

This section has considered the contemporary context of health care in the UK including the structure, organization and delivery of services, and how this has influence on the development of ANP roles. In order to explore the concept of 'advanced nursing practice' further it is necessary to consider the development of these roles from a historical perspective.

HISTORY AND DEVELOPMENT OF ADVANCED NURSE PRACTITIONER ROLES

The circumstances that led to the initial development of nurse practitioner roles in the USA and UK are comparable. In the 1960s, American nurse practitioners were employed in response to a shortage of doctors and inaccessibility to health care, especially for disadvantaged groups (Harris and Redshaw 1998, Ketefian et al. 2001, Furlong and Smith 2005). In the UK the first nurse practitioner was employed in the 1980s as a pilot project to address the health care needs of Muslim women in primary care (Stilwell 1982). In the late 1980s nurses in accident and emergency departments (A&E) extended their skills to attend to the needs of patients presenting with 'minor injuries' to reduce excessive waiting times (Marsden et al. 2003). The potential for utilizing nursing skills further was recognized in policy documents at that time.

New patterns of treatment and care will stimulate changes in professional practice in both hospital and community settings. Carefully evaluated innovations to change traditional boundaries of clinical and professional practice need to be encouraged. New nursing concepts are being tested and evaluated; they include the primary nurse, the nurse practitioner and the nurse consultant.

DoH (1989: 13)

The development of those roles coincided with the Government facing criticism of neglect towards the NHS (Read et al. 2001). The response was publication of *The Patient's Charter* (DoH 1991a) and this initiative, together with funding, resulted in further opportunities for role development. Workforce restructuring also resulted from the Department of Health's directives to reduce the working hours of junior doctors (DoH 1991b), which was felt acutely in areas such as A&E.

The nursing profession itself also contributed to advanced role development, and in 1992 the United Kingdom Central Council (UKCC), the nursing profession's statutory body at that time, issued its *Scope of professional practice* document, which sanctioned further progress. Although it did not clarify the competencies required for 'advanced practice', nurses were no longer required to gain certificates for tasks and practice was limited only by personal competence. A pilot project, Higher Level Practice, was undertaken by the UKCC in an attempt to test and set a standard (UKCC 1999), although neither an agreed definition nor title resulted. This lack of clarity led to confusion and ambiguity about the role (Torn and McNichol 1998, Smithson 1999, Walsh 1999, Read and Roberts-Davis 2000, Castledine 2003, Daly and Carnwell 2003, Czuber-Dochan et al. 2006) and inconsistent approaches to education preparation (Ketefian et al. 2001, Cox 2002).

In 1996 the Royal College of Nursing (RCN) led the direction by agreeing the definition of nurse practitioner practice in the UK (RCN 1996), and setting standards for educational preparation (RCN 2002). The competencies agreed were based on those produced by the National Organisation of Nurse Practitioner Faculties (NONPF) in North America and embraced the traditional ideals of nursing within a specific role identity. These competencies have informed the definition of advanced nursing practice subsequently agreed by the NMC, and the requirements for this are now clearly defined (Furlong and Smith 2005).

Coxhead (1993) proposed that nurses themselves were key drivers in the development of advanced roles, frustrated by their inability to have their knowledge, skills or expertise recognized. A decade later Colyer (2004) suggests that the value and potential of advanced nursing roles were more widely acknowledged and had become 'embedded' in the NHS.

A survey conducted in 2006 revealed that nurse practitioners have established roles in both primary and secondary care in a wide variety of settings (Ball 2006). Examples include general practice, walk-in centres, out-of-hours services, A&E departments, minor injury units, pre-assessment clinics, medical assessment units and areas such as paediatrics and ophthalmology (RCN 2008). However, because the role was unregulated, educational preparation has been variable and there is risk that nurses may be using the title 'nurse practitioner' without undertaking the appropriate level of study to underpin the knowledge and competence required (RCN 2008).

In 2004 the NMC acknowledged this concern and launched a consultation regarding a framework for the regulation of advanced practice. It stated:

> The NMC shares the concerns of both the public and the profession that some nurses may hold job titles that imply an advanced level of knowledge and competence that may be beyond the level they hold. There has been a rapid growth in the number of titles that suggest practice at a higher level. The concern is that currently the public cannot be sure that the level of expertise and competence of the nurse providing care is commensurate with their title.
>
> NMC (2004: 3)

The final report presented to the council showed considerable support for the proposal, and in June 2005 the Council agreed that 'advanced nurse practitioner' should be a registrable qualification and that the NMC should seek approval from the Privy Council for opening a further subpart to the nurses' register for advanced practice. A policy was also agreed for accommodating existing practitioners, including those who had completed RCN-approved programmes and those who had undertaken alternative routes. Personal portfolios of evidence prepared for recognition would require demonstration of competence in each of the domains of practice.

This section has reviewed the development of ANP roles in the UK. It is evident that some confusion and inconsistency exists but, despite this, ANPs have led service delivery and innovation. In the first of four scenarios an advanced nurse working in secondary care presents his perspective.

Scenario 1.1

Geoffrey is a Modern Matron for Medicine in a Foundation Trust hospital. His role incorporates both management and clinical skills, and he is actively engaged in patient care via his own nurse-led cardiology clinic. Previously he was a nurse practitioner in coronary and intensive care.

My position is fairly unique in that I am a matron with budget-holding and management responsibilities, and also an ANP – running my own clinic for cardiology patients. I have always been an advocate for ANPs – whether at ward level or in specialized areas. My ethos has always been to encourage professional development in my staff – and this is key to recruitment and retention. I currently have responsibility for 350 staff in nine clinical areas. I observe nurses undergoing nurse practitioner training and I can see the difference in their ability – I see the different ways in which medical colleagues relate to them, I see the difference it makes to patient care.

When I began my training I didn't want to be a 'good' nurse I wanted to be the 'best'. I have reached the level I have because I've worked hard within my Trust, I've gained the necessary qualifications – albeit in a fragmented way (as I haven't done a nurse practitioner degree). In some ways this has been the drawback of unregulated 'advanced' roles – in that my skills are not necessarily transferable outside this Trust. I certainly have the experience and can demonstrate my competence – but this may not be recognized elsewhere. And this is unsatisfactory for the NHS – even if you are a qualified nurse practitioner with a degree – individual Trusts may well set their own standards for what they want or do not want you to do and this is what I hope that the NMC registration for ANPs will sort out. What I hope is that now the NMC has set a standard – that this will regulate practice, protect a recognizable title and improve transferability of qualifications. This is what is needed, because in the NHS at the moment we have variability between Trusts – even within the same region – and that could compromise patient care.

How do we gain credibility as advanced practice nurses? We gain credibility by enhanced knowledge, communication and team-working. Using language that reveals clinical knowledge improves credibility. Nurses working at advanced level think at an advanced level – they see patients in a different way. In my clinic I do things that would be expected of a doctor: patients are referred directly to me either from a GP or from a consultant. I see them, assess them, cannulate them, I treat them and monitor them through the investigation, and I then discharge them. I manage the complete patient pathway. I feel very competent to do that because I've been trained and can demonstrate my competence. I believe the service has improved since I took over the clinic because, in the past, a doctor would be asked to cover the clinic – perhaps without much prior experience – whereas I have developed expertise in this specialty and patients appreciate this. I believe the patient experience is central to service development and I am driven in this respect. In terms of improvement, I have reduced the waiting list from 26 weeks to 2–3 and there is now another ANP working with me.

I have a fundamental belief that when you're ill you deserve the best possible care – second best will not do. ANPs have great potential as well as demonstrable competence in delivering high-quality care. But regulation is important – and although I would find compiling a portfolio of evidence time-consuming and a challenge, the incentive is there. So I would want to go on to the advanced register, not because I have to, but because I want to.

In this scenario Geoffrey raises important issues for consideration. He draws attention to the impact that unregulated titles and non-standardized education and preparation have had on transferability within the NHS. The next section will explore the complexity of defining ANP practice.

DEFINING THE PRACTICE OF ADVANCED NURSE PRACTITIONERS

There is much ongoing debate regarding the definition of 'advanced practice' (Woods 1999, Castledine 2003, Carnwell and Daly 2003, Bryant-Lukosius and DiCenso 2004, Colyer 2004, Furlong and Smith 2005), complicated further by the huge variation in clinical contexts and settings in which advanced nursing roles have evolved (Lloyd Jones 2005, Mantzoukas and Watkinson 2006). The rapid rise in the number of ANPs has resulted in different models of practice emerging (Woods 2006) and challenges to those who are expected to work beyond the traditional nursing role. Confusion is also compounded in that some trusts have not distinguished clearly between specialist, advanced and nurse practitioner roles (Williams et al. 2001).

Although the debate is likely to continue, many authors have agreed that autonomy is a defining element of advanced practice (Castledine 2003, Bryant-Lukosius et al. 2004, Ball and Cox 2004). Ulrich et al. (2003: 319) describe autonomy as the 'freedom to make binding decisions based on discretion, expertise, and clinical knowledge within the scope of practice'. Legal accountability is an important consideration for advanced practitioners who are professionally autonomous and these concepts are discussed more fully in Chapter 2. However, the reference point for all ANPs is the Code (NMC 2008), which dictates that practice is bound by an ability to demonstrate personal competence.

In 2001 Ormond-Walshe and Newham analysed the discrete differences between clinical nurse specialist (CNS) and nurse practitioner (NP) roles and proposed that the specialist role utilizes a narrower knowledge and skills base within a defined area. Daly and Carnwell (2003) presented a framework for transition to competence, emphasizing another clear difference, in that ANPs deal with undiagnosed patients and conduct comprehensive health assessments, diagnosis, intervention and discharge or referral. The authors propose that the degree of expertise and autonomy differentiates the two levels. Castledine (2003) explains that confusion between the terms specialist and advanced exists because both were used synonymously to refer to practice beyond initial registration. He acknowledges that the role of the ANP differs in terms of advancement.

In 2002 the RCN agreed a definition for ANPs and made recommendations for their educational preparation (RCN 2008). They defined an ANP as:

> A registered nurse who has undertaken a specific course of study of at least first degree (Honours) level and who:
> Makes professionally autonomous decisions, for which he or she is accountable
> Receives patients with undifferentiated and undiagnosed problems and makes an assessment of their health care needs, based on highly developed nursing knowledge and skills, including skills not usually exercised by nurses, such as physical examination
> Screens patients for disease factors and early signs of illness
> Makes differential diagnosis using decision-making and problem-solving skills
> Develops with the patient an ongoing nursing care plan for health, with an emphasis on preventative measures
> Orders necessary investigations, and provides treatment and care both individually, as part of a team, and through referral to other agencies
> Has a supportive role in helping people to manage and live with illness
> Provides counselling and health education
> Has the authority to admit or discharge patients from their caseload, and refer patients to other health care providers as appropriate
> Works collaboratively with other health care professionals and disciplines
> Provides a leadership and consultancy function as required
>
> RCN (2008: 3)

The key components of the RCN competencies correlate with those that have been approved by the NMC (Table 1.2). The NMC's (2005) decision to open a subpart of the nursing register is significant for the nursing profession as a whole. For the first time a clear outline of the core standard of proficiency for advanced practice has been defined by the regulatory authority. Furthermore, a precise definition for ANPs has been agreed, with indication that the title will be protected, and criteria for educational programmes will be established. There is optimism that this policy will facilitate implementation of future advanced nursing roles, and resolve the role ambiguity that hindered development in the past (Lloyd Jones 2005). Additionally, regulation will ensure that safety, effectiveness and quality of practice are monitored, leading to further 'legitimacy' of the role (Bryant-Lukosius et al. 2004).

At an international level there is little differentiation between advanced practice and the role title of 'nurse practitioner' as is evident in the following definition from the International Council of Nurses (ICN):

> A Nurse Practitioner/Advanced Practice Nurse is a registered nurse who has acquired the expert knowledge base, complex decision-making skills and clinical competencies for expanded practice, the characteristics of which are shaped by the context and/or country in which s/he is credentialed to practice. A master's degree is recommended for entry level.
>
> ICN (2002)

This also supports a recommendation in the broader literature that advanced practitioners should demonstrate 'masters level ability' (Hughes 2005). The recommended academic level for programmes of education will be discussed in the next section. However, the NMC have agreed that ANPs should demonstrate 'masters level thinking' (NMC 2005).

An additional aspect that appears in the literature is related to personal attributes of advanced practitioners such as self-motivation, capability and determination for professional development (Read and Roberts-Davis 2000, Griffith 2004, Elsom et al. 2005, Gardner et al. 2008). Fulbrook (1998) suggests that advanced nursing practice is 'a complex composite of knowledge and experience applied in a unique way according to each situation through the medium of self' (p. 100). Advanced practitioners require an ability to engage in critical reflection on the nature of nursing and the beliefs, judgements and values that underpin it (Elsom et al. 2005). Furlong and Smith (2005) describe the personal 'challenge' that ANPs face. Self-awareness is a powerful attribute that enhances consultation, collaboration and communication skills, all of which are fundamental to the ANP role. Authors agree that it is the combination of these personal attributes together with all, rather than some of, the specified skills that distinguishes advanced practice from other nursing roles (Castledine 2003, Carlisle 2003).

In summary, this section has considered the definition of ANP practice and presented issues of contention. In the second of the scenarios included in this chapter, the perspective of an advanced practitioner working in primary care is presented.

Scenario 1.2

Rosemary is employed in a general practice on the south coast of England. She worked as a practice nurse for 19 years before undertaking a nurse practitioner degree and states that her practice has changed immeasurably as a result.

I had been a practice nurse for 19 years and had done many courses, including family planning, asthma, COPD, A51 Practice Nurse, Advanced Life

Support, CHD training, etc., and I wanted to formalize what I'd done. My role was continually evolving and the nurse practitioner (NP) degree offered me the opportunity to consolidate my skills and develop them further. With the skills from the NP degree I could be more autonomous and offer patients a 'one-stop-appointment' and deal with any other problems that arose during their consultation. For instance, in the asthma clinic, if the patient had a chest infection I would have had to refer to a GP for examination, investigation and prescribing. Now I'm able to do this myself.

I didn't call myself a 'nurse practitioner' until I'd completed my training and had a job as an NP. Changing identity from a practice nurse to a nurse practitioner was challenging. Even though I had completed the training there was a steep learning curve once I started to practise as an NP. The NP degree opens your eyes to what you don't know ... the more you learn the more you realize what there is to learn – my role is now totally different.

I work autonomously as an NP and Independent Nurse Prescriber – and I am accountable for my practice. I work 35 hours a week in clinical practice – much of that open access. I can request and interpret my own investigations. Patients book directly to see me and I don't know in advance what problems they're going to see me about – I have to be equipped to deal with anything. The role is well evaluated and patients choose to come and see me. I have never had a problem in being accepted by patients – they are happy to book to see a NP. The only difficulty I encountered initially was having my referrals accepted by some of the local consultants, but this is no longer a problem. I hope in the future that I will be able to request X-rays when the necessary changes to local policy have been made.

Advancing my skills is also about collaborating with colleagues – I manage the nursing team, which comprises two nurse practitioners, three practice nurses and one health care assistant. Within the team I have developed nurse protocols and training. I am the mentor for our health care assistant and trained as an NVQ 3 assessor (A1/A2) in order for her to gain her NVQ3 in Care. It's also about managing my role: because when I do need to refer a patient to see a GP there has to be a system in place to support that. I have regular clinical supervision and meet with my GP mentor every 2 weeks for case note analysis and review of clinical decision-making.

I'm very pleased that the NMC are planning to protect the Advanced Nurse Practitioner title. This will protect the public by ensuring that only nurses that are registered with the NMC and have achieved the competencies will be allowed to use the title. Importantly it will ensure public safety and give guidance to other nurses and health care professionals about the role.

Rosemary reveals the impact of education in support of her developing role and ongoing clinical supervision. In the next section the issues surrounding educational preparation are discussed.

EDUCATIONAL PREPARATION OF ADVANCED NURSE PRACTITIONERS

Currently in the UK there is no regulatory framework for the education of advanced practice nurses, and as a result there is inconsistency in the academic preparation of

ANPs (Woods 1999, Bryant-Lukosius et al. 2004, Laurant et al. 2004a). In the early 1990s, the RCN developed a specific programme of education at honours degree level based on NONPF guidelines (RCN 2008) and this has been viewed by some as a 'minimum standard' for the education of ANPs. Since 2002 the RCN Accreditation Unit has accredited programmes offered at Higher Education Institutes that have attained the required standards. Simultaneously, a number of universities have developed programmes designed to prepare students for advanced practice, often at master's degree level, but have not sought RCN accreditation. Regardless of the route undertaken, it is the demonstration of clinical competence against each of the specified advanced level outcomes that is the key requirement (Furlong and Smith 2005). Specific guidance on collating evidence of personal practice is given in Chapter 10.

The NMC has yet to clarify precise details of the standards for educational programmes, although it is likely that 'masters-level thinking' will be a required outcome (NMC 2005). This correlates with consensus within the literature internationally and within the UK regarding academic level (ICN 2002, Hughes 2005, NES 2007), although the current NMC proposal does not specify a complete master's programme.

One additional benefit of achieving standardized training for advanced practitioners is the prospect of increased validity in future research. Few studies reviewed by Laurant et al. (2004a) specified detail about the educational preparation that the practitioner under investigation had for their advanced practice role. It could be argued that validity of results may be jeopardized given the tremendous variability that exists among advanced nurses.

There is no doubt that educators will need to respond to the emerging requirements for advanced practice, and foremost of these will be the consideration of patient and service needs. Opportunities for interprofessional learning will facilitate collaborative working in the modernized NHS (NES 2007). Emphasis should be placed on the learning environment and mentor support (Griffith 2004, Pauly et al. 2004, Williamson et al. 2006), and curriculum content and assessment processes must reflect regulator requirements. It is interesting to note that the NMC expect ANPs to 'prescribe medications' (Table 1.2), yet currently the Independent Nurse Prescribing programme is not consistently incorporated within advanced practice programmes. Research suggests that prescriptive authority is an integral aspect of advanced practice and should not be overlooked in curriculum development (Furlong and Smith 2005, Williams and Jones 2006).

Continuing professional development (CPD) is an essential feature of advanced practice (Ketefian et al. 2001) and is exemplified in the scenario that follows.

Scenario 1.3

Tracy is a British Heart Foundation (BHF) heart failure specialist nurse and is also an independent prescriber. She completed an NP programme (post-graduate diploma) 2 years ago and is currently working on her dissertation to complete an MSc Nurse Practitioner degree. Although originally funded by the BHF, she is now employed by her local Primary Care Trust. She is the principal research investigator for Better Together, a new supportive and palliative care service for patients with heart failure. She is also a facilitator on the advanced communication skills course for BHF nurses, for which she recently received an award.

My role involves managing patients in the community with a diagnosis of heart failure and preventing their admission to hospital. Patients are referred to me by cardiologists, GPs, community nurses and nurse practitioners – there is a high prevalence of confirmed heart failure in elderly people and my goal is to improve their quality of life and improve life expectancy. I review and optimize their treatment and in order to do that I have to take a detailed history, physically examine them and then make decisions about their medications. Frequently this involves taking patients off inappropriate medicines before optimizing the drugs they should be on. Originally my role was funded by the BHF and during the first 3 years it was evaluated by York University. This research revealed that the Trust can't afford not to have us – because every patient we see saves the Primary Care Trust around £2600. But it's not just about saving money – it's also about improving patient care. Patients say to me 'I wish I'd known you a long time ago' – because they previously hadn't heard about the heart failure service. That's a lesson for us really – to promote the service more.

Patients value my role because I visit them in their own homes – I can spend time listening to their anxieties, discussing their symptoms and reviewing their medications. I also provide support for their families or carers. If blood tests are required I can do these, interpret the results and amend drug dosage if necessary. I would say about 80 per cent of my work is home visits and I generally see the high-intensity patients – those with stage three or four heart failure. Unfortunately mortality rates are high and palliative care is an important aspect of my role. I manage this through liaison with health care team members such as the Marie Curie nurses.

Frequently I am phoned by GPs who may ask for advice about medicine management of specific patients. They may phone and say 'this patient is still breathless and I've done this with the diuretics and I don't know where to go next' and I'll take over and monitor the patient as medication is titrated or adjusted. They don't refer straightforward patients – it's often the ones with complex problems: with co-morbidities and/or multiple medications. I am a link between primary and secondary care – and I often reinforce that to patients. It's reassuring for them to know that if their next cardiology review is booked in 3 months time I will see them before this, if necessary. Patients appreciate this – they see me as a link between their GP and their consultant.

I have a very rewarding job. Just over 3 years ago I was a staff nurse on the critical care unit, but I knew I could do a more autonomous role and be responsible for my professional decisions. That is what led me to further education. I wanted to do the nurse practitioner course because I'd seen the programme and thought 'this is exactly what I need to know and want to learn' – I wanted to be autonomous. But prior to this I'd worked on a medical ward where my manager didn't agree that this was an appropriate course – mainly because I wouldn't be able to use the skills in that particular role. So it took a move to a new department where I was supported in my desire to advance my skills – and I was put forward for training.

I couldn't do the job I have now without the skills I learned on the nurse practitioner programme. Everything I studied is important for my current role. Even areas that I'd studied before – such as health promotion theory – I've applied and use daily. In particular the 'entrepreneurial skills' we were taught

> helped me to have a broader understanding of the context of health care, and I was able to write a proposal for my current job. I'm always setting myself goals – learning never stops does it? And I now lecture at conferences all over the country – and I enjoy that – sharing good practice.
>
>   I think the NMC's decision to protect and regulate the ANP role is extremely important. There need to be explicit standards for advanced practice roles in order that patients and health care colleagues are assured of 'fitness to practice'.

This scenario illustrates an ANP with expert knowledge and skills, providing a valuable service greatly appreciated by the patients for whom she cares. Effort to audit and quantify her work in terms of measurable outcomes has revealed cost benefits, but this is only part of the picture. There is a need to consider how future research will capture the 'essence' of advanced nursing practice.

FUTURE ISSUES

The development of new roles is often contentious, with perceived threats to existing health care professionals and standards of patient care, but the NMC's proposal for advanced practice regulation will provide structure and clarity for the NHS workforce. However, there is legitimate concern that advanced nursing roles developed to undertake skills previously undertaken by doctors will be medically driven rather than grounded in nursing (Bryant-Lukosius et al. 2004). This is illustrated in recent debate within the USA regarding American NPs in which the American Medical Association (AMA) Young Physicians' Section voted to seek change in legislation, in order that regulation of NPs came under medical, rather than nursing, jurisdiction (AMA 2007). This has been robustly defended by the American College of Nurse Practitioners (ACNP 2007) but clearly illustrates that contention remains despite 40 years of established NP practice. Collaborative interprofessional working will require strategic planning to facilitate greater understanding and acceptance of advanced practice roles (Reay et al. 2003, Bryant-Lukosius and DiCenso 2004). Hughes (2005) anticipates that practice-based commissioning, designed to support development of local services, is an opportunity for reshaping and redesigning patient-focused care, but managers must utilize leadership strategies to fully implement the skills and realize the potential of ANPs (Reay et al. 2003, Jasper 2005). And it is imperative that nurses themselves engage at organizational level to influence and lead health care policy.

  There is good support in the literature that ANPs make significant contributions to health service delivery, offering more holistic care than medical colleagues (Seale et al. 2006), which results in increased patient satisfaction (Horrocks et al. 2002, Laurant et al. 2004a). Coxhead (1993) established that ANPs exhibit more personal interest, provide more information, health promotion and psychosocial support, and possess better communication and interviewing skills than other health care providers. This evidence supports the opinion that advanced nurses retain a strong nursing orientation (MacDonald et al. 2005) but more evidence is required to illustrate the unique contribution of the nursing components in advanced practice roles (Ketefian et al. 2001, Carlisle 2003, Bryant-Lukosius et al. 2004). Pauly et al. (2004) proposes that new 'nurse-sensitive' outcome indicators should be developed rather than replicate existing research that compares ANPs with doctors. Aranda and Jones (2008) call for greater focus on the social and cultural processes that influence ANP roles, rather than more evaluative studies that merely add 'description' of function. There is, however, a reluctance among ANPs to participate in research (Hayes 2005) and this must be overcome if ANPs are to demonstrate their true aptitude and value.

Cost-effectiveness is an important consideration in a climate where NHS finances are limited. In a Cochrane Review of studies evaluating the impact of doctor–nurse substitution in primary care on patient outcomes, process of care and resources (including costs), there was no appreciable difference in any area although patient satisfaction was increased with ANP consultations (Laurant et al. 2004a). The expectation that savings on nurses' salaries would demonstrate cost reduction was offset by increased consultation times, increased tests ordered and further use of services. However, the study by Sibbald et al. (2006) demonstrated that the detailed advice and enhanced information about treatment resulted in higher patient satisfaction when compared with general practitioner (GP) consultations (and the measurement of the effect of 'self-management strategy' or 'health advice' as a health outcome for patients is difficult to quantify). Additionally, gains will not be achieved while GPs continue to provide services that are within the scope of ANPs. In an author's response to commentary regarding their research Laurant et al. (2004b) clarify:

> The fact that we found no impact on doctors' workload is, in our opinion, not a reflection on the capability of the nurses. Rather, it reflects an inability on the part of the doctors to stop doing the type of work which should have been delegated to the nurses.
>
> Laurant et al. (2004b)

The 'solution', they argue, is to introduce better management systems to ensure doctors stop doing the work that nurses have been prepared to take over.

In the final scenario a consultant nurse reveals her perspectives on ANP developments.

Scenario 1.4

Mandy is a Consultant Nurse in Urgent and Unscheduled Care. She completed an MA in Interprofessional Heath and Community Care while holding the position of Lecturer Practitioner/Clinical Nurse Specialist in A&E. Ten years ago she established and managed one of the first nurse practitioner-led minor injury units. She is also one of the Non-Medical Prescribing Leads for a rural primary care trust.

As a consultant nurse 50 per cent of my work is clinical practice. I currently spend 1 day a week in a general practice: seeing, treating and discharging patients with a wide range of presenting complaints – whether it is a minor ailment, chronic condition or an acute problem. In order to do that I use every skill associated with advanced practice: one minute I may be dealing with a minor skin wound that requires suturing, and the next I may have to deal with a paediatric emergency, such as a child presenting with scalded skin syndrome.

Of course, this would require urgent referral to a paediatrician. But it reflects the broad range of health problems I have to deal with. But despite my background in acute care, I am also able to treat people with chronic conditions, such as diabetes, or give advice to a newly diagnosed patient with hypothyroidism.

I learned my physical examination skills in London many years ago – on a course run by an American Nurse Practitioner teacher, so my training didn't follow a conventional 'nurse practitioner degree'. (Although my physical examination skills were assessed by means of an OSCE at a later date – which I think adds to my credibility.)

I absolutely think that the decision to protect the title of ANP is important. It is vital, in fact. Because my overwhelming concern is that there are nurses out there working with a title that implies an advanced level of ability – yet they don't possess the skills and competencies to do that job. And not only that, but for someone like me in the position of Consultant Nurse, holding a masters degree with many years of experience, but without an RCN-accredited nurse practitioner degree – where's my protection? I know that I can demonstrate my personal competency within the framework of the NMC Code – but I see the opening of a register for advanced practice as an important development. I want to go on that register – and I think all nurses working in advanced practice should strive towards that. I was involved in the Higher Level of Practice (HLP) project many years ago – as an assessor – and what that revealed to me was that there were many nurses working competently in extended roles who could demonstrate their ability, yet there were some who could not. And that's what we need to sort out. Another real strength of that HLP assessment process was that nurses were observed in their clinical practice areas – and that isn't done objectively enough by some universities today.

One of the single most important elements for advanced practice is personal vision. If you don't have the vision for the role – or you see it as very narrowed – how can you develop your vision? That's when you get lost along the way. Masters level thinking is about planning and developing personal practice – and nurses need support in that. You know, I'm always striving to learn more. I think there is a real danger in that advancing your practice you could become complacent about your knowledge base – thinking you know sufficient for a particular job, then losing that drive to further your knowledge.

In my opinion to be an ANP you need to be able to prescribe independently. I think that's integral to an advanced nursing role. But I don't think 'independent prescribing' in isolation makes a nurse an advanced practitioner: it's important also to have the physical examination skills, the health assessment skills, the knowledge of physiology and pathophysiology, diagnostic reasoning and disease management. I studied neuro-behavioural biology – and this grounding in physiological processes has underpinned my subsequent knowledge. I don't think that I could do my job without that knowledge – not that I think all ANPs need to study this in depth! But I do think that generally this is an aspect of advanced nurse education that needs to be strengthened.

I also think clinical reasoning is an area which, for some nurses, needs to be developed further. I'm making complex decisions about care management – and I have to be fully accountable for those decisions. Now to some extent all nurses use clinical reasoning skills to a greater or lesser degree. But the difference is considerable when you move into advanced practice and are providing care to patients with complex health problems and making decisions about their medications. And understanding risk management is vital too.

I know that building a portfolio of evidence to support my competency – against all the standards the NMC has proposed – will be time-consuming. But I will do it. Because it will show my proficiency in the role that I do, and in that respect it's important for the nursing profession as a whole. As a consultant nurse I am required to submit a portfolio of evidence, on a yearly basis, against the four competencies – and it takes time to do that. But it verifies my scope of practice and I know that every other nurse holding the title of 'consultant' could do the same. It's about setting standards that are nationally agreed and therefore recognized – we operate on the same level, and this leads to better understanding for patients and colleagues.

One of the strengths of advanced nursing practice is enhanced patient care – in which patients are viewed as partners who should be actively involved in decisions about their treatment. In every patient encounter I'm promoting health; I'm preventing ill health; I'm supporting them in their homeostasis and supporting them in maintaining their social networking. To me that's the essence of what makes this advanced role 'nursing'. But I do remember that, at first, as I moved into advanced practice I focused on the medical skill acquisition, and the 'nursing' element can slip into the shadows for a while. It's only when you are confident in those skills that the nursing, which is inherent, becomes integrated into your practice once again.

I think this book will be important – because it will enable nurses like me, who haven't had 'traditional' nurse practitioner training to demonstrate the strengths of their advanced practice, by producing personal evidence in a portfolio. There are many different nursing titles now, and a variety of roles that hint at 'advancement', but now is the time to have consensus on the level of expert practice.

CONCLUSION

This chapter has considered the concept of advanced practice in relation to contemporary developments regarding professional regulation in the UK. The contextual influence of current health care policy has been described and the prospective issues surrounding the NHS Careers Framework discussed. It is evident that ANPs are expert nurses who provide high-quality care that is valued by patients and widely accepted in a variety of health care settings. There is significant opportunity for all nurses who want to move forward to advanced practice, and the four scenarios have exemplified this. Each of their journeys has been unique in terms of professional development, experience and training, but their narratives reveal harmony in their strong nursing philosophy and commitment to enhance patient care. They are also united in their desire to seek registration on the NMC professional register and share determination to achieve this.

Advanced practice nursing … represents the future frontier for nursing practice and professional development. It is a way of viewing the world that enables questioning of current practices, creation of new nursing knowledge, and improved delivery of nursing and health care service ..., therefore, continued development is of paramount importance for society and the nursing profession.

Bryant-Lukosius et al. (2004: 520)

ACKNOWLEDGEMENT

I would like to extend my sincere thanks to the four contributors for their inspirational stories.

REFERENCES

American College of Nurse Practitioners (ACNP) (2007) Letter. http://www.acnpweb.org/i4a/pages/Index.cfm?pageID=3633 (accessed on 14/03/08).

American Medical Association (2007) Resolution. http://www.acnpweb.org/i4a/pages/Index.cfm?pageID=3631 (accessed on 14/03/08).

Aranda, K. and Jones, A. (2008) Exploring new advanced practice roles in community nursing: a critique. *Nursing Inquiry* 15 (1): 3–10.

Ball, J. (2006) *Nurse Practitioners 2006 – the results of a survey of nurse practitioners conducted on behalf of the RCN Nurse Practitioner Association*. Hove: Employment Research Ltd.

Ball, J. and Cox, C. (2004) Part 2: The core components of legitimate influence and the conditions that constrain or facilitate advanced nursing practice in adult critical care. *International Journal of Nursing Practice* 10: 10–20.

British Medical Association (2002) *Health policy and economic research unit discussion*. London: The Future Healthcare Workforce, BMA.

The Bristol Royal Infirmary Inquiry (2003) *Learning from Bristol: the report of the public inquiry into children's heart surgery at the Bristol Infirmary 1984–1993*. London: Stationery Office.

Bryant-Lukosius, D. and DiCenso, A. (2004) A framework for the introduction and evaluation of advanced practice nursing roles. *Journal of Advanced Nursing* 48: 530–540.

Bryant-Lukosius, D. DiCenso, A. Browne, G. and Pinelli J. (2004) Advanced practice nursing roles: development, implementation and evaluation. *Journal of Advanced Nursing* 48: 519–529.

Carlisle, C. (2003) *Moving on: education for advanced practice in nursing*. Glasgow: NES.

Carnwell, R. and Daly, W. (2003) Advanced nursing practitioners in primary care settings: an exploration of the developing roles. *Journal of Clinical Nursing* 12: 630–642.

Castledine, G. (2003) The development of advanced nursing practice in the UK. In *Advanced nursing practice*, 2nd edn. McGee, P. and Castledine, G. (eds), pp. 8–16. Oxford: Blackwell.

Colyer, H. (2004) The construction and development of health professions: where will it end? *Journal of Advanced Nursing* 48: 406–412.

Cox, C. (2002) Advancing practice for practice nurses. *Practice Nursing* 13: 406–408.

Coxhead, J. (1993) United we stand – divided we fall. *The Australian Journal of Rural Health* 1: 2.

Czuber-Dochan, W. Waterman, C. and Waterman, H. (2006) Atrophy and anarchy: third national survey of nursing skill-mix and advanced nursing practice in ophthalmology. *Journal of Clinical Nursing* 15: 1480–1488.

Daly, W. and Carnwell, R. (2003) Nursing roles and levels of practice: a framework for differentiating between elementary, specialist and advancing nursing practice. *Journal of Clinical Nursing* 12: 158–167.

Department of Health (1989) *A strategy for nursing.* London: DoH.

Department of Health (1991a) *The patients charter.* London: DoH.

Department of Health (1991b) *Hours of work of doctors in training – the New Deal.* (Executive Letter: EL (91) 82). London: DoH.

Department of Health (2000a) *The NHS plan.* London: DoH.

Department of Health (2000b) *Meeting the challenge: a strategy for the allied health professions.* London: DoH.

Department of Health (2002) *Liberating the talents: helping primary care trusts and nurses deliver the NHS Plan.* London: DoH.

Department of Health (2004a) *Agenda for change: final agreement.* London: DoH.

Department of Health (2004b) *The NHS knowledge and skills framework and the development review process.* London: DoH.

Department of Health (2005a) *The implementation and impact of hospital at night pilot projects: an evaluation report.* London: DoH.

Department of Health (2005b) *Health care scientists career framework: supporting agenda for change documentation.* London: DoH.

Department of Health (2006) *Modernising nursing careers – setting the direction.* London: DoH.

Department of Health (2007) *Trust, assurance and safety – the regulation of health professionals in the 21st century.* London: DoH.

Elsom, S. Happell, B. and Manias, E. (2005) Mental health nurse practitioner: expanded or advanced? *International Journal of Mental Health Nursing* 14: 181–186.

Fulbrook, P. (1998) Advanced practice: the 'advanced practitioners' perspective. In *Advanced nursing practice,* Rolfe, G. and Fulbrook, P. (eds), pp. 87–102. Oxford: Butterworth-Heinemann.

Furlong, E. and Smith, R. (2005) Advanced nursing practice: policy, education and role development. *Journal of Clinical Nursing* 14: 1059–1066.

Gardner, A. Hase, S. Gardner, G. et al. (2008) From competence to capability: a study of nurse practitioners in clinical practice. *Advanced Nursing Journal of Clinical Nursing* 17: 250–258.

Griffith, H. (2004) Nurse practitioner education: learning from students. *Nursing Standard* 18: 33–41.

Harris, A. and Redshaw, M. (1998) Professional issues facing nurse practitioners and nursing. *British Journal of Nursing* 7: 1381–1385.

Hayes, E. (2005) Promoting nurse practitioner practice through research: opportunities, challenges, and lessons. *Journal of the American Academy of Nurse Practitioners* 18: 180–186.

Horrocks, S. Anderson, E. and Salisbury, C. (2002) Systematic review of whether nurse practitioners working in primary care can provide equivalent care to doctors. *British Medical Journal* 324: 819–823.

Hughes, J. (2005) Advanced practice roles in primary care: a critical discussion of the policy and practice implications. *Work Based Learning in Primary Care* 3: 119–128.

International Council of Nurses (2002) *Definition and characteristics for nurse practitioner/advanced practice nursing roles.* Geneva: ICN Geneva. http://www.icn.ch/networks_ap.htm (accessed on 07/05/08).

Jasper, M. (2005) New nursing roles – implications for nursing management. *Journal of Nursing Management* 13 (2): 93–96.

Kendall, L. and Lissaur, R. (2003) *The future health worker.* London: Institute for Public Policy Research.

Ketefian, S. Redman, R. Hanucharurnkul, S. et al. (2001) The development of advanced practice roles: implications in the international nursing community. *International Nursing Review* 48: 152–163.

Laurant, M. Reeves, D. Hermens, R. et al. (2004a) Substitution of doctors by nurses in primary care. *Cochrane Database Systematic Review* 5: CD001271.

Laurant, M. Reeves, D. Hermens, R. et al. (2004b) *Author response.* http://www.bmj.com/cgi/eletters/bmj.38041.493519.EEv1#62886 (accessed on 28/03/08).

Lloyd Jones, M. (2005) Role development and effective practice in specialist and advanced practice roles in acute hospital settings: systematic review and meta-synthesis. *Journal of Advanced Nursing* 49: 191–209.

MacDonald, M. Schreiber, R. Davidson, H. et al. (2005) Moving towards harmony: exemplars of advanced nursing practice for British Columbia. *Canadian Journal of Nursing Leadership* 20: 39–44.

Mantzoukas, S. and Watkinson, S. (2006) Review of advanced nursing practice: the international literature and developing the generic features. *Journal of Clinical Nursing* 16: 28–37.

Marsden, D. Dolan, B. and Holt, L. (2003) Nurse practitioner practice and deployment: electronic mail Delphi study. *Journal of Advanced Nursing* 43: 595–605.

National Assembly for Wales. (1999) *Realising the potential: a strategic framework for nursing, midwifery and health visiting in Wales into the 21st century.* Cardiff: NAfW.

NHS Education for Scotland (NES) (2007) http://www.nes.scot.nhs.uk/nursing/recent_events/documents (accessed on 04/04/08).

National Health Service Executive (NHSE) (1999) *Agenda for Change: Modernising the NHS pay system.* London: HMSO.

Northern Ireland Practice and Education Council (2005) *An exploration of nursing and midwifery roles in Northern Ireland's health and personal social services.* Belfast: NIPEC.

Nursing and Midwifery Council (2004) *Consultation on a framework for the standard of post-registration nursing.* London: NMC.

Nursing and Midwifery Council (2005) *Advanced nursing practice – council strategy.* http://www.nmc-uk.org/aFrameDisplay.aspx?DocumentID=1669 (accessed on 09/09/07).

Nursing and Midwifery Council (2007) *Advanced nursing practice – update.* http://www.nmc-uk.org/aArticle.aspx?ArticleID=2528 (accessed on 09/09/07).

Nursing and Midwifery Council (2008) *The code: standards of conduct, performance and ethics for nurses and midwives.* London: NMC.

Ormond-Walshe, S. and Newham, R. (2001) Comparing and contrasting the clinical nurse specialist and the advanced nurse practitioner roles. *Journal of Nursing Management* 9: 205–207.

Pauly, B. Schreiber, R. MacDonald, H. et al. (2004) Dancing to our own tune: understandings of advanced nursing practice in British Columbia. *Canadian Journal of Nursing Leadership.* 17 (2): 47–59.

Read, S. Lloyd Jones, M. Collins, K. et al. (2001) *ENRiP: Exploring new roles in practice: final report.* Bristol University: Kings Fund Development Programme.

Read, S. and Roberts-Davis, M. (2000) *Preparing nurse practitioners for the 21st century.* Sheffield University: RSANP.

Reay, T. Golden-Biddle, K. and Germann, K. (2003) Challenges and leadership strategies for managers of nurse practitioners. *Journal of Nursing Management* 11 (6): 396–403.

Royal College of Nursing (1996) *What is a nurse practitioner?* London: RCN.

Royal College of Nursing (2002) *Nurse practitioners: an RCN guide to the nurse practitioner role, competencies and programme accreditation.* London: RCN.

Royal College of Nursing (2008) ANPs: *an RCN guide to the advanced nurse practitioner role, competencies and programme accreditation.* London: RCN.

Seale, C. Anderson, E. and Kinnersley, P. (2006) Treatment advice in primary care: a comparative study of nurse practitioners and general practitioners. *Journal of Advanced Nursing* 54: 534–541.

Scottish Executive Health Department (2005) *Framework for developing nursing roles.* Edinburgh: SEHD.

Skills for Health (SfH) (2005) *NHS careers framework.* http://www.skillsforhealth.org.uk/page/career-frameworks (accessed on 04/04/08).

Sibbald, B. Laurant, M. and Reeves, D. (2006) Advanced nurse roles in UK primary care. *Medical Journal of Australia* 185: 1.

Smithson, J. (1999) Nurse practitioners: the need for recognition. *British Journal of Community Nursing* 4 (2): 65–69.

Stilwell, B. (1982) The nurse practitioner at work. 1. Primary care. *Nursing Times* 78: 1799–1803.

Torn, A. and McNichol, E. (1998) A qualitative study utilizing a focus group to explore the role and concept of the nurse practitioner. *Journal of Advanced Nursing* 27: 1202–1211.

Ulrich, C. Soeken, K. and Miller, N. (2003) Predictors of nurse practitioners' autonomy: effects of organizational, ethical, and market characteristics. *Journal of the American Academy of Nurse Practitioners* 15: 7.

United Kingdom Central Council for Nursing and Midwifery (UKCC) (1992) *Scope of professional practice.* London: UKCC.

United Kingdom Central Council for Nursing, Midwifery and Health Visiting (UKCC) (1999) *A higher level of practice, the report of the consultation.* London: UKCC.

Walsh, M. (1999) Nurses and nurse practitioners. 1. Priorities in care. *Nursing Standard* 13 (24): 38–42.

Wanless, D. (2002) *Securing our future health: taking a long term view. Final report.* London: Stationery Office.

Williams, A. McGee, P. and Bates, L. (2001) An examination of senior nursing roles: challenges for the NHS. *Journal of Clinical Nursing* 10: 195–203.

Williams, A. and Jones, M. (2006) Patients' assessments of consulting a nurse practitioner: the time factor. *Journal of Advanced Nursing* 53 (2): 188–195.

Williamson, G. Webb, C. Abelson-Mitchell, N. and Cooper, S. (2006) Change on the horizon: issues and concerns of neophyte advanced healthcare practitioners. *Journal of Clinical Nursing* 15: 1091–1098.

Woods, L. (1999) The contingent nature of advanced nursing practice. *Journal of Advanced Nursing* 30: 121–128.

Woods, L. (2006) Evaluating the clinical effectiveness of neonatal nurse practitioners: an exploratory study. *Journal of Clinical Nursing* 15: 35–44.

2

THE LEGAL AND REGULATORY IMPLICATIONS OF ADVANCED NURSING PRACTICE

CAROLINE PENNELS

INTRODUCTION

This chapter sets out to clarify the extent and nature of the legal and regulatory framework that underpins the practice of the advanced nurse practitioner (ANP).

It will identify the elements of the legal and regulatory framework surrounding advanced nursing practice and illustrate its effect on selected aspects of the advanced nurse's clinical role. Many of the principles and concepts described apply to both 'ordinary' and 'advanced' practice. Differences in relation to advanced practice will be explained later in the chapter.

A feature of advanced nursing practice is the wide variety of clinical environments where such nursing takes place. This is not always viewed as a positive characteristic, and it can be seen as difficult to create standardized practice when both the clinical specialty base is so wide and the qualifications and experience of the practitioners so variable.

Advanced nursing practice is not necessarily as difficult to regulate as anticipated, however, and the legal controls in particular are effective because they are robust. Throughout the chapter, a key theme will be the checklist in Table 2.1, showing the broad categories of regulatory controls that are universally applicable to all areas of nursing practice, whether it is defined as 'advanced' or not.

The assignment of a 'level' indicates the degree of nursing-specific principles or instruction contained in that type of regulatory control. For some areas of nursing (e.g. nurse prescribing), statutory controls will be in place and can be very nursing specific; others may be less so. Statutes (level 1) represent the highest level of mandatory instruction that applies to that particular advanced nursing practice, and in a nursing sense statutes are generally enabling rather than instructive or prescriptive in terms of nursing practice. There should be no variation in the application of statute law between organizations.

Far more commonly, the bulk of legal guidance for ANPs will be found in common law (level 2). This relates to the legal principles established through individual cases which have been litigated in court and whose outcomes either become comparative principles to be applied to similar situations or binding judgements. The English

TABLE 2.1   *Types of legal and regulatory control*

Level 1 Statute Law
Level 2 Common Law
Level 3 Professional regulations (NMC)
Level 4 Local organizational policies

legal system requires that courts operate the 'doctrine of precedent'. When hearing cases that have factual similarities with other, previously decided cases, the courts must follow those previous decisions. In other words, where the legally significant facts of a case match those of a previously decided case, the final outcome must be decided in the same way.

Common law sits at level 2 because the principles established within it may be generally applicable to health care practice (especially medical) rather than specific to nursing. The principles in common law are mandatory as far as the interpretation of them is agreed.

The third level of detail refers to the professional, regulatory component, represented for ANPs by the Nursing and Midwifery Council (NMC). Within this, ANPs are bound by the code of professional conduct and other official guidance and standards. This sits at the third level because it reflects nursing law only – and often in some detail.

The greatest level of detail with respect to the legal and regulatory framework of nursing practice (level 4) is in the local policy structure laid down by the practitioner's employer. This element will offer the greatest amount of instruction on clinical and organizational practice and procedure. It will have been developed locally to reflect a chosen organizational direction but must nonetheless be constructed upon the principles of statute and common law and incorporate professional ethical guidance.

Every branch of advanced nursing practice, therefore, in whatever variation it exists, will be subject to the range of regulatory measures shown in Table 2.1. Local policy controls (level 4) will, of necessity, be of the greatest specificity to a given clinical area but these may show a variation between organizations in terms of implementation. Even so, they will be based upon the general legal principles established in statute and common law (levels 1 and 2).

It is sound professional practice to have at least a working knowledge of how these various levels of control apply to the particular clinical area where the practitioner works, to allow informed and confident professional practice to develop. Appreciation of these controls should not hinder or limit professional advanced practice but should encourage practice freedom through an understanding of the boundaries of the professional role.

Within advanced nursing practice there should be frequent occasions when advanced practitioners should ask the question: 'Do I know if my practice is underpinned by any particular statute or principles derived from case law and, in addition to the usual professional guidance, are there any relevant local policies within which I should be working?'

THE REGULATORY ENVIRONMENTS APPLYING TO CLINICAL PRACTICE

For advanced practitioners, as discussed, there are four areas which regulate practice:

- civil law;
- criminal law;

- employment law;
- professional law.

Civil law

This provides the case and civil law principles in the law of tort (i.e. 'civil wrongs' compared with 'criminal wrongs'), which is known as professional (or clinical) negligence. This section deals with the detail of the process of establishing negligence and the conditions that have to be satisfied for negligence claims to succeed.

Four criteria must be fulfilled in order for a negligence claim to be actionable, described below. The actions will be subject to proof on the 'balance of probabilities'; i.e. whether the case is 'more likely than not' to have happened in the way alleged by the claimant. This is known as the civil standard of proof.

Duty of care

The first of these criteria is that a duty of care is owed by the professional to the individual. This duty is defined for doctors and nurses in the case of *R. v. Bateman* [1925], when it was stated 'if a person holds themselves out as possessing special skill and knowledge and is consulted as possessing such by or on behalf of a patient, he then owes a duty to that patient'.

This has been professionally acknowledged and incorporated into the code of conduct.

A duty is owed to the following:

1 Any person, if a nurse's actions are reasonably likely to cause them harm (*Donaghue and Stephenson* [1932]). This could include relatives and visitors.
2 A patient personally, when they are under the care of a nurse, but not to all patients universally.
3 Any patient admitted by a hospital trust or health authority.
4 Any person voluntarily attended by a nurse in an emergency situation (*Skelton* v. *London North West Railway* [1867]).

The last of these applies where a nurse is acting as a volunteer offering assistance outside her usual course of employment. Here there is no legal duty to assist, and a nurse cannot be sued for breach of duty in deciding not to help in an emergency situation. However, there is a professional duty to assist in these circumstances. Once a nurse does assist, the expected reasonably competent standard of care must be given, and a breach in this standard is actionable if damage can be shown to have resulted.

A duty of care is owed under the following circumstances:

1 When an implied or expressed professional relationship exists between the patient and the nurse.
2 When a patient presents himself or herself to hospital and nurses have knowledge of that patient (*Barnett and Chelsea and Kensington HMC* [1968]).
3 When help is sought from nurses within their employment, even if facilities are not ideal; for example, in an emergency where there is no A&E department. This is different from the emergency circumstances described above, where the nurse is outside her course of employment.

The duty of care is owed by the following people:

1   individual doctors looking after the patient;
2   individual nurses caring for the patient;
3   the employing trust or health authority (*Cassidy* v. *Ministry of Health* [1951]).

Standard of the duty of care

The second criterion is that the duty of care must have been discharged to the required standard. For an ordinarily skilled practitioner, the standard of this duty of care is that defined in *Bolam* v. *Friern HMC* [1958] (see Box 2.1). For specialist practitioners the standard is that defined in *Wilsher* v. *Essex AHA* [1988] (see Box 2.2). Both these cases are considered in some detail later in this chapter.

Box 2.1   *Bolam* v. *Friern Hospital Management Committee* [1958]

John Bolam was admitted to Friern Hospital suffering from depression. He was treated by electroconvulsive therapy (ECT), given by attaching electrodes to each side of his head and passing an electric current through the brain. His doctors did not warn him of the side-effects of the treatment and when the treatment was given, no relaxant drug was administered or manual constraint used to contain any violent or convulsive movements. The only precautions taken were manual support for the chin and shoulders and a gag placed in the mouth. Nurses were present on either side of the couch to prevent him from falling. During the treatment Mr Bolam's movements were so violent that bilateral fractures of the acetabula were caused. Mr Bolam alleged negligence in failing to warn him of the risks, failing to give him relaxant drugs and failing to control his convulsive movements.

At trial, the defendants were found not negligent. The judge stated, 'Where you get a situation which involved the use of some special skill or competence, the test as to whether there has been negligence is judged against the standard of the ordinary, skilled man exercising and professing to have that special skill. A man [doctor] need not possess the highest expert skill. It is sufficient if he exercises the ordinary skill of an ordinary competent man [doctor] exercising the particular art.'

Box 2.2   *Wilsher* v. *Essex Area Health Authority* [1988]

Martin Wilsher was born 3 months prematurely. He could not breathe effectively and needed extra oxygen such that an umbilical arterial catheter was required to monitor his oxygen saturations. The senior house officer (Dr Wiles) accidentally and unknowingly inserted the catheter into a vein instead of an artery, providing false oxygen saturation readings. The readings were questioned. Dr Wiles requested a radiograph of the catheter and asked the registrar to check its position. As a result, the registrar replaced the catheter but again, a vein was cannulated instead of a artery, this time by the registrar. Despite further radiographs, the error was not noticed. Consequently, Martin Wilsher received excessive levels of oxygen for 8–12 hours and developed retrolental fibroplasia (RLF).

It was held at trial and on appeal that there was no dispute about negligence. A doctor's (and nurse's) duty of care is related to the post he or she holds. The registrar was found negligent but Dr Wiles was not as he was entitled to rely on his work being checked by the more experienced doctor. Whether the raised oxygen in the baby's blood actually caused or contributed to the RLF was not decided because of conflicting expert opinions.

Other cases also comment on the issue of competency and the level of skill required. For example, if you possess special skills you must also exercise the ordinary skills of your job (*Maynard* v. *Midlands RHA* [1984]). It is also understood that to be inexperienced in a role is never a defence to incompetence or poor performance (*Jones* v. *Manchester Corporation and Others* 1952, *Nettleship and Weston* 1971).

It is also essential to appreciate that the standard of care required is that agreed to be of acceptable and current practice at the time of the incident (*Roe* v. *Ministry of Health* 1954) and not the practice at the time the incident is investigated or litigated.

Breach in the standard of care

The third criterion to be met is that a claimant must show that there has been a breach in the required standard of care. A breach in the duty of care can arise either because a duty was owed to an individual but the duty was not discharged because the care was not given at all, or because care was given but alleged to have been of substandard quality.

It is usually clear to the patient and the nurse involved that a professional relationship exists between them for the purposes of carrying out nursing care. Therefore, the more common cause of a breach in the duty of care occurs where that care and treatment is allegedly negligent. At this point, even if the care is negligent, it is possible that no harm has resulted.

A negligent breach in the standard of care (whether the ordinary standard or the specialist standard) can result from either an action which was not properly or adequately undertaken, or a failure to act when reasonably expected to have done so. The classic description of negligence was explained in *Blythe* v. *Birmingham Waterworks* [1987] (not a medical case) as 'the omission to do something which a reasonable man, guided upon those considerations which ordinarily regulate the conduct of human affairs, would do, or doing something which a prudent and reasonable man would not do'.

There are many clinical examples of failures to act or actions that cause a breach in the standard of care and which are enshrined in classic textbook cases. Examples are listed here.

- Failure to get advice or a second opinion (*Payne* v. *St Helier Group HMC* [1952]). A patient was seen in A&E after being kicked by a horse. The attending doctor noted bruising but considered internal injuries unlikely and discharged the patient. He returned 18 days later with peritonitis and died shortly afterwards following two operations. The court decided that the doctor had ignored important clinical signs and should not have discharged the patient, and failed to exercise reasonable care in the diagnosis.
- Departure from normal practice for no good reason (*Clarke* v. *McKlennan* [1983]). In this case, a woman found she was suffering from stress incontinence 2 days after giving birth.

She was offered corrective surgery and this was performed 4 weeks after delivery. Subsequently, the patient suffered a substantial haemorrhage and the surgical site also broke down. Despite two further remedial operations, the incontinence became permanent. The patient brought a case claiming that the initial surgery was performed too soon. She won her case and the court decided that the doctors had unreasonably and unjustifiably departed from usual gynaecological practice, which was to offer this surgery 3 months after birth, as the passage of time reduces the risk of haemorrhage and increases the chance of successful wound healing.

Examples of actions that should not constitute a breach include:

- Any action which is supported by a responsible body of similarly qualified nurses (a 'Bolam' defence). For example, an individualized wound dressing regime devised by a tissue viability nurse to meet the particular requirements of a patient, and based on guidelines drawn up by the National Institute for Health and Clinical Excellence (NICE) and informed by her clinical experience.
- Any accepted, approved and justifiable nursing practice; for example, any clinical practices described in current textbooks of nursing care and which may be additionally repeated in employers' local policies.
- Any action that was reasonable in all the circumstances, even if there is no supporting opinion available; for example, a decision not to fit anti-embolitic stockings to a mobile patient who did not meet the criteria for such stockings, against the view of the relatives that stockings should have been offered as a preventative measure, regardless of lack of clinical need. The supporting opinion in these circumstances is whether or not damage would be caused by applying the stockings where there is no apparent clinical requirement.
- Any failure to follow accepted practice but for which a justifiable and good reason can be made (*Maynard* v. *West Midlands RHA* [1984]); for example, for a post-operative knee replacement patient, a failure to fit foot pumps for deep vein thrombosis (DVT) prophylaxis as prescribed by the doctor, when a deformity of the patient's feet prevented the foot pumps working, and in circumstances where the patient was also receiving appropriate oral prophylactic medication.

In some situations, even where there is a division of nursing opinion, the questionable action carried out may not necessarily represent a breach in the standard of care.

Absolute knowledge of a process, treatment or procedure is also not demanded (see Box 2.4 *Crawford* v. *Charing Cross Hospital* [1953], p. 43). This case also established that 'failure to know' does not necessarily constitute negligence, but given the date of the case and the changes in nursing practice and expectations since, it would be prudent not to rely on this without a responsible professional approach. It is also fair to say that precautions can only be taken against reasonably known risks (*Roe* v. *Ministry of Health* [1954]) and that a pure error of clinical judgement is not necessarily negligent (*Whitehouse* v. *Jordan* [1981]).

Causation and harm

The fourth criterion for a successful claim is that the claimant is able to prove recognizable physical and/or psychological harm and that they cannot claim compensation for something they did not suffer. Importantly, and in addition, it is essential that there is a direct and causal link between the alleged negligence and the harm.

It is possible, however, that as in *Wilsher* above, the negligence is just one possible cause of the harm (*Kay* v. *Ayrshire and Arran HB* [1987]), although it may be sufficient in some circumstances to show that the negligence 'substantially contributed' to the harm (*Hotson* v. *East Berkshire AHA* [1980]). In these cases it can be very difficult to apportion the cause of the harm between several, simultaneously occurring possible causes (*Sindell* v. *Abbott Laboratories* [1980]).

In some cases it may seem unlikely for the incident to have occurred without negligence (e.g. the amputation of the wrong leg or retention of surgical swabs) and these are known as *res ipsa loquitur* decisions (meaning the facts speak for themselves). The claimant would have to show that what happened would not have occurred if a reasonable standard of care had been given. For their part, the defendant would have to show how the circumstances could occur without negligence (*Ward* v. *Tesco Stores* [1976]).

Reasonable forseeability

Even if the harm can be shown to have resulted from the negligent act, that harm must also have been reasonably foreseeable. Precautions can only be taken against reasonably foreseeable risks (*Roe* v. *Ministry of Health* [1954]). If the harm that occurred was not reasonably foreseeable, even if the act causing it was negligent, there will be a defence to the claim.

Connection between the negligent act and the alleged harm

Harm alleged to have been caused by the negligent act can be challenged if the harm can be shown to be more extensive or generally not of the kind expected as a result of that particular alleged act of negligence. As an obvious example, if there was an allegation of negligence in an ANP applying the incorrect technique to bandage a leg ulcer, a patient who also alleges that development of subsequent recurrent toothache is also a result of the negligent nursing actions is likely to have that particular allegation challenged.

Breach of duty of care but no causation

It is also possible that there may be shown to be a breach of duty of care, but that the negligent act may not have caused any harm. For example, a patient falls off the operating table in theatre having been unattended by nursing staff following the reversal of an anaesthetic. Subsequent radiographs show what seems to be a fracture of a bone in the arm. Expert radiological opinion, however, shows that the fracture was an old one, pre-dating the fall in theatre. In addition, there are no injuries as a result of the fall. Thus in this case, there is a breach of the duty of care in allowing this patient to fall off the operating table, but the negligence did not cause any damage.

Defences

An important part of assessing whether a claim for clinical negligence will succeed is an examination of whether there are any substantial defences to all or part of the claim. These defences will commonly be contributory negligence, voluntarily taking a risk (*volenti non fit injuria*) or factual inadequacies.

Contributory negligence occurs when the damage suffered can be wholly or partly attributed to the actions of the claimant. An example may be when an important part of the claimant's treatment is to take certain medication and she/he chooses not to take it. The resulting harm could be said to be due to some extent to the failure to follow medical instructions.

Voluntarily taking a risk (*volenti non fit injuria*) describes cases where a particular proposed treatment carries known risks to the claimant who is informed of those risks. If the consent process is correctly completed, no action can follow if the risks do materialize and cause harm. This value of this defence is dependent upon the quality of the consenting process. Where a difference of opinion exists between one professional and another, one professional is not negligent merely because his conclusion differs from another.

Finally, it is not unknown for the facts of a particular case to be absent or incomplete in the documentary record. If essential facts are unable to be determined, the claimant may fail to bring their claim because they cannot establish the facts of their case. This can be without fault on the part of the defendant.

Criminal law

In contrast to civil claims for clinical negligence, criminal prosecutions are proven on the basis that the guilt of the accused person is proven 'beyond reasonable doubt', rather than 'on the balance of probabilities'. This higher test reflects the significance of the penalties for some criminal offences. The burden of proof to this standard rests with the prosecution.

Crime connected with health care practice is either that committed by someone who happens to be a health care worker by profession, or a crime that is professionally connected to their work. Of greater professional interest are those offences or crimes where the intention of the health care worker was to harm or kill patients. In terms of clinical practice, one of the distinctions between civil and criminal law is the interface concerning whether or not it can be proven that the accused individual intended to cause the harm or not. In clinical negligence, it is accepted that there is no such intention. Where any intention is suspected, this directs the case into the arena of criminal law.

Alternatively, there are instances when the intention to harm the patient cannot be proven (and may even be agreed to be unlikely), but when the standard of care is so low and the outcomes so serious that a criminal penalty is considered. For example, when a patient has died and the standard of care is shown to have been grossly negligent, such that a prosecution for manslaughter is appropriate. The involvement of a criminal penalty reflects the fact that the professional standard of care was so reprehensible that the health care practitioner involved deserves punishment.

Employment law

Every nurse working in an employed capacity (as distinct from being 'self-employed') will have contractual conditions of employment as specific terms within their contract of employment, whether an ANP or not. Through these terms of employment the practitioner is accountable to his/her employer. Each contract of employment contains the implied or express terms that nurses will 'obey' the employer (by adhering to hospital policies and organizational practices) and 'use reasonable care and skill in their work' that sets a competency standard. A breach in either of these terms could lead to implementation of the employer's disciplinary process and appropriate action thereafter.

Employer's responsibility

Employers are responsible for failures in care within the hospital services which they provide. These arise out of statutory responsibilities delegated to them by the Secretary of State for Health. This is a non-delegable duty and cannot be passed on to staff working in the hospital.

The second type of responsibility that employers have is known as indirect or vicarious responsibility. This arises out of the direct liability described above and means that the employing organization will accept legal responsibility for the alleged acts or omissions of any employee.

Under the principle of vicarious liability, in a situation where any individual nurse is involved in an allegedly negligent incident, the employer assumes responsibility for the allegedly negligent act and can be sued in place of the employee.

Certain conditions need to be in place for this to happen:

- the allegedly negligent individual must be an employee;
- he/she must have been acting in the course of his/her employment;
- he/she must have used due care and skill at the time;
- he/she 'obeyed' the employer by working within hospital policies.

If any of these conditions do not apply, the employee is at risk of losing this cover and may be vulnerable to being sued personally.

Reasons why these conditions may not apply relate to the status of an individual as an 'employee' as seen in the first of the criteria above. In particular, the law is not settled on the status of individuals who work through employment agencies, that is, the law is not clear whether that individual is an employee of the recruitment agency, an employee of the place where they are working or indeed an employee at all (*Brook Street Bureau (UK)* v. *Patricia Dacas* [2004]).

This uncertainty applies specifically to agency nurses, where the practical outcome is that the legal benefit arising from the employer being vicariously liable for the acts and omissions of the agency nurse may *not* be available to the agency nurse, or may not be available without some analysis of the employment relationship. Furthermore, it is not safe to assume that without an express term in the employment contract, that there is some implied term that indemnity is offered by the employer (*Lister* v. *Romford Ice and Cold Storage Co Ltd* [1957]) or that in any particular set of circumstances, the employer will automatically be liable for the tortuous acts of an employee (*L and Others (AP)* v. *Hesley Hall Ltd* [2001].

Professional regulation

It is not the purpose of this chapter to deal in detail with the workings of the Nursing and Midwifery Council (NMC) as there are many texts which deal comprehensively with this. However, reference needs to be made to their professional regulatory authority as part of the advanced practitioner's regulatory framework and to the main elements of their function.

The principal functions of the NMC are to establish standards of education, training, conduct and performance for nurses, midwives and health visitors, to ensure the maintenance of those standards and to safeguard the health and well-being of persons using or needing the services of the registrants.

The NMC is also required to prepare and maintain a register of qualified nurses whose education, training, conduct and performance it will record, to add nurses to the register on qualification and to remove them from the register where appropriate.

Recognizing that nurses' practice was moving into extended, advanced roles, and in the interests of improving standards of public protection, the NMC took the decision in 2005 to set up and maintain a separate part of the register for advanced practitioners. Full consultation on this is currently in process, but providing it is approved by parliament and the Privy Council, ANPs will be listed on this subpart of the nursing register if they meet the required standards and competencies described in detail in subsequent chapters.

Nurses can be removed from the register because of impaired fitness to practise, because there is an error connected with the entry on the register or because there is a suspicion that this has been fraudulently obtained.

Reasons for removal from the register due to questionable fitness to practise arise from:

- allegations of misconduct;
- allegations of lack of competence;
- conviction or caution for a criminal offence or conviction elsewhere which would constitute a criminal offence in England and Wales;
- questionable state of physical or mental health. Any suggestion from a body in the UK responsible for the regulation of a health or social care professional that fitness to practice is impaired.

The outcome for any of these conditions is that the individual can be removed from the register. Alternatively an individual can be suspended from the register for a specified period of time which will not exceed 1 year.

ADVANCED NURSING PRACTICE

What's in a name?

As discussed, one of the defining features of advanced nursing practice is the wide range of clinical specialties in which this type of practice will be found, and the wide range of skills and qualifications of the practitioners within it (Carroll 2002). There is a continual and unresolved debate about the inequalities and inaccuracies arising from the extensive range of titles that are created and used in advanced practice (Nazarko 2004).

This is seen to be a problem because it allegedly gives neither comparative fairness to those who have got the qualifications to be considered appropriately qualified for advanced practice and who should be allowed to call themselves 'advanced' or 'specialist' on the basis of their knowledge and expertise, nor recognition to those who lack the academic qualifications but compensate by virtue of their experience – which can be less easy to evidence and to accredit (Scott 2005).

This concern has been the subject of regulatory investigation through the NMC consultation (NMC 2004) around the standards required for advanced nursing practice. If this is a real difficulty, it is primarily one of defining a standard of achievement in practice which can be correlated with an expected standard of care. The regulatory authorities are concerned to accurately label the standard of care that is given, reliant upon the practitioner being able to demonstrate a level of practice-based competence. The value of ANPs in many roles has been described and acknowledged (Jolly 2002, Jones 2002, Palmer et al. 2003, Hekkink et al. 2005).

The law sees this situation in an alternative, if not opposite, way. Instead of taking the standard of practice and assigning the agreed title, the law will see the title and have an expectation of the standard of care which will be demonstrated. The law is quite clear that whatever the practitioner's title says the practitioner does, that is precisely what the law will expect them to be able to do.

For example, a specialist nurse who has arrived at that position by gaining several academic qualifications will be judged in law by exactly the same criteria as a specialist nurse who has none. Both will be expected to deliver a specialist level of care, regardless of the precise nature of their skills, simply because of the title they use.

Similarly, a consultant nurse will be required to provide evidence of the level of her standing that allows her to be regarded as a senior colleague to whom colleagues may make referrals for advice, and an ANP will be assumed to be able to deliver an advanced level of practice.

The law will not look behind what your title says you are. Your title will be taken at face value and will be interpreted on the basis of the meaning which an ordinary member of the public would place upon it. In practice, this also means that if your practice has fallen short of the standard expected by your title, the law may not tend to leniency with regard to reasons and explanations for that failure. Rather, it will rely on the reasonable expectations created in an ordinary member of the public who is treated by a practitioner with a particular title. The rule of thumb is that in a situation where the quality or standard of care is under question, to claim inexperience (that is, experience which is less in quality, length or qualification to that implied by your title) will not be a defence.

Higher standard of care

In situations where the quality of care given is alleged to be substandard, there are different legal standards that define the acceptable level of care. For example, an 'ordinary' nurse (one who neither calls herself a specialist of any type, nor holds a title of broadly that description, nor professes to be one in any other way) is measured by a different standard from a nurse who has the title of a 'specialist', 'consultant' or 'advanced' nurse. The last one is higher and more demanding and can be analogous with the medical standard if the care given requires a medical standard of knowledge and/or skill.

The legal tests and case law defining the two standards of care are found in *Bolam v. Friern HMC* [1957] (Box 2.1 on p. 24) and *Wilsher v. Essex Area Health Authority* [1988]. This is an example of the application of the level 2 regulatory control described in Table 2.1 whereby binding law has been created by common law cases.

Bolam v. Friern HMC [1958] (see Box 2.1 on p. 24)

The question of what constitutes a generally acceptable standard of care has been described in this case, which ultimately defined the standard to be expected of 'a reasonably skilled and competent doctor (nurse)'.

In directing the jury in this case, the judge stated: 'where you get a situation which involves the use of some special skill or competence then the test is to whether there has been negligence or not. It is not the test of the man on the top of a Clapham Omnibus because he has not got this special skill. The test is the standard of the ordinary skilled man exercising and professing to have that special skill. A man need not possess the highest expert skill, it is a well established law that it is sufficient if he exercises the ordinary skill of an ordinary competent man exercising that particular art'.

Bolam based his claim partially on the fact that no relaxant drugs were given and that staff had failed to restrain his movements. However, expert witnesses agreed there was a large body of competent medical opinion that was opposed to the use of relaxant drugs for ECT. It was also the view of some competent and respected doctors that the more restraint that was used the more likelihood there was of a fracture occurring. There was also a conflict about whether or not a warning should have been given, whereby the doctors attending Mr Bolam took the view it was not desirable to warn a patient unless he specifically asked about the risks, in contrast with the experts who say the patient should have been warned.

With respect to the warning about risks, the judge commented: 'Having considered the evidence you [the jury] have to make up your mind whether it has been proved to your satisfaction that when the defendants adopted this practice [namely the practice of saying very little and waiting for questions from the patient] they were falling below a proper standard of competent professional opinion on this question of whether or not to warn'.

The judge went on to say that even if it is decided that it is good practice to give some warning, the real question is whether that would have made any difference to Mr Bolam's acceptance or refusal of the treatment. Unfortunately, the only man who could answer that question was Mr Bolam and he was never asked. The result of the case was that the judge stated: 'a doctor is not guilty of negligence if he has acted in accordance with the practice accepted as proper by a responsible body of medical men skilled in this particular art. Putting it another way round, a doctor is not negligent if he is acting in accordance with such practice merely because there is a body of opinion that takes a contrary view'.

Translating this to nursing practice, the Bolam case confirmed, therefore, that it is sufficient to exercise an ordinary level of nursing skill and competence, and that the highest standard of nursing is not necessary to practise in a lawful manner if you are an 'ordinary' nurse.

Wilsher v. Essex AHA [1988] (see Box 2.2 on p. 24)

This case illustrates an extremely important principle for ANPs. Although the standard of competence for an ordinary skilled nurse has been established by the Bolam test, the standard expected of specialist nurses – those who profess a particular or special skill – is different and higher.

This case illustrates the contrast in the accountability and standard of care expected from a junior and senior practitioner. The main principle established was that in comparison to a non-specialist, a specialist practitioner is expected to deliver a higher standard of care which reflects their additional training and experience, and the fact that he or she occupies a specialist position. The case also illustrates the difference in the standard of the duty of care between a senior and a junior practitioner.

Principles that arise from this which are significant to ANPs are that:

- the standard of care required is related to the post and not to the individual;
- the standard of care is related to the skills needed for the job, not what skills the individual doing the job can offer;
- specialist practitioners are expected to give a higher standard of care than more junior nurses because a registrar is expected to correct the work of the junior doctor.

R. v. *Adomako* [1995] (Box 2.3)

Box 2.3   *R.* v. *Adomako*: manslaughter by an anaesthetist

Dr Adomako was an anaesthetist in charge of a patient during a surgical procedure. He failed to realize during the early part of the operation that part of the equipment had been disconnected and failed to remedy the problem. He became aware that something was amiss when an alarm sounded on the machine monitoring the patient's blood pressure. The supply of oxygen to the patient ceased and led to a cardiac arrest at 11.14 a.m. From the evidence it showed that some 4.5 minutes had elapsed between the disconnection and the sounding of the alarm. When the alarm sounded, the defendant responded in various ways by checking the equipment and administering atropine to raise the patient's pulse. But at no stage before the cardiac arrest did he check the integrity of the endotracheal tube connection. The disconnection was not discovered until after resuscitation measures had been commenced. The patient subsequently died.

Dr Adomako accepted at his criminal trial that he had been negligent. The issue was whether his conduct was criminal. He was convicted of involuntary manslaughter, but appealed against conviction. He lost his appeal in the Court of Appeal and a subsequent appeal to the House of Lords was also dismissed.

This case is of extreme importance to all nurses but has a particular significance to ANPs, providing the clearest indication of the way in which the law regards fatalities which arise from negligent professional care.

The case makes important clarifications about how seriously low the standard of care has to be in order to place it into the realm of criminal behaviour. The interaction of civil law and criminal law is interesting at this point.

Civil law provides that an individual who can show that if on the balance of probability (i.e. more likely than not) some negligent act or omission by an advanced practitioner caused some physical or psychological damage, monetary compensation can be recovered by the patient. This reflects the intention that the patient should, as far as is possible, be put back into the position they were in before the negligence happened. Because the only compensatory mechanism available is money, this is what a damaged patient is offered.

In circumstances where there is also a potentially criminal component to the incident (as in *Adomako*) a criminal prosecution as well as a negligence claim can be made. The involvement of criminal law indicated that the professional behaviour which caused the problem is viewed as being so serious that a jury would class it as being 'gross' (and this is a decision for a jury) and is worthy not just of offering monetary compensation but the individual accused of grossly negligent care ought to be punished.

Manslaughter has traditionally been one of the offences where gross negligence can form a sufficient basis of liability for prosecution. However, the question remains as to how bad the negligent actions have to be in order to meet this threshold for prosecution. A helpful test was given in *R* v. *Bateman* [1925] which is still relevant:

> the facts must be such that in the opinion of the jury the negligence of the
> accused went beyond a mere matter of compensation between subjects and

showed such disregard for the life and safety of others as to amount to a crime against the State and conduct deserving punishment.

Having established that negligent professional conduct can fall as low as the criminal threshold, what then are the ingredients of manslaughter by gross negligence? An answer was provided in a recent case whereby two junior doctors were convicted of manslaughter (Dyer 2006) but received suspended prison sentences. The doctors were treating a young patient admitted for routine knee surgery. The patient developed toxic shock syndrome which the doctors were accused of failing to treat, and he died four days later. The doctors failed to take blood samples, give antibiotics or seek senior review of the patient in a timely manner. Although account was taken of the fact that the case had exceptional circumstances and those were not of the doctor's making, that is, the orthopaedic ward was understaffed and both doctors were under pressure, the case confirmed that, nevertheless, the criteria for gross negligence is:

> the offence [of gross negligence or manslaughter] requires first, death resulting from the negligent breach of the duty of care owed by the defendant to the deceased, second, that in negligent breach of that duty the victim was exposed by the defendant to the risk of death and, third, that the circumstances were so reprehensible as to amount to gross negligence.

The final question to consider is whether the conduct was 'gross' in its seriousness. This is regarded as a question for the jury to decide at the time of the trial and this is confirmed in *Adomako*:

> the essence of the matter – which is supremely a jury question – is whether, having regard to all the risk of death involved, the conduct of the defendant was so bad in all the circumstances as to amount in their judgement to a criminal act or omission.

There is therefore no criminal definition of 'gross' to describe the negligent act or omission except to confirm that it will be made in accordance with the jury's understanding of the word 'gross', which does, after all, have a comprehensible meaning and needs no sophisticated legal definition.

Boundaries of the advanced nursing practice role

For any advanced nursing role to be successfully integrated into a multidisciplinary team, the boundaries of the role and what is contained within it must be agreed, as far as possible, at its inception, by the members of that team who might be affected by it. In particular, it must be agreed by medical colleagues who should accept and support the extended role specifically on the point that it is likely that the advanced practitioner will be contributing to the medical assessment and treatment of the patient. In this respect it is vital that all parties understand where the boundaries of the advanced role are and where nursing and medical responsibilities begin and end.

Initiated by the employing organization

It is also very important that the advanced practitioner role is initiated and authorized by the employing organization, as only by these means will the acts or omissions of the ANP be vicariously indemnified. In this way the employer has asked the nurse to undertake certain tasks by virtue of creating the job description and recruiting the nurse to that job. The employing organization, through its recruitment process, has made an assessment of the skills of the nurse and, by implication, has decided that this meets the competencies required. Therefore the organization assumes responsibility for the standard of care offered by that nurse.

Skill-matching

It is therefore very important to match the individual nurse to the job very carefully in terms of experience, qualifications and skills and to take account of the principle in the *Wilsher* case (Box 2.2 on p. 24). Here it was confirmed that the person undertaking the role must be fit to practise in that role. The boundaries of the job must not be set too wide (or allowed to become too wide) to encompass skills which the practitioner cannot offer, just because they are the only practitioner available to fulfil that particular post.

Setting the boundaries

The support of other members of the multidisciplinary team is also important in that whenever the advanced practitioner approaches the boundaries of the role, reaching a point which is becoming beyond their area of expertise, the other members of the team need to accept that it is professionally appropriate for the nurse practitioner to refer onwards and upwards to other colleagues, if the nurse practitioner feels it necessary. This again refers back to the *Wilsher* case, where the junior doctor who had not been able competently to fulfil a post had escaped negligence by referring upwards to a more senior member of the team.

For a practitioner to feel they are regularly exceeding the boundaries of the post would indicate that there is a legal and professional risk for them in doing so and also that the job has not been adequately assessed. For the nursing practitioner, accountability will follow whatever the practitioner has agreed to undertake. Again, if the boundaries of the post are too wide, this will create areas of practice for which the nurse cannot really be held accountable.

Although many ANP roles are unusual and even innovative, the legal principle of adhering to common and accepted nursing practice should be uppermost in the minds of those creating and undertaking these roles. If the boundaries of the role are significantly beyond what might be seen as common practice, an area of risk is being created in justifying why these boundaries are so wide and also for the individual practitioner who has to account for his/her practice.

Competent advanced nursing practice

Other chapters in this book will explain the professional view of competent advanced practice. However, according to the law, competent practice will involve the following components.

- On an ordinary level and for ordinary nursing skills the practitioner must be able to demonstrate 'reasonably competent' practices (*Bolam*).
- As an advanced nurse or a practitioner with advanced nursing skills, the standard of care must be shown to be that of a specialist practitioner as described in the case of *Wilsher*.
- ANPs must have both ordinary and advanced skills. It is not an acceptable defence to have lost basic, ordinarily competent nursing skills or to have those basic skills but to practise advanced skills infrequently.

- For both ordinarily competent practitioners and ANPs the standard of competent practice can fall so far short of what is expected that the level of care may be judged to be criminally grossly negligent, in which case it becomes a matter of criminal prosecution rather than civil procedure (*Adomako*).

In deciding what makes up competent practice, three areas can be considered – the standard of care, what constitutes common or accepted practice and evidence-based practice.

Standard of care

First, the employing organization needs to decide the standard that the advanced practitioner needs to meet and this will be based on what is broadly expected of the role. These expectations will be created by what the organization expects of the role and what is commonly offered in other similar circumstances. This must be in line with what is widely accepted as required of the job and research may be required into comparable posts. Even if parallels are to be found in other organizations, there may still be an element of risk in the organization deciding where to draw the line in terms of the training, skills and experience needed to be competent in that particular advanced practice role.

For a defence of substandard practice to be effective, the practitioner's standard of care must conform with the *Bolam* and *Wilsher* cases; that is, the ANP must be able to show that he/she can offer the standard of care expected by a specialist practitioner, and in so doing is operating at a level which would be supported by a group of similarly trained and qualified advanced practitioners.

Common and accepted practice

The second component of competent practice is that the care and standards offered by the advanced practitioner must be in accordance with the current, common and accepted practice of other individuals doing that particular job. This connects with the standard of care in that both refer to there being a certain safety in numbers. If any advanced nursing practice is challenged it must be able to be shown that the practice under scrutiny is the same as that offered by a group of practitioners doing that job and is representative of common and accepted practice at that time.

Evidence-based practice

The third component of competent practice is a demonstration that it is in line with available evidence relating to those practice issues. There may not be a great depth of evidence available but where there is, it may be incompetent not to comply with what the evidence base demonstrates. It may also be that the evidence base does not refer specifically to nursing practice but may originate from research into the practice of other health care professionals. It is generally recommended that the advanced practitioner has a wide knowledge of these various practices and gives careful consideration to what applies in their particular role. It may be seen as less competent to be acting in contravention of some evidence base, where this is available, and to do so would mean taking accountability for giving the reasons why this was done.

Keeping up-to-date

As previously mentioned, the classic case of *Crawford* v. *Board of Governors Charing Cross Hospital* [1953] (Box 2.4) makes it clear that the law does not demand absolute

Box 2.4   *Crawford v. Board of Governors Charing Cross Hospital* [1953]

In this case, a patient was admitted to hospital for treatment of a cancerous bladder growth and was duly operated upon. During the surgery, the anaesthetist extended the patient's left arm at approximately 80 degrees to enable a blood transfusion to be given. Subsequently, the patient discovered that he was suffering from loss of power in the left arm due to brachial palsy. This was particularly problematic for the patient as he had lost the use of his right arm in childhood. The patient sued the anaesthetist for negligence on the basis that 6 months before his operation an article had been published in the *Lancet* journal on the subject of the operation, and the anaesthetist had not read the article. The trial judge held that failure to be familiar with clinical journals amounted to negligence. However, the anaesthetist appealed the decision and the Court of Appeal subsequently held that there was no negligence because it would place an unreasonably high burden on medical professionals to require them to read every article available in the medical literature.

nursing knowledge of all procedures or treatments. This case also introduced the principle that a 'failure to know' is not necessarily negligent, meaning that a nurse is not expected to know of every development in nursing care.

However, when previously new or innovative nursing practice and procedures reach the point where they may be considered reasonably well accepted, and increasingly grounded in nursing research and practice, the defence that an advanced nurse did not know about that development may be challenged. Although it is not possible to keep up to date with every aspect of nursing development, advanced nurses should ensure that they are familiar with those developments in the areas of their own practice. This applies with particular respect to high profile guidelines such as those produced by NICE.

Although advanced clinical practice allows a measure of judgement about the applicability of guidelines in the treatment of every patient, in a case where a problem arises as a result of nursing care given outside accepted guidelines, there would at best be a weighty burden on the advanced nurse to justify why guidelines had not been adhered to in the circumstances.

Clinical supervision

Another required element of competent practice is for the practitioner to undergo clinical supervision. Although it is acknowledged that this is often a personally directed reflective activity, there may be occasions when it would be valuable to show that supervision or reflective practice had taken place.

It is not necessary to show that the clinical supervision was offered by a colleague working in precisely the same area. The appropriate clinical supervisor may well be a doctor or another member of the multidisciplinary professional team. In this way it would be responsible practice to seek clinical supervision of the best and most appropriate quality from whoever is best placed to offer it. It is appropriate to be imaginative about where the supervision can be obtained, and to prioritize the maintenance of safe practice rather than unnecessarily to emphasize a nursing input into the supervisory process.

Awareness of limits of competence

A critical part of competent practice is to know where your boundaries of competence lie and to apply the principles in *Wilsher*. It is not a weakness to pass on the problem to another practitioner better placed to resolve the difficulty, and the *Wilsher* case was very clear that this is the most professionally appropriate course of action and can act to deter any allegations of negligence.

Whistleblowing

Part of professional practice at all levels is not only possessing the ability to identify when one's own practice is being drawn into unfamiliar areas, but also to see and act when this is happening to colleagues. It may be necessary to report colleagues who do not reach levels of competence or do not refer onwards when their own boundaries of competence have been reached.

It is important to know what whistleblowing policies are in existence in your organization. There would be a difficult area of accountability to satisfy if it was shown that substandard practice of one practitioner was known about by others and not acted upon.

Entrepreneurial activities

It is accepted that there have been many reports of innovative practice by ANPs and indeed the role itself is an example of the boundaries being pushed back in terms of how highly qualified and experienced nurses are prepared to develop (Faugier 2005). There are tremendous opportunities available for practice to continue to develop and this is also in the best interests of patients (Harrison 2006). Entrepreneurial activities can take place where the advanced practitioner is employed to develop an individual service for patients, for example in a general practice surgery where a particular nurse-led clinic is devised. In this situation, the requirements of indemnity and other statutory requirements of employment are the responsibility of the employer.

Where the advanced practitioner is the employer

However, opportunities are now developing for the advanced nurse to become an employer in his/her own right, for example setting up a clinic or clinical services to provide nursing and/or prescribing care independently of the NHS, or private nursing clinics caring for patients with particular nursing needs matched by the skills of the advanced practitioner. Such arrangements could potentially present opportunities for these care settings to operate on a commercial basis, part of which may involve the employment of other qualified or unqualified nursing staff. The business owner who is an ANP could employ any professional colleagues, whether qualified nursing or not, or medical or therapy staff. In these circumstances, the legal and regulatory framework extends beyond medical law into company and commercial law, the detail of which is outside this chapter.

However, within this scenario the following are important considerations. The advanced nurse as employer can employ colleagues on a permanent basis with a 'contract *of* service' (i.e. they are contracted to work for the company set up by the advanced nurse employer) or colleagues who are contracted to perform certain services for the employer, a 'contract *for* services', and these have different implications for the employer. In the first situation, the advanced nurse as the employer would have vicarious liability for the acts and omissions of the employed staff. If, however, staff are contracted to provide services, the professional responsibility to provide a competent service rests with the individual nurse or doctor, while the business owner who contracts the services has a responsibility to reasonably ensure that the contracted professional is competent. In all instances, the ANP, who may be the owner of such a business, remains professionally accountable for his/her own clinical practice.

Personal indemnity

If the ANP is an employer but also continues to work in a clinical capacity, an adequate amount of insurance cover will be required. This may mean that the nurse will have to take out new professional indemnity cover with an insuring organization, and this may be the first time in his/her clinical career when this has been necessary. The amount of indemnity cover required should be carefully assessed, both in relation to the clinical activities currently being undertaken, and those which may be undertaken with any future development of the role. Some medical defence organizations (that is, organizations providing indemnity to doctors) for example Medical Defence Union (MDU) or Medical Protections Society (MPS) extend their indemnity cover to non-medical professionals in circumstances where additional indemnity is required, thus nurse practitioners, practice nurses, assistant practitioners and consultant nurses can source additional indemnity where needed. Subscription rates for indemnity for such categories of ANP are based on the actual clinical tasks undertaken, hence the need for careful and realistic assessment of the role.

Vicarious liability for permanent employees (full-time or part-time)

It may be the intention of the ANP to employ other clinical colleagues and to offer contracts of employment and in this situation, the advanced nurse as employer needs to investigate how this indemnity will be provided. At the moment, members of the Royal College of Nursing (RCN) who employ other clinical staff can offer vicarious liability cover to those staff only if they are also RCN members. If not, this cover will not be effective. This is a commercial decision on behalf of the insurance company.

This is currently a developing situation and enquiries need to be made by any prospective employer to ensure that indemnity practices are up to date. Any prospective advanced nurse employer needs to ensure that this is clear in the terms and conditions of the contract of employment. This is clearly important as the employee will be relying upon the vicarious liability to cover their practice.

Liability for practitioners who are not permanently employed

It is possible that an advanced nurse employer may recruit or hire colleagues to perform particular roles on specific occasions. In these instances the individuals recruited may be employed by other agencies, or may be self-employed. In the first instance, it is vital to check whether the other agency offers indemnity. If not, the individual needs to understand that they are responsible for providing their own cover. Where the individual is self-employed, there will be no option but to have their own cover, and the employing advanced nurse needs to be sure this is appropriate and functioning.

Additional insurance cover

As an employer, the advanced nurse has obligations under health and safety laws for the protection of employees and the public. This means that both employer's liability (to have cover for employees suffering personal injury during the course of their work) and public liability cover (for the protection of the public on the employer's premises) need to be in force. If the premises are not owned by the advanced nurse employer, then occupier's liability cover is the alternative.

Health and safety requirement for employers

There are many requirements under health and safety legislation that need to be put in place in order to act lawfully as an employer, and professional advice must be taken on these aspects.

Where the advanced practitioner is a partner in a practice

It may become an increasingly attractive proposition for nurses to become full or conditional partners in general practices. In these working environments, conditions for indemnity cover and other implications of professional practice are different, principally in the manner in which indemnity cover may be organized. The practitioner needs to be clear whether there is whole-practice cover, or whether individuals are expected to arrange their own indemnity.

It is also a feature of partnerships that there is 'joint and several liability' between the partners. This means that each partner is asked to take on part of the liability of a practice partner and liability for claims is shared between the partners. This can sometimes put pressure on the quality and competence of the partners, as each partner is partly responsible for the acts and omissions of the other partners. Again, specific legal and professional advice must be taken on all these issues.

Common and accepted practice

Because ANPs are often operating in areas where there are few colleagues doing the same thing, or few examples of nursing services being run in the same way, it can be difficult to satisfy the important legal test of adhering to common and accepted practice.

To be entrepreneurial is deliberately to push the boundaries beyond common practice. It may be that the activity being developed will be accepted as appropriate for an advanced practitioner and something which similarly trained colleagues would undertake if the opportunity were available to them. In this instance, if the new activity is set up correctly it should not attract risk simply because it is not an activity frequently practised by nurses. The greater risk is attached to whether the new activity would be supported by a body of practitioners if the opportunity were given to them to undertake it, whether or not they are nurses. For example, if the activity involves an element of medical skill, the body of practitioners whose common and accepted practice was to be considered would be doctors.

Justification

In order to set up any entrepreneurial activities in a safe manner, a good case needs to be constructed about why it is appropriate, safe and professional to practise in a way which may be approaching the boundary of common and accepted practice. Any such developing practice needs to have an accurate basis of reasoning why the practice has been allowed to develop, what the intended benefits are and how likely it is that those benefits can be realized. It is also important to have reasonable safeguards put in place and to demonstrate that appropriate practitioners are undertaking the roles and that they have the right skills, qualifications and experience.

Accountability

Developing practices for ANPs can mean that they are solely responsible for a patient caseload without recourse to medical care. This can occur in some specialist, nurse-led areas where patients may not have a nominated medical consultant for the entirety of their care.

These situations are new and unusual. They also illustrate the level of accountability that may be put upon the advanced nurse, whereby they fulfil the role of the medical consultant in retaining complete responsibility for the patient's clinical care. They are also responsible for the delegation of care to other clinical (medical and nursing) staff and for the quality of that care.

It is also prudent to continue to check the set-up parameters of any new activity at regular intervals. This is not only to ensure that the new practice is still operating within the originally defined guidelines but also to monitor any feedback from patients or from the advanced practitioner undertaking the duties.

Confidentiality and access to health records

This section is included not because the dangers of poor practice concerning health records apply only to advanced practitioners – indeed they apply to all health care professionals – but because ANPs may have a more sophisticated and closer relationship with a patient and relatives (which may continue for a significant period of time) and thus may have access to a considerable quantity of confidential information. ANPs may also find themselves involved not simply with the patient but holistically with several members of the patient's close family. The burden to respect the confidentiality of this information is considerable. A careful path has to be taken between maintaining the relationship and confidence of those supporting the patient and at all times knowing which information the patient wishes to remain entirely confidential and which information the patient is happy to share with those close to her/him.

Access to confidential information comes not only by reading the medical or health record but also through conversation with and physical treatment of the patient. In these circumstances the ANP may have more information to protect than ordinarily skilled members of the nursing staff. It is therefore of paramount importance that the advanced practitioner regularly assesses which information patients are happy to make freely available and which they are not.

In some situations, advanced nursing practice allows patients to be treated in the community or their own home. In such cases, confidentiality needs greater protection than is automatically available in a hospital and advanced practitioners must be aware of this and act professionally and ethically.

Regarding access to written records, the legal rules are clear but not often easily applied. For living patients, access to their health records is only by their consent. In practice this means that health care professionals use and pass on health care information about the patient on a need-to-know basis only. This procedure and ethical duty is explained in the Department of Health guidance document *Confidentiality – the*

NHS Code of Practice (2003). It is commonly understood by health care professionals that information relevant for treatment by professionals in other disciplines can be freely exchanged. This is necessary for safety and continuity of care and is accepted practice, although it may be prudent to ensure the patient is aware of this.

Under the Data Protection Act 1998, access to health records can only be made by the living patient her/himself or with her/his express written consent. This means that in any situation of advanced practice, the patient must be consulted before any information from health records is shared. Access to the written record will not be given by the data controller (i.e. the organization holding and using the medical record) to any other individual. This includes any member of the family who for any reason assumes that they have an entitlement to see the health records of the patient.

This can be a difficult situation, and a high level of communication skills is required from the advanced practitioner to explain that the information requested by the relatives or next of kin will not be disclosed without express consent from the patient. It would be dependent upon the skills of the advanced practitioner to balance the rights and wishes of the patient with the expectations of those close to the patient. Some verbal explanation can be given to the relative or next of kin, but confidentiality must be uppermost in the mind of the ANP. It may be appropriate to make reference to a document, but visual or physical access to the medical records should not be given. A general guide is to ask the reason why the relative or next of kin wishes to see the medical records. It may be that the records will not answer their query, and the relative or next of kin can be satisfied by other means, such as careful discussion with a doctor, nurse or other staff involved in the care of the relative.

After the death of a patient, the ANP may continue to have a therapeutic relationship with those close to the patient, possibly for a considerable time. During this period, the relatives may wish to discuss the care and treatment of the deceased or indeed access their health records. The Access to Health Records Act 1990 provides clear legal rules on who can have access to such records and who cannot.

Because the legal duty of confidentiality extends into death, only individuals who have a potential or actual claim (e.g. of clinical negligence or personal injury, or an insurance claim or a claim on the estate which is reliant in some way on information in the medical record of the deceased) may have access to that record. To gain access to the records, such individuals do not necessarily have to be the personal representative of the deceased, or the executor of the estate, but they do have to prove that they have an actual or contemplated legal claim.

The ANP's professional and ethical duty of confidentiality to the patient continues, therefore, after the death. Even when a documentary authority is validated, it is the responsibility of the organization holding the notes to continue to protect the confidentiality of the deceased patient by deciding which notes are relevant for release and which are not.

It is interesting to note that the Mental Capacity Act (2005) provides that an Independent Mental Capacity Advocate (ICMA), where appointed, can have access to the records of an incapacitated patient. This seems to conflict with the Access to Health Records Act, where only those who can demonstrate the basis of a claim arising out of a patient's death can obtain relevant parts of the records.

In situations where the ANP is dealing with a living patient who does not have the capacity to give or withhold consent (e.g. because of dementia or confusion), these patients are wholly protected and their medical records will not be released as their consent cannot be given. Again this may present a very difficult communication responsibility for the advanced practitioner and again they will have to balance the rights of the patient with the expectations of the relatives.

Leadership and responsibility

By the nature of the role, the ANP will be in a position of leadership. This may take the form of personal, professional leadership in individual decision-making or it may involve managing teams and working within them.

On the issue of personal leadership and decision-making, previous points relating to standards of care and competence are relevant. In addition, the legal rules relating to the boundaries and parameters of individual practice will also dictate where leadership within individual practice will end.

Leading the team

Leadership for the advanced nurse is also commonly seen in terms of leading a team or being one of several senior members of a team. This is manifest in decisions related to prioritizing care for individuals, delegating tasks to team members and supervising team members. Prioritizing care, whether on a one-to-one basis, or between a team, requires accurate and competent clinical assessment and diagnosis skills. These will need to be demonstrably in compliance with both *Bolam* (see Box 2.1, p. 24) and *Wilsher* (see Box 2.2, p. 24) in the sense that the skills expected of an advanced practitioner will need to be representative of the decisions made by a body of similar colleagues. When those decisions are felt to be beyond the knowledge of the advanced practitioner, they will need to be referred onwards.

Delegation

Similar skills will be needed when prioritizing that care among the staff available in the team, when the effective delegation of duties becomes important. An advanced nurse, the team leader will be expected to know accurately the skill mix of staff available so that the workload can be appropriately divided between them.

This may range from health care assistants and student nurses to other qualified staff. A wide skill mix may lead to easier decisions about the delegation of tasks than where there is a rather more limited range of staff available. In either situation, the advanced practitioner must be fully aware of the importance of appropriate delegation, to ensure that no member of staff is allocated a task which falls outside their skills or experience.

Advanced nurses are often in a position in which delegation to qualified and unqualified staff is routine. There are two potential hazards connected with this. First, advanced practitioners can be guilty of wrongful delegation in circumstances where the nurse to whom the job has been delegated is not competent to carry it out. The delegating nurse is consequently accountable for his or her actions in wrongly delegating the task, although the individual nurse who is at fault remains personally liable for his or her own acts or omissions. Unqualified staff and students do not carry the same accountability and the delegating nurse retains complete responsibility for the work given to them.

Second, ANPs must be careful not to allow misuse of their specialist position by undertaking work wrongfully delegated to them by doctors who have not ensured that the nurse in question has the requisite skills to carry out the particular task. There is an equal burden on the practitioner to whom the work has been delegated to make it known if he/she is not able to safely carry out the task.

Team liability

Many advanced practitioners work in small mixed teams of doctors and nurses together with unqualified staff and students. In law there is no concept of team liability, whereby accountability for an incident can be apportioned to the whole team. It will always be the case that the team members involved in the incident are individually liable for their actions or inactions connected with the incident.

It is possible that multiple liability can exist, whereby several members of the team can simultaneously be individually liable for their part in the incident. Consequently, it is extremely important to be aware of the skill mix and competence level of your colleagues.

Consent

ANPs are increasingly involved in the consent process, either as a patient advocate or by themselves obtaining consent from the patient. This is a welcome and appropriate professional development and has arisen from the recognition that the taking of consent does not have to be carried out by a medical practitioner. The Department of Health *Reference guide to consent for examination or treatment* (2001) recognizes that

> the task of seeking consent may be delegated to another health professional as long as that professional is suitably trained and qualified, in particular they must have sufficient knowledge of the proposed investigational treatment and understand the risks involved in order to be able to provide any information the patient may require.

This has opened the way for many patients to have consent for procedures obtained in outpatient and pre-assessment clinics by ANPs.

For the advanced practitioner there are three particular issues concerned with the consent process. First, they must meet the criteria stated in the guidance above and be suitably trained and qualified to take the consent. This refers to previous explanations with regard to the boundaries of their role; it is not an automatic assumption that advanced practitioners should be required to take consent for procedures and this should only be undertaken if the advanced practitioner thinks he/she is competent to do so.

Second, the advanced practitioner must have sufficient knowledge of the proposed investigation or treatment and understand the risks involved. This again corresponds to the points raised about making the boundaries of the role entirely clear and within that being certain of the skills required to do the job. If the advanced practitioner does not feel he/she has sufficient knowledge to be able to inform the patient, taking consent should be referred on to a member of the medical team.

Third, the practitioner must be able to answer all questions put to them by the patient, or find a colleague who can answer them. The amount of information which should be given to a patient in order for a valid consent to be obtained is often a difficult one. Advanced nurses are often at the forefront of providing information and education to patients and as such have a considerable responsibility to ensure sufficient meaningful information is offered and to consider how this information is given.

The question of what information should be imparted to the patient is addressed in the cases of *Sidaway and Bethlem Royal Hospital* [1985] and the case of *Blythe* v.

Bloomsbury HA [1987]. The guidelines derived from these cases were that the information given must conform with that which a responsible body of similar professionals in the same speciality would tell the patient (i.e. it must be 'Bolam compliant').

The information must tell a patient about the 'material risks of agreeing to the treatment and also the material risks of not having the treatment'. In this respect material risks are those to which a 'reasonable patient' would attach some significance.

A doctor can withhold information (even if there is a material risk) if in his or her clinical opinion it would be detrimental to the patient to inform him or her of those material risks. This is commonly referred to as the therapeutic privilege and it is important to understand that this is a concept unique to the medical profession and does not extend to ANPs. If situations arise where the ANP has concerns about the effect that certain information will have on a patient, it is recommended that they refer this on and discuss it with the medical team concerned, since a doctor does not have to tell a patient all that he/she knows about a subject and will not be criticized for not doing so, even if the patient specifically asks.

The amount of information provided can be related to the specific circumstances. For example, more comprehensive information is expected in an outpatient clinic environment or pre-assessment clinic than in a situation where there is some urgency, such as A&E. Emergency treatment is often limited and there is every possibility that further treatment will be required, so there will be the opportunity to add any further information necessary.

This illustrates the disadvantage ANPs experience when called upon to obtain consent. ANPs do not have the same or any therapeutic or professional right to withhold information. In order to protect against the allegation that inadequate information was given for some risky procedures it may be prudent to ask the patient to sign a form to confirm receipt of relevant information. Giving a patient information leaflets can be very helpful in this situation.

Consent and mental incapacity

With regard to consent, it is also important to have a good working knowledge of the Mental Capacity Act (MCA) 2005, which came into force in full in October 2007. The MCA makes provision for the treatment of individuals who lack the capacity to make decisions for themselves, and is directly applicable to the health and social care of such patients (Bartlett 2005). Those provisions within the MCA which directly impact upon the ANP's decision-making process are considered below.

The capacity principles

The MCA sets out a clear set of principles explaining how professionals are required to approach patients who have no or fluctuating capacity (Box 2.5). Where an ANP has been delegated the task of obtaining consent from a patient, a capacity assessment is part of consent process and will identify whether a patient has the capacity at that particular time to give consent to treatment. The statutory test for capacity is the commonly used two-stage test (Box 2.6).

'Best interests' decision

Where the patient lacks capacity, it is up to the medical staff to confirm that the proposed treatment is in the patient's best interests. It is entirely likely that an ANP

Box 2.5   The five capacity principles

- A person must be assumed to have capacity unless it is established that he lacks capacity.
- A person is not to be treated as unable to make a decision unless all practicable steps have been taken to help him to do so without success.
- A person is not to be treated as unable to make a decision merely because he makes an unwise decision.
- An act done, or decision made, under this Act for or on behalf of a person who lacks capacity must be done, or made, in his best interests.
- Before the act is done, or the decision made, regard must be had to whether the purpose for which the act is needed can be effectively achieved in a way that is less restrictive of the person's rights and freedoms.

Box 2.6   Two-stage capacity test

Stage 1

Is there an impairment of, or disturbance in, the functioning of the person's mind or brain?

Stage 2

If so, is the impairment or disturbance sufficient that the person lacks the capacity to make that particular decision?

Test for capacity – the individual must then be able to do the following:

- Understand the information relevant to the decision
- Be able to retain that information
- Be able to use or weigh up that information as part of the process of making that decision
- Communicate his decision (by talking, using sign language or any other means)

will be involved in multidisciplinary discussions about the choice of treatment for such patients and the ANP must be aware of the statutory checklist which exists to guide such decisions (Box 2.7). It is now a legal duty to make any such best-interest decisions in accordance with this checklist.

Duty to consult

The MCA places a legal duty upon clinical decision-makers to consult with anyone who has an interest in the patient's welfare. These interested persons have no decision-making powers, and could be relatives, next-of-kin, friends or acquaintances, but the ANP may be an important link in identifying and supporting any such individuals, while also satisfying her/his own professional advocacy responsibilities. This must, of course, be carried out with the usual care to safeguard the patient's confidentiality.

Where the incapacitated patient has no known individuals interested in their welfare, the MCA requires that an independent advocate is provided – an ICMA.

Box 2.7   Checklist for determining best interests

- Avoid making assumptions about someone's best interests on the basis of age, appearance, condition or behaviour
- Consider all the relevant circumstances – the checklist is not inclusive of all possible factors
- Consider whether the person will at any time have capacity, and if so, when that could be? Can the decision be put off until then?
- Permit and encourage the person to participate as fully as possible in the decision-making process
- Proposed treatment relating to life-sustaining treatment must not be motivated by a desire to bring about death
- Consider what is known about the person's past and present wishes and feelings, any beliefs and values that could influence any decision of his and any other factors, particularly any relevant statements written while he had capacity
- Must take into account (where practical) the views of any person nominated by the person as one to be consulted in these circumstances, any carers, any donee of a lasting power of attorney or any court deputy
- Take account of the views of any appointed independent advocate
- Record clearly the decision-making process that leads to the proposed treatment in best interests
- Take the least restrictive treatment option

In the acute and community setting, these will commonly be supplied through the ANP's employing organization.

There is a legal duty on all clinical staff to source an ICMA for any patient they regard as being unsupported by an individual interested in their welfare, where the clinical decision can wait the short period of time it takes to provide an ICMA. Where the proposed treatment is time critical, the treatment must be carried out as usual in the patient's best interests.

CONCLUSION

This chapter has attempted to set out the legal and regulatory requirements for advanced nurse practice. More detailed texts about the legal aspects of nursing are referenced so that points of particular interest can be followed up. The key points covered are as follows:

- practice is subject to statute law, common law, professional law and local policies;
- these types of regulatory controls appear in different forms in the different levels of accountability which apply to ANPs, that is, accountability to the patient through civil and criminal law, to the employer through contractual and employment law, and to the nursing profession through the Nursing and Midwifery Council;
- the title the nurse has as a practitioner determines the standard of care expected;
- a higher standard of care is expected for the ANP than for the 'ordinary' nurse;
- general nursing skills practised by ANPs will be expected to be carried out at a higher level of skill and knowledge;
- entrepreneurial activities for ANPs carry specific risks which need to be understood and particular advice obtained.

This chapter is not written defensively, but in the spirit that responsible ANPs will want to be shown clearly where the professional and legal dangers to themselves lie, so that these can be accounted for to the benefit of their patients.

CASES

Barnett v. *Chelsea HMC* [1968] 1 All ER 1068.
Blyth v. *Bloomsbury Health Authority*, The Times, 11 February 1987; [1993] 4 Med LR 151.
Bolam v. *Friern Barnett HMC* [1958] 2 All ER 118; 1 WLR 528.
Brook Street Bureau (UK) v. *Patricia Daces* [2004] EWCA Civ 217.
Cassidy v. *Ministry of Health*; [1939] 2 KB 14.
Clark v. *MacLennan* [1983] 1 All ER 416.
Crawford v. *Board of Governors Charing Cross Hospital*, The Times, 8 December 1953.
Donoghue v. *Stevenson*; [1932] AC 562.
Hotson v. *East Berkshire HA* [1987] AC 750.
Jones v. *Manchester Corporation CA*; [1952] 2 All ER 125.
Kay v. *Ayrshire and Arran Health Board*; [1987] 2 All ER 417.
L and Others (AP) v. *Helsey Hall* [2001] UKHL 22.
Lister v. *Romford Ice and Cold Storage Co Ltd* [1957] AC 555.
Maynard v. *W. Midlands RHA*; [1984] 1 WLR 634.
Nettleship v. *Weston*; [1971] 3 All ER 581.
Payne v. *St Helier HMC* [1952] CLY2442 Times, December 12.
R.v. Bateman [1925] 19 CrApp Rep 8.
R. v. *Adomako* [1995] 1 AC 171; [1994] 3 All ER 79.
Roe v. *Minister of Health*; [1954] 2 QB 66.
Sidaway v. *Bethlem Royal Hospital Governors and Others*; [1985] 1 All ER 643.
Sindell v. *Abbott Laboratories* 26 Cal 3d 588 163 Cal Rptr.
Skelton v. *London North West Railway* [1867] LR2 CP 6321.
Ward v. *Tesco Stores Ltd*; [1976] 1 WLR 810 HL.
Whitehouse v. *Jordan*; [1981] 1 All ER 267.
Wilsher v. *Essex Area Health Authority*; CA [1986] 3 All ER 801 HL; [1988] 1 All ER 871 CA.

REFERENCES

Bartlett, P. (2005) *Blackstones guide to the Mental Incapacity Act 2005*. Milton Keynes: OUP.
Carroll, M. (2002) Advanced nursing practice. *Nursing Standard* 16(29).
Department of Health (2001) *Reference guide to consent for examination or treatment*. London: DoH.
Department of Health (2003) *Confidentiality – NHS code of practice*. London: DoH.
Dyer, C. (2006) Hospital Trust prosecuted for not supervising junior doctors. *BMJ* **332**: 135.
Faugier, J. (2005) Developing a new generation of nurse entrepreneurs. *Nursing Standard* 19(30).
Harrison, S. (2006) The tide has turned for specialists as trusts try to balance their books. *Nursing Standard* 20(39).
Hekkink, C. Wigersma, L. Yzermans, C. and Bindels, P. (2005) HIV nursing consultants: patients preferences and experiences about quality of care. *Journal of Clinical Nursing* 14: 327–333.
Jolly, L. (2002) The role of the specialist nurse. *Heart* 88(Suppl. II): ii33–ii35.
Jones, P. (2002) Consultant nurses and their potential impact upon healthcare delivery. *Clinical Medicine* January/February: 39–40.

Nazarko, L. (2004) We need to define advanced practice. *Nursing Times* 100(20): 18.

NMC (2004) *Consultation on a framework for the standard for post registration nursing.* London: Nursing and Midwifery Council.

Palmer, N. Appleton, B. and Rodrigues, E. (2003) Specialist nurse-led intervention in outpatients with congestive heart failure. *Manage Health Outcomes* 11: 693–698.

Scott, H. (2005) NMC is to set standard for advanced nursing practice. *British Journal of Nursing* 14(1): 5.

3 DOMAIN 1: THE NURSE–PATIENT RELATIONSHIP

RENATE THOME

INTRODUCTION

Good communication and interpersonal interactions underpin and form the foundation of advanced practice. Higgs and Jones (2000) view communication as one of the multiple dimensions that contribute to clinical expertise. Without skilled communication the practitioner, however knowledgeable or technically skilled, remains a mere technician. Stilwell uses the analogy of the pianist to illustrate this point.

> A pianist can perform with technical brilliance, but to be a truly great performer she also needs to combine technical competence with sensitive interpretation, and an understanding of and feeling for the music.
>
> Stilwell (1998: 44)

This chapter considers the domain of the 'nurse–patient relationship'; the competencies of the domain will be explored in terms of their meaning for advanced practice. One main case study provides the anchor to illustrate different aspects of the domain and links the ideas to practice; other smaller vignettes illustrate specific points. The focus of the chapter will be in helping the practitioner to construct a portfolio of evidence to demonstrate competence in the domain discussed.

SCENARIO 3.1

Mary, aged 49 years, presented to me in surgery describing symptoms of a muzzy head, dizziness, tingling in her forearms and one episode, 3 weeks previously, of loss of strength in one leg that lasted for 10 minutes. While telling me this she became tearful and told me she had lost her husband suddenly 3 months ago but she was 'coping very well'.

I explained that I would need to take a detailed history and Mary was very pleased that I took her seriously as she was afraid she was having a stroke. My immediate thoughts were that she had been in shock which had enabled her to 'cope very well' with her bereavement, but that she was now experiencing a bereavement reaction that was manifesting itself in anxiety and physical symptoms.

Her medical history revealed nothing of any note, but I found Mary to be very guarded in her responses to questions about her personal situation and feelings. With her consent, I proceeded to undertake a thorough cardiovascular and neurological examination. This activity enabled me to explore her feelings about her husband's death without the need to maintain eye contact, which she might have found overly intrusive. Mary became very tearful and explained that she had no siblings, her children lived away, her neighbours had been very good but she had no one to grieve with. She also revealed other symptoms of anxiety, such as inability to concentrate and poor sleep.

My only physical finding was of elevated blood pressure and although I felt increasingly confident in my initial hypothesis I had to remain aware that it was not possible at this stage for cerebrovascular pathology to be conclusively excluded. I explained this to Mary and arranged for fasting lipids to be taken. In the meantime, having ensured there were no contraindications, I advised her to take 75 mg of aspirin daily. I also discussed with her the possible use of medication for anxiety, a course of action I was not keen to pursue but I wanted to give her a sense of choice. Her response to my suggestions also enabled me to assess her ability to cope with decision-making, even in her distress. Mary was quite clear that she did not want medication to lift her mood and with this decision she regained control of her feelings and actively negotiated a plan with me.

Mary was travelling to stay with her son in 2 days' time. I asked her to come and see me on her return so we could re-check her blood pressure and discuss the results of her blood test. Mary told me she felt much better, partly from relief that I had found 'nothing wrong', but mainly because I had encouraged her to talk about her husband. When I saw her 2 weeks later her blood pressure and blood lipid results were normal, making the likelihood of cerebrovascular pathology very low. Indeed, Mary had accepted that her symptoms were due to anxiety and had independently developed coping strategies so that her symptoms began to improve. I mentioned the bereavement counselling service but she declined.

I followed Mary up over the ensuing months and after a time she became depressed. At this point she accepted the need for treatment with anti-depressants, which she took under my supervision for a period of 6 months. During this time she found a job and her social life improved.

SPECIFIC COMPETENCIES

Creates a climate of mutual trust and establishes partnerships with patients, carers and families

This is one of several competencies in the domain that emphasize the building of a working partnership between practitioner and patient. The concept of partnership means that the nurse is not the sole decision-maker, the patient, too, has a part to play. This particular competence focuses on building mutual trust as a basis for working together.

Good and effective relationships are built on trust and mutual understanding. In health care this kind of relationship has to be established quickly and often within difficult circumstances for the patient, who finds him/herself in an alien and threatening environment, afraid and anxious.

In acute settings, much of this initial rapport is established through good eye contact, reassuring body language and the ability of the practitioner to remain calm and confident in highly anxiety-provoking situations. In other settings the practitioner needs to remain relaxed and flexible, and be able to adapt her/his communication through subtle reading of the patient's signals as they first present. All of this happens very quickly and is not often made explicit.

Body language and eye contact are important in all situations. However, the following example demonstrates their particular importance in building a rapport when two-way verbal interaction is difficult or impossible and body language becomes the main means of communication.

Scenario 3.2

'How can I analyse my communication skills with someone having an acute asthma attack!' was my outraged reaction to being asked to video a routine consultation in my practice.

It was only when I had done the video that I realized how much communication did go on. How much I worked with eye contact, gestures and body language. Using the video I was able to analyse what was happening between me, my colleagues and the patient in a busy A&E department. Our team used the video to change some aspects of our practice, for example making sure we did not turn our back on a very distressed patient (this involved changing the rooms around), and making sure we made eye contact at the level of the patient. I learnt so much about how I communicate, things I was not aware of until I saw myself on the video (Nurse practitioner student 2005).

This scenario illustrates a number of points about creating trust:

- the crucial role of body language and non-verbal communication in the nurse–patient relationship;
- the difficulty of being aware of these issues without feedback;
- the unwitting contribution of the environment to poor communication.

The student in this scenario learnt to observe her practice and the team reconsidered how they worked together to improve the contact with patients in this environment. Understandably, everyone had been focused on the acute care and paid less attention to the communication issues. It was only when they saw the video that they became aware of how they might have built mutual trust through body language and eye contact. Regular observation of practice or video recording can help you to give evidence to the skills in the competency as well as generate useful information for changing practice. Video recording is a powerful tool, which, given careful consideration of the ethics involved, can be used to improve practice (Royal College of General Practitioners 2003).

Effective communication is easy to recognize when observed, but hard to define and describe in detail. Titchen's (2001) work on the expert practitioner goes some way towards articulating some of the more elusive aspects of skilled communication.

Her work on skilled companionship, although initially difficult to read, is very helpful in thinking about and naming expert practice, and the communication skills that are usually left unspoken.

Titchen (2001) suggests that communicating effectively is about entering into a relationship with another person or persons to establish a rapport that will support the relationship, however long- or short-lived it may be. Creating this rapport demands a willingness from the practitioner to be open and receptive to the world and understanding of the other person. It requires the practitioner to develop an awareness of their own judgements, prejudices and preoccupations, and letting them go so that they are open to the other person and their needs. Competency 9 in NMC Domain 1 explores the practitioner's self-reflection in greater depth.

Core skills required in this crucial stage of relationship-building are good listening skills and patience, conveying a sense of having time and not being preoccupied with the next task. This idea of 'being there for the patient' is discussed in Competency 4. Listening requires fluency and competence in the technical aspects of the practitioner's work. Without this fluency the space to listen is simply not available.

Scenario 3.1 demonstrates some of this process, in that the practitioner hears and is sensitive to the patient's reluctance to talk. However, the discussion is facilitated by using the physical examination to allow the patient to release the feelings that are of concern to her. A less experienced practitioner might be preoccupied with technical skills and reaching the correct diagnosis. Such preoccupations would make the practitioner less available and less sensitive to the patient's signals.

In the scenario, the practitioner remains open to the patient, noting that the initial reluctance to talk is part of a process of building rapport and trust and testing out the evolving relationship. The sense of timing is demonstrated by the practitioner not pushing the patient to reveal feelings when she is reluctant to do so, and yet giving the patient time and space to do so later when ready. The practitioner is sensitive to the patient's needs and this helps build mutual trust; the parctitioner's interactions go beyond the tasks to be completed and include what Sellman (2006) calls the essential component of nursing practice, 'trust'.

The skill of the advanced practitioner is to select appropriate interventions for each encounter, not only through physical clues but also by establishing the kind of relationship that will allow wider issues and emotional concerns to be considered (Stilwell 1998). This practitioner was aware of the reluctance of the patient to talk about her recent bereavement. Having noted this, a different approach was used, allowing the patient to relax and tell her story in that 'space between'. The practitioner's confidence and experience made it possible to work in this way.

KEY POINTS

- Trust is fundamental to the nurse–patient relationship.
- The importance of non-verbal communication, body language and eye contact in the initial and ongoing relationship with the patient.
- The sensitivity of the practitioner to both verbal and non-verbal cues given by the patient.
- A sense of timing – not being rushed and putting other preoccupations aside.
- Fluency in practical skills to allow space for listening and 'being there'.
- The importance of the physical environment in facilitating effective communication.

Building rapport and establishing a trusting relationship are the foundations of the nurse–patient working relationship (Sellman 2006). Without these, the encounter remains superficial and frequently unsatisfactory (Freshwater 2002). The experienced practitioner is able to assess a situation and quickly tune in to the patient, using all the skills inherent in building rapport and trust, consciously and purposefully with the intent to help and support the patient.

Validates and checks findings with patients

Validating and checking findings with patients is an important element in building the working partnership between practitioner and patient. It enables the practitioner to start bringing the patient into the decision-making process and to improve the patient's understanding of the course of treatment prescribed.

The emphasis on consultation and history-taking skills in nursing is new and is covered in detail in Domain 3. In broad terms, however, there is a threefold process. First, the practitioner needs to listen to the patient without early interruptions. Second, they gather further evidence by taking a history and carrying out a relevant physical examination. Finally, they provide feedback to the patient about their thinking and possible conclusions.

The conduct of a consultation is a relatively new concept for nurses. Nurses have always assessed patients and made care plans but have tended not to take an active role, asking the pertinent questions required by a 'consultation'. Nurse practitioners now bring their nursing skills to the consultation and combine these with the skill of history-taking and physical examination and case-presentation (Connie and Coralli 2006).

However, in the process of taking a history it is easy to become caught up in clinical reasoning and intense questioning of the patient. This approach tends to silence the patient and put the practitioner in control of the consultation. The results of failing to give a patient adequate opportunity to tell their story can have a surprisingly powerful and detrimental impact on patient care (Silverman et al. 2005).

Research demonstrates that if patients are given the opportunity to give their narrative without interruption, the practitioner is much more likely to come to the correct diagnosis. In contrast, if patients are not given this opportunity and are interrupted, they frequently do not actually reveal the reason for attending the consultation (Kurtz et al. 2004).

Validating and checking findings starts, therefore, with allowing patients to explain their concerns. It is then possible to focus, take a more detailed history and come to a diagnosis. This thinking process can then be checked with the patient to ascertain their view as well as their cooperation with any suggested treatment plans (Pendleton et al. 2003).

In Scenario 3.1 the practitioner engages with the patient, while at the same time drawing on their own professional knowledge and expertise to formulate ideas as to diagnosis. The nurse practitioner integrates their internal thinking and their interaction with the patient. They involve the patient in their thinking and are able to do so fluently. They manage their time well and conduct the consultation within the allocated time. This fluency is built on experience and takes a confidence developed over time and through numerous patient encounters.

Inexperienced practitioners often fear that allowing a patient to tell their story will take too much time and that it will then be impossible to conduct the consultation within the required timeframe. This is not usually the case, given sufficient practice.

Skills required include careful listening, observing the patient for non-verbal cues and sensitive questioning. Both open and closed questions can be used, moving from an open approach to more focused closed questions in order to form a clear picture about the issue presented by the patient. The practitioner needs to focus on the patient and not be preoccupied with other concerns (Pendelton 2004).

Based on these foundations, the practitioner is much better able to validate and check findings with the patient. The patient will then hopefully feel that their story has been heard and may be able to take a more active part in their treatment decisions.

KEY POINTS

- Listening to the patient's story is the first step in taking a good history.
- Checking that the patient's narrative has been correctly understood supports good diagnostic skills.
- Taking a history based on the patient's narrative moves from broad open questions to more closed and focused questions.
- Validation and feeding back findings to the patient helps to retain partnership and cooperation for treatment planning.

Creates a relationship with patients that acknowledges their strengths and knowledge and assists them in addressing their needs

Two patients manifesting exactly similar symptoms may differ radically in terms of their abilities to cope with their condition, their knowledge about it and indeed their level of interest in finding out. This competence asks the practitioner to assess each patient's unique combination of strengths and knowledge and to tailor his or her relationship with each patient accordingly.

This approach ties in with the overall theme of forming a working partnership between practitioner and patient. In addition, it encourages patients to recognize their own strengths, thereby allowing them to move on and regain a sense of control that may have been lost through illness (Nordgren and Fridlund 2001).

To recognize and acknowledge a patient's strengths requires both attention and a level of creativity from the practitioner. On a simple level it means being sure to listen to the patient and to ascertain what their level of knowledge might be and what they expect and wish from the consultation. Although this sounds obvious, practitioners can forget to allow the patient to share their experience and knowledge about their illness (Neighbour 2003).

On a more complex level, ascertaining a patient's strengths might require a great deal more imagination and creativity on the part of the practitioner (Mattingly 1991). For example, patients who are suffering a serious life-threatening illness or a condition that will limit their lives may not initially see how they will be able to cope. This is where the advanced practitioner can take care a great deal further, and work with the patient to create a new and different future, one that reintegrates the new life circumstances of the patient into the present and future (Haidet et al. 2006).

Mattingly (1998) calls this way of working 'practical' or 'narrative reasoning'. The practitioner is mindful of the change that has taken place and, without losing her own hope and courage, joins with the patient in bearing the pain and loss that the patient has to face (Mattingly 1998, Naef 2006). This process allows the practitioner to understand the person that the patient used to be and to help the patient construct the new person that he/she will be.

A glimpse of this kind of work is visible in Scenario 3.1. Here the practitioner was able to give the patient sufficient space and respect to tell her story, initially of the worrying symptoms and then the loss of her husband and the loneliness of grieving, away from family and friends. Over time this patient did reconstruct her life, rebuilding her social network. The quiet and unobtrusive support given by the practitioner no doubt played a part in that process. The practitioner could have discharged the patient once they had established that there was no physical problem. However, they remained available for long enough to allow the patient to recover and determine in her own time when it was right to leave.

The following scenario illustrates this creative way of working in a different setting.

Scenario 3.3

I was working with a man who had suffered a stroke which affected his short-term memory in particular. He was no longer able to carry out his normal job as a business person. He had lost his sense of identity, had become very depressed and did not want to participate in rehabilitation. Through talking with him I realized that the one thing he had some interest in was his grandson. We talked a lot and I came up with the idea to teach him to juggle to impress the grandson. He took up the challenge and has now become 'grandad the extraordinary juggler' to the delight of his grandson. He constructed for himself a new identity and role in the family that defines him differently from his stroke and illness (Physiotherapist 2004).

This may sound easy but to work in this way requires imagination and the ability really to 'be with' a patient, to enter their world without fear, to be able to recognize strength and courage at times when patients themselves are unable to see the future. It requires the practitioner to sustain his or her belief in recovery and to support the patient in their journey towards redefining themselves (Heath 1998).

It also demands of the practitioner that they step back and let go once the patient is able to take control. Campbell (1984) captures this idea in the analogy of the nurse accompanying and assisting a patient on a journey. It suggests working together for a time and parting at the end of the journey, each going their own way.

KEY POINTS

- Each person possesses a unique combination of strengths and knowledge.
- Acknowledging a patient's strengths and knowledge is more than just listening.
- Holding hope for the patient at times when they cannot see a future.
- Walking alongside the patient on their journey bearing the pain with them.
- Creative and imaginative thinking are integral to this competency.

Communicates a sense of 'being there' for the patient, carers and families and provides comfort and emotional support

Being there for a patient and others, also called 'presence', is a rather elusive quality that is easily recognized by those who are at the receiving end, but more difficult to explore and make explicit. It is completely different from the practitioner being in the same physical location as the patient. It is much more to do with being genuinely interested in the viewpoint of patient, carer and family member, and indeed it is quite possible to achieve this during a telephone call.

In the phrase 'being there for', it is the word 'for' which is perhaps the most important but is often overlooked. It says why the practitioner is there. It is for the patient, their carers and family – rather than from any notion of having a duty to dispense standard and convenient treatment solutions on a one-size-fits-all basis. Again this moves away from the practitioner being in sole charge and towards the concept of partnership (Jonsdottir et al. 2004).

Patients frequently comment on this quality of presence, and they are quick to recognize when it is missing. They might say, 'She was with me' or 'I did not have to explain all the time. She knew what I needed' or 'She seemed to always have time for me' or 'She listened to me and understood'.

These comments touch on various aspects of presence. 'She was with me' highlights the idea of being fully engaged with the other person and focused on their needs without distraction. 'She listened to me and understood' expresses the ability of the practitioner to listen empathically and imagine herself in the place of the patient. It also indicates her ability to feed this back in a way that allows the patient to feel heard and understood.

'She seemed to always have time for me' suggests that, despite the time-limited nature of many nurse–patient interactions, the experienced practitioner is able to create the feeling of time and space focused on this particular patient. With sensitivity the practitioner paces the interaction, giving the patient the sense that he or she is the most important concern for the practitioner in that moment (Jacobs 1993).

'I did not have to explain. All the time she knew what I needed' suggests the practitioner is attentive to the patient's needs and that this attention is underpinned by her experience and expertise, fluently woven into the consultation.

Campbell (1984) encapsulates these ideas when he says that:

> We feel cared for when our need is recognised and when the help which is offered does not overwhelm us but gently restores our strength at a pace which allows us to feel part of the movement to recovery. Conversely, a care which imposes itself on us, forcing a conformity to someone else's ideas of what we need, merely makes us feel more helpless and vulnerable.
>
> (Campbell 1984: 107–108)

Two phrases from Campbell's words are particularly powerful: 'our need is recognised' and 'conformity to someone else's ideas'. Being there entails the former rather than the latter.

The quality of presence is often observed in less experienced health care professionals. However, the advanced practitioner is able to use these skills more consciously and with intent, using and adapting their skills to work in partnership with the patient (Hardy et al. 2002).

In Scenario 3.1 the practitioner is sensitive to the patient's needs and allows the patient time to relax and feel comfortable to tell her story. Although concerned to exclude physical problems the practitioner remains open to the broader issues in the patient's life.

It is easy enough to be 'present' with a patient we like and feel positive towards. It is much more difficult to bring the same quality to a patient who challenges us and whom we may not like. Gallant et al. (2002) point out that this aspect of the nurse–patient relationship is largely ignored in the literature. Being present at this level is very skilful and demanding. To build and sustain a therapeutic relationship requires self-knowledge and the ability to use empathic understanding consciously, even when the situation is difficult and anxiety inducing.

It requires the practitioner to be willing to explore and develop his/herself and to examine his/her own feelings and emotions about difficult issues. Fear of not being able to cope with the emotions or feelings the patient may present is a frequent block to good communication and the ability to build meaningful relationships (Sandgren et al. 2006, Sheldon et al. 2006). It is for this reason that self-reflection, as discussed in Competency 9, is so important for a practitioner.

KEY POINTS

- Having a sense of timing and pacing, giving the patient space to build trust.
- Good time management and the ability to focus on the patient despite other pressures.
- Being genuinely interested to understand the viewpoint of each patient, their carers and their family.
- Being able to listen with empathy and feed this back to the patient.
- Paying attention to the patient's needs and having the experience and confidence to contain and hold the patient's concerns and feelings.
- The ability to give of self and to be physically and emotionally present for the patient and family.

Evaluates the impact of life transitions on the health/ illness status of patients and the impact of health/ illness on patients' lives (individuals, families, carers and communities)

This competency is concerned with change, with life transitions and their effect on health and illness, as well as transitions that are unexpected and which traumatically affect the lives of those involved. Being mindful of transitions is part of the idea of practitioners approaching each patient as an individual with a view to building a working partnership.

Transitions are a normal part of the process of life and occur throughout the lifespan. Most transitions are expected and managed as part of the normal rhythm of life, for example puberty and menopause. Nevertheless, such transitions can be difficult to navigate and may cause temporary difficulties even when foreseen. For example, a young person might find it challenging to adapt to university life, despite looking forward to leaving home and being independent, or an older person could become depressed following retirement despite looking forward to the freedom (Meleis et al. 2000).

Illness impacts powerfully on people's lives. Any illness demands some level of adaptation and adjustment in the life of a patient, and this kind of transition is mostly unexpected and unwelcome. Even a short illness can affect a person powerfully and a practitioner needs to remain sensitive to this. Practitioners who are routinely exposed to a great deal of human suffering need to be aware of the danger of underestimating the impact of what may appear to be a 'minor problem' in a patient's life.

Illness sometimes coincides with major life transitions and this can complicate the adaptation process, for example an adolescent who is diagnosed with diabetes. In contrast, life transitions can sometimes be responsible for bringing about illness, such as the physical symptoms of fatigue experienced by a patient who is losing her role in the social world as her children move away into adult life. Keeping the broader aspects of a patient's life in mind will help the practitioner to work more effectively (Meleis et al. 2000).

In Scenario 3.1, the patient is negotiating the transition from wife to widow state, her body betraying the pain and anxiety she is unable to express openly. The practitioner recognizes this process and the stress that the bereavement and adjustment to a new life role brings. They give the patient permission to talk about it, unafraid of the emotions that may spill out in the process. They are aware that they cannot 'make it better' for the patient, and know that the adaptation may take some time. They anticipate this by not discharging the patient as soon as the physical symptoms are dealt with.

KEY POINTS

- Transitions are a normal part of life.
- Illness can complicate normal life transitions.
- Difficult transitions can manifest as physical and psychological symptoms.
- Practitioners need to have an understanding of normal transitions and remain sensitive to these when working with a patient.
- Taking account of transitions is part of working in partnership with patients as individuals and understanding their unique viewpoints.

Applies principles of empowerment in promoting behaviour change

This competency focuses on the empowerment of patients. Taken literally, empowerment means granting real power to patients in terms of decision-making and taking control over their care. However, it is only possible for practitioners to empower patients if the practitioners themselves feel empowered.

True partnership and empowerment of patients and their families presupposes a person-centred approach to care, an approach where patients are truly consulted and their decisions accepted, even if they do not necessarily fit with the ideas of the practitioner. This does entail some element of risk, and a willingness on the part of the practitioner to be an advocate for a patient's choice, even if it goes against normally accepted views (Wheeler 2000).

'Advocacy' is another term used in nursing literature to denote empowerment (Mallik 1997). It has been variously defined. For example Baldwin (2003) chose three main and useful attributes of patient advocacy:

- a therapeutic nurse–patient relationship in which to secure a patient's freedom and self-determination;
- promoting and protecting the patient's rights to be involved in decision-making and informed consent;
- acting as an intermediary between patients and their families and between them and health care providers.

In Scenario 3.1 the practitioner meets the first two criteria of advocacy. They offer the patient an option of treatment with anti-depressants, even though they themselves do not feel this to be the best option at that moment. They have the power to withhold this treatment option. By giving the patient the choice they put aside their view of what is 'best', giving the patient real choice. It was possible that the patient might have opted for anti-depressants contrary to the practitioner's initial clinical judgement. But this willingness to share power with the patient helps build mutual trust and opens the opportunity to get to know the patient, to understand the unique details of this person's illness within the context of her life, building a real partnership.

Central to the discussion surrounding advocacy and nursing practice is the concept of moral agency. To act as moral agent, nurses must have the power of decision and action (Wilmot 1993). Advanced nurses are increasingly gaining more control over their clinical decisions and actions. Moral agency is linked to personal agency and has been defined by Bandura (1995) as a person's self-belief in their ability to achieve control over situations. Some authors believe that the higher a person's self-esteem the higher their moral practice (Arthur and Thorne, 1998).

The stronger a nurse's sense of self the more they will be able to influence and affect care positively (Randle 2002). Acting as moral agent for patients and their families is not easy in the light of the pressures inherent in modern health care, such as resource constraints, staffing shortages and low morale. It requires self-confidence and leadership skills.

The advanced practitioner needs to develop their practice and at the same time develop themselves. The Royal College of Nursing leadership programme demonstrated that learning to manage uncertainty, handling negative feelings and developing self-confidence are essential prerequisites to improve and influence patient care issues, and at the same time empower patients to take control over their care (Cunningham and Kitson 2000).

Evidence from the literature seems to indicate that in order to help other people, nurses need to be aware of themselves and to develop their self-confidence and

---

KEY POINTS

- Empowering patients to make decisions about their care is part of a good nurse–patient relationship.
- To empower others the practitioner needs to have a sense of self and a measure of power over her own decisions and practice.
- To act as advocate for patients and families is not easy in the present climate of health care.

self-esteem (Higgs and Titchen 2001, Pask 2003). Freshwater (2002) also posits that self-awareness not only benefits the nurse–patient relationship but is also important to the well-being and efficacy of the practitioner.

Preserves the patient's control over decision-making, assesses the patient's commitment to the jointly determined plan of care and fosters personal responsibility for health

This competency is concerned with giving patients some control over the decision-making about their care. It touches on the notion of who holds the power in this relationship and how decisions are made or negotiated. It is central to the key theme for this entire domain, encouraging practitioners to allow patients to play an active part in decisions about their own care.

Government policy advocates patient involvement in care decisions. Consumers of health care should experience choice and express opinions about the care they receive. This view challenges the traditional paternalistic approach to health care, which believed that 'the professional knows best'. Nurses have long espoused the idea of holistic patient-centred care, which by definition involves the patient in the decision-making. Most nurses would express this as part of their core philosophy of nursing.

However, the reality of shared decision-making with patients is complex, fraught with difficulties and often misunderstood (Charles et al. 1997). As nurses increase their decision-making power and gain more control over their own practice, involving the patient in this decision-making process becomes more urgent.

Much of the literature on shared decision-making relates to medicine, as diagnostic and treatment decisions have mostly lived in the medical realm. Nursing literature has tended to promote the importance of a nurse–patient relationship that fosters the involvement of the patient in negotiation and decision-making regarding care, and tends to be less focused on diagnostic or treatment options. This is changing with the advent of the role of advanced nurse practitioner (ANP).

The scenario illustrates the type and level of diagnostic and treatment decisions nurses and patients will now need to negotiate. It also demonstrates the level of autonomy in decision-making of the ANP. This will be further enhanced with the advent of independent prescribing. The practitioner here remains sensitive to the patient's perspective and offers treatment choice but does not impose it nor withhold it, despite their own views and feelings.

Concern with shared decision-making has come about largely because of a shift in the power relationship between doctor and patient. In particular, patients are becoming more informed and are able to access specialist knowledge. Increased consumerism and patient autonomy is challenging medical authority and forcing a more equal relationship. As the asymmetry of information between patient and medical practitioner diminishes, so the power of the medical profession decreases.

In addition, the changing nature of medical practice with ever-increasing speed and the need for long-term care and monitoring has altered some of the focus of treatment from cure to long-term care and management. Complex treatment options and increased choice options require more discussion and negotiation between practitioner and patient (Elwyn and Glyn 1999).

The ANP operates under the impact of all these changes; indeed, advanced practitioners, with more autonomy and prescribing power, may well be perceived by patients as more powerful now than nurses who do not function at that level. This creates an interesting reversal. ANPs need to be aware how powerful they may appear to patients and will need to temper this in the way they construct the relationship with the patient.

The partnership relationship between practitioner and patient is crucial in shaping how decisions are made in the consultation. In a shared decision the process, outcome and responsibility are truly shared and negotiated by the patient and the practitioner. This way of working implies a commitment on both sides to engage fully in that relationship and share responsibility for the outcome.

Sharing decisions in this way does imply a positive and trusting relationship between health care professional and patient. It is a model that necessitates some of the skills discussed earlier and a level of insight into one's own process as a practitioner, as it can be challenging and disturbing fully to take on board the wishes and context of patients' lives (Greenhalgh 2002).

It is important to remain sensitive to the patient's wishes (Elwyn et al. 1999, Levinson et al. 2005). Some patients may not want to be so involved in the decision-making process and prefer to leave the decision to the professionals, others may want more or less involvement depending on the decisions being made (Whitney 2003). Gwyn et al. (2000) suggest that inherent in the interaction between health professional and patient there is a power imbalance and a knowledge asymmetry that cannot be entirely eliminated. They go on to say, however, that the quality of the relationship can temper and reduce the power imbalance; a view that is supported by Rundqvist and Lindstrom (2005), who argue that a caring relationship is not mutual since nurse and patient cannot change places as they are on different levels, nor can responsibility be delegated from nurse to patient.

Sharing decisions with patients often entails sharing the uncertainties about the outcomes and involves exposing the fact that data are often unavailable or not known; this can cause anxiety to both patient and practitioner. To accept that some patients choose not to do the things we would see as imperative to their health, to be able to sustain the relationship and to support the patient in their choices, some of which might challenge our deeply held beliefs, demands a great deal of confidence and humility.

KEY POINTS

- True shared decision-making requires the building of a meaningful partnership between practitioner and patient.
- Shared decision-making has become more current because of changes in health care and the shift in power relationships between practitioners and patients.
- Not all patients want to be that closely involved in the decision-making process.
- The level, complexity and timing of the decision may inform how much the patient wants and is able to be involved.
- Compliance with treatment tends to be improved if the patient has some input into the decision-making process.

Maintains confidentiality while recording data, plans and results in a manner that preserves the dignity and privacy of the patient

This competency addresses the issues of recording and keeping records of the patient's care. This includes how a record is made, where it is stored and who has sight of it. The specific points discussed here are based on the Nursing and Midwifery Council guidelines (NMC 2005) and the *NHS confidentiality code of practice* (DoH 2003).

Record-keeping is an important and necessary part of nursing work. Records provide continuity and safety of care for the patient. The NMC (2005), in its guidelines for record keeping, states that:

> Accurate record-keeping is essential to protect the welfare of clients, to maintain high standards of care and to afford continuity of care. Good record-keeping should give an accurate account of treatment care planning and delivery of care, thus increasing the ability to detect problems such as changes in patient condition at an early stage. Good records increase the communication and dissemination of information between members of the inter-professional team.
>
> NMC (2005)

To review the NMC guidelines you can access the NMC website at http://www.nmc.uk.org.

The way care is delivered in the NHS is changing. In the past, patients would receive treatment from one GP or a hospital doctor. Today, owing to the reduction in junior doctors' hours and an increasing number of specialists involved in care, patients are most likely to be treated by a team of health care professionals, both in primary and in secondary care. Although this delivers great benefits in terms of the quality of treatment, it also means that professionals from different disciplines need to communicate effectively with each other.

Record keeping, in this changed environment, becomes ever more crucial to ensure continuity and patient safety (Dimond 2005). Nurse practitioners will be contributing to medical records as well as nursing records and will need to be sure that they are able clearly to outline the work they have done with the patient and the action they have taken or wish to be taken.

In some settings ANPs will only see a patient when called in on a consultancy basis. The practitioner may not initiate the care actions and needs to be sure that their advice is clearly recorded in the patient notes, both for their own protection as well as to enable continuity of care for the rest of the team. Sometimes it may not be clear which patient records the practitioner needs to use. Clarity within the organization as to which set of records are to be used is essential when developing a new ANP role.

The way the records are written is also important. Depending on the setting of care, the input of patients should become the norm in record keeping. This is more possible in primary care where the record of the consultation can form a normal part of the summary and closure of the nurse–patient encounter.

The practitioner reviews the findings, the plan for the future and the treatment decisions with the patient and carer if appropriate, when they are recorded in the notes. This process requires some fluency in the mechanics of recording as well as maintaining the connection with the patient. In sharing the content with the patient the practitioner ensures that the record remains respectful and is written in such a way as to be understandable to the patient and carer.

This immediate participation and involvement of the patient may not be possible in different settings, although it should always be considered. Sharing records allows for good communication with the patient, with both parties being clear about planned action and treatment options. It avoids confusion and mistakes and supports the idea of shared decision-making.

Confidentiality of records is another important consideration. Patients entrust us with sensitive information relating to their health. They do so in confidence and they have the legitimate expectation that staff will respect their privacy and act appropriately (DoH 2003).

The *NHS confidentiality code of practice* (DoH 2003) suggests three main requirements for confidentiality. First, protecting patient information entails looking after the patient's information. This is achieved at individual level in keeping accurate and consistent records and at organizational level in the safe storage and retrieval of records. Equally, all staff need to be aware of their responsibility regarding the confidentiality of records. Second, informing the patient involves making sure that patients know how and in what way information is used and that there are no surprises at any stage. Third, providing choice allows the patient to decide whether information can be disclosed and used in a particular way. It is important to remember that different people have different sensibilities.

These same principles apply to the use of patient material in the construction of the portfolio. Permission needs to be sought for the use of patient material and the patient should never be identifiable.

KEY POINTS

- Records are an important aspect of patient care.
- Sharing records with patients whenever possible is good practice.
- The habit of sharing records ensures the notes are written respectfully and in a way that patients can understand.
- The principles of confidentiality apply to all use of patient information, including the portfolio material.

Monitors and reflects on own emotional response to interactions with patients' carers and families and uses this knowledge to further therapeutic interaction

This competency deals with the ideas of reflection, reflection on self and reflection on practice, in order to grow and develop as a person and as a practitioner. It touches on the ideas of therapeutic use of self and intentional practice.

This is possibly the most challenging and difficult aspect of advanced practice. To be able to reflect on one's own process and to allow others to challenge long-held beliefs and familiar patterns is not easy. Nurses have traditionally found it hard to explore themselves. In many ways, it is easier to help others than to delve into our own motivations and feelings (Freshwater 2002).

Nurse culture has, and to some extent still does, sustained this attitude, and self-exploration is often described as 'navel gazing'. However, in the last few years there has been a much greater focus on reflection in nurse education, and the implementation of clinical supervision in many clinical areas has brought about some change in this way of thinking (Rolfe et al. 2001).

It can be difficult to make time to examine one's own feelings and thoughts in a busy clinical practice. Yet unless reflection becomes part of nursing practice, the level of development and growth a practitioner can achieve remains limited. In particular, advanced practitioners who often work alone and autonomously need to reflect and to participate in clinical supervision. The idea of 'presence' and 'being there' explored earlier as part of the relationship with patients requires a level of investment of self that demands time and space for reflection (Graham et al. 2005).

The Scenario 3.1 demonstrates some of the process of reflection. The practitioner has written down their encounter with the patient. As they explore some of the reasons for their actions, the practitioner reflects on the idea that the patient was reluctant to make direct eye contact. The practitioner then uses the physical examination to build trust and make a safe space.

This realization of the intent of their actions may have happened 'in action', in that they had experienced this before and knew the examination would offer another opportunity to help the patient to talk. Or it may have been a 'reflection on action', in that in writing the encounter down they then unpicked the process and realized or made conscious what it was they had done, without being aware of it at the time (Schon 1991). They made the invisible part of their practice visible by reflecting critically on what happened and how they acted.

This practitioner also makes explicit in their account the thinking they are engaged in during the consultation, their diagnostic reasoning, the type of knowledge they bring to their decision-making process, and the conclusions they draw from this. All of this is captured in the writing and reflection, allowing the reader and themselves a glimpse into their thinking.

The writing of scenarios is a useful tool for constructing a portfolio. One scenario, carefully written and reflected on, can be evidence for a number of competencies. That process in itself demonstrates the practitioner's ability to reflect and think critically about practice.

In teaching reflection I am frequently asked why it is so important and what difference it really makes. Scenario 3.4, recounted to me by a colleague, will help answer this.

Scenario 3.4

I was teaching one of the nurses in our team to carry out cervical smears. She was finding it really difficult to do and was hesitant and shaky at every attempt. This surprised me as she was quick to learn in other situations. We struggled and tried different approaches without success. It then occurred to me to ask her how she felt about having a smear taken herself. Her response was explosive: 'I hate it, it is awful and always painful.' We were both left a little breathless after this outburst. We then sat and talked, I asked if she assumed that every woman felt the same about having a smear and she admitted that she did, realizing in that same moment that this was an unreasonable assumption and the impact it had on her ability to perform the smears.

Amazingly the next smear she performed went smoothly and well. She never looked back. I reflected on the powerful influence our own assumptions and experiences have on our practice and I was grateful to have thought to explore this with her and not dismiss her as 'useless at smears'. I was also glad to have realized that it was not of necessity my poor teaching skills that were at fault. Two thinking patterns I could easily have fallen into to explain the inexplicable difficulties my colleague was having in acquiring this practical skill.

This story illustrates the power of reflecting on what we do, paying attention to the reactions that seem different and outside our usual behaviours. Doing this alone can be difficult, but writing and keeping a diary is helpful.

Working with others in supervision is another positive way to talk about and critically examine our practice. Jill Down's writing in Chapter 3 of *Therapeutic nursing* (Freshwater 2002) is a useful example of how supervision can be used to explore in depth some of the tensions around the care of an acutely ill patient. She struggles with the tension between technology and retaining the human element of care in a highly technical setting. The process of clinical supervision enables her to begin to unravel some the complex issues that face her as a nurse and as an individual.

KEY POINTS

- Critical reflection is an integral part of working as an advanced practitioner.
- Reflection develops self-knowledge and moves practice forward.
- Writing about one's practice is an important part of the process of reflection.
- A reflective group or clinical supervision should be part of every advanced practitioner's life and practice.

Considers the patient's needs when bringing closure to the nurse–patient relationship and provides a safe transition to another care provider

This competency is concerned with endings, boundaries and the skill of knowing when and how to close a relationship. As with other competencies in this domain, it is a question of understanding each patient as an individual and working with them in partnership.

Some relationships with patients end naturally. These time-limited encounters do not usually present a problem. The care setting often determines the length of involvement with a patient. In acute care the patient's discharge usually heralds the end of the relationship. Even in these settings it may be important to plan the ending and to have a pre-discharge consultation to ensure the patient has all the resources and information they require.

Today, with the increase in chronic illness, even in the acute setting, there may be relationships that last over a number of years, some ending only when the patient dies.

Nurses need to acknowledge the importance of these relationships to themselves and to the family and allow time for that bond to dissolve. In many instances the practitioner will have become a familiar and trusted figure in the lives of the patient and the family and they may feel the need to seek support even after the patient has died. Whether this is appropriate depends much on the individual situation and requires some reflection on the nurse's part. In primary care a nurse practitioner will develop relationships that span years and involve close knowledge of the patient and the family. Some of these relationships never end entirely. Only different episodes of care come to closure.

It is important to know when to close the relationship and when to refer to other care providers. This is not always easy to achieve, as some patients may want to continue the contact with the practitioner for reasons other than the health needs they presented with initially. Loneliness and a need to receive attention may motivate the patient to continue seeking advice and help when they could manage on their own. Gently helping the patient to let go and to seek resources elsewhere is a skill many nurses find difficult to manage. Discussing cases with peers can be helpful in finding solutions to some of these dilemmas.

Appropriate referrals are important but negotiating the referral with the patient without jarring their trust can be difficult. For example, if a patient has been telling the practitioner their difficulties, a referral to a counsellor may seem like a rejection of the patient. The reverse may also be the case where the practitioner finds it hard to let the patient go. The nurse may find it hard to accept that the patient has the resources to manage their own problems. Repeated appointments to make sure the patient is all right should alert the practitioner to their own needs and lead to reflecting on who is being served by these actions.

In some situations endings can be left in the patient's control and in Scenario 3.1 the practitioner left the patient the choice and once she had built up her resources and moved on to another phase of her life she was able to close the relationship herself. This is not always appropriate and some endings need to be managed more actively by the practitioner.

KEY POINTS

- Endings need careful planning.
- Ending a relationship can be difficult for the patient and the practitioner.
- Referrals need to be negotiated sensitively taking into account the patient's feelings.
- Building the patient's resources throughout the relationship helps facilitate endings.

CONCLUSION

This domain of nurse–patient relationship underpins every aspect of the work carried out with patients. Technical know-how and up-to-date knowledge are the basis for good practice; however, knowledge and technical skills alone are not sufficient to bring about a successful nurse–patient encounter. Sensitivity, empathy and a willingness to give of oneself are essential elements of advanced practice. In this domain we have explored issues such as trust and the elusive quality of 'presence' and have focused on skills and qualities that can be refined and honed in the service of the patient. This work is arduous and demanding but it is also immensely rewarding and enriching to the practitioner. It is a journey taken with each patient; it is also a journey of self-discovery and growth for the nurse. Working in this way in the busy and demanding context of today's health care is not easy; it is hard to remain steady and focused faced with the conflicting demands of this rapidly changing environment. Being an advanced practitioner is about keeping the human and caring elements of working with patients at the forefront of practice, to role model and advocate for it, and thus support others to follow in their footsteps.

REFERENCES

Arthur, D. and Thorne, S. (1998) Professional self-concept of nurses: a comparative study of four strata of nursing students in a Canadian university. *Nurse Education Today* 18(5): 380–388.

Baldwin, M.A. (2003) Patient advocacy: a concept analysis. *Nursing Standard* 17(21) 33–39.

Bandura, A. (1995) *Self-efficacy in changing societies.* Cambridge: University Press.

Campbell, A.V. (1984) *Moderated love.* London: SPCK.

Charles, C. Gafni, A. and Whelan, T. (1997) Shared decision-making in the medical encounter: what does it mean? (or it takes at least two to tango). *Social Science & Medicine* 44: 681–692.

Connie, H. and Coralli M. (2006) Effective case presentation: an important clinical skill for nurse practitioners. *Journal of the American Academy of Nurse Practitioners* 18: 216–220.

Cunningham, G. and Kitson, A. (2000) An evaluation of the RCN clinical leadership development programme, part 2. *Nursing Standard* 15(13–15): 34–40.

Dimond, B. (2005) Legal aspects of documentation: exploring common deficiencies that occur in record-keeping. *British Journal of Nursing* 14(10): 568–571.

DoH (2003) *The NHS confidentiality code of practice: guidelines on the use and protection of patient information.* London: DoH publications.

Elwyn, G. and Glyn, R. (1999) Stories we hear stories we tell: analysing talk in clinical practice. *British Journal of Medicine* 318: 186–188.

Elwyn, G. Edwards, A. and Kinnersly, P. (1999) Shared decision-making in primary care: the neglected second half of the consultation. *British Journal of General Practice* 49: 471–482.

Freshwater, D. (ed.) (2002) *Therapeutic nursing: improving patient care through self awareness and reflection.* London: Sage.

Gallant, M. Beaulieu, M. and Carnevale, F. (2002) Partnership: an analysis of the concept within the nurse–client relationship. *Journal of Advanced Nursing* 40(2): 149–157.

Graham, I. Andrewes, T. and Clark, L. (2005) Mutual suffering: a nurse's story of caring for the living as they are dying. *International Journal of Nursing Practice* 11: 277–285.

Gwyn, R. (2002) *Communicating health and illness.* London: Sage.

Gwyn, R. Edwards, A. Kinnersley, R. and Grol, K. (2000) Shared decision-making and the concept of equipoise: the competencies of involving patients in health care choices. *British Journal of General Practice* 50: 892–899.

Haidet, P. Kroll, T. and Sharf, B. (2006) The complexity of patient participation: lessons learnt from patients' illness narratives. *Patient Education and Counselling* 62(3): 323–329.

Hardy, S. Garbett, R. Titchen, A. and Manley, K. (2002). Exploring nursing expertise: nurses talk nursing. *Nursing Inquiry* 9: 196–202.

Heath, I. (1998) *Following the story: continuity of care in general practice.* In *Narrative Based Medicine. Dialogue and discourse in clinical practice,* Greenhalgh, T. and Hurwitz, B. (eds), pp. 83–92. London: BMJ publications.

Higgs, J. and Jones, M. (2000) *Clinical reasoning in the health professions.* Oxford: Butterworth-Heinemann.

Higgs, J. and Titchen, A. (2001) *Practice knowledge and expertise in the health professions.* Oxford: Butterworth-Heinemann.

Jacobs, M. (1993) *Still small voice: an introduction to pastoral counselling,* 2nd edn. London: SPEC.

Jonsdottir, H. Litchenfield, M. and Dexheimer Pharris, M. (2004) The relational core of nursing practice as partnership. *Journal of Advanced Nursing* 47(3): 241–250.

Kurtz, S. Silverman, J. and Draper, J. (2004) *Skills for communicating with patients,* 2nd edn. Oxford: Radcliffe Medical Press.

Levinson, W. Kao, A. Kuby, A. and Thisted, R. (2005) Not all patients want to participate in decision-making: a national study of public preferences. *Journal of General Medicine* 20: 531–535.

Mallik, M. (1997) Advocacy in nursing: a review of the literature. *Journal of Advanced Nursing* 19: 947–953.

Mattingly, C. (1991) The narrative nature of clinical reasoning. *American Journal of Occupational Therapy* 45: 998–1005.

Mattingly, C. (1998) In search of the good: narrative reasoning in practice. *Medical Anthropology Quarterly* 12: 273–297.

Meleis, A. Sawyer, L. Im. E. Hilfinger, M. DeAnne, K. and Schumacher, K. (2000) Experiencing transitions: an emerging middle-range theory. *Advances in Nursing Sciences* 23(1): 12–28.

Naef, R. (2006) Bearing witness: a moral way of engaging in the nurse–patient relationship. *Journal of Advanced Nursing* 40(2): 149–157.

Neighbour, R. (2004) *The inner consultation: how to deliver an effective and intuitive consultation style*. Oxford: Radcliffe Medical Press.

NMC (2005) *Guidelines for records and record keeping*. London: NMC.

Nordgren, S. and Fridlund, B. (2001) Patient's perceptions of self determination as expressed in the context of care. *Journal of the Royal Society of Medicine* 35: 117–125.

Pask, E. (2003) Moral agency in nursing: seeing value in the work and believing that I make a difference. *Nursing Ethics* 2003 10(2): 165–174.

Pendleton, D. Schofield, T. Tate, P. and Havelock, P. (eds) (2003) *The new consultation: developing doctor–patient communication*. Oxford: Oxford University Press.

Randle, J. (2002) The shaping of moral identity and practice. *Nurse Education in Practice* 2: 251–256.

Rolfe, G. Freshwater, D. and Jasper, M. (2001) *Critical reflection for nurses and the helping professions: a user's guide*. London: Sage.

Royal College of General Practitioners (2003) *Examination for membership (MRCGP). Regulations for 2003. Patients' consent to video-recording*. Royal College of General Practitioners. Available from: http://www.rcgp.org.uk/rcgp/exam/regulations/regu14.asp (accessed on 27/06/06).

Rundqvist, D. and Lindstrom, U. (2005) Empowerment and authorization who provides and who receives meta-study of empowerment in nursing research: a caring science perspective. *International Journal of Human Caring* 9(4): 24–32.

Sandgren, A. Thulesius, H. Fridlund, B. and Peterson, K. (2006) Striving for emotional survival in palliative cancer nursing. *Qualitative Health Research* 16(1): 79–96.

Schon, D. (1991) *The reflective practitioner: how professionals think in action*. Aldershot: Avebury Publications.

Sellman, D. (2006) The importance of being trustworthy. *Nursing Ethics* 13(2): 106–115.

Sheldon, L. Barrett, R. and Ellington, L. (2006) Difficult communication in nursing. *Journal of Nursing Scholarship* 38(2): 141–147.

Stilwell, B. (1998) The search for meaning in advanced nursing practice. In *Advanced Nursing Practice*, Rolfe, G. and Fulbrook, P. (eds), *Advanced Nursing Practice*, pp. 43–49. Oxford: Butterworth-Heinemann.

Titchen, A. (2001) Skilled companionship in professional practice. In Higgs, J. and Tichen, A. (eds), *Practice knowledge and expertise in the health professions*, pp. 69–79. Oxford: Butterworth-Heinemann.

Wheeler, P. (2000) Is advocacy at the heart of professional practice? *Nursing Standard* 14(36): 39–41.

Whitney, S. (2003) A new model of decisions: exploring the limits of shared decision-making. *Medical Decision-making* 23(4): 275–280.

Wilmot, S. (1993) Ethics, agency and empowerment in nurse education. *Nurse Education Today* 13: 189–234.

FURTHER READING

Bonnie, M. Haggerty, K. and Patusky, L. (2003) Reconceptualizing the nurse–patient relationship. The theory of human relatedness is useful in nurse patient relationships. *Journal of Nursing Scholarship* 35(2).
This is a brief but useful article raising some interesting ideas around the changing nature of nurse–patient relationships in a fast-moving environment. The authors challenge some of the assumptions traditionally made about nurse–patient relationships and offer a different framework to explore nurse–patient relationships. Thought provoking.
Campbell, A.V. (1984) *Moderated love*. London: SPCK.
Again a classic that bears reading and re-reading. Campbell sensitively and searchingly explores the relationship between professional helpers and those who seek their help; his theological perspective offers a different and refreshing glimpse of the ambiguities and joys of helping and healing. This book is also useful background to the work of Angie Titchen.
Freshwater, D. (ed.) (2002) *Therapeutic nursing: improving patient care through self awareness and reflection*. London: Sage.
Chapters 1 and 2 are particularly helpful in drawing out some of the issues of self reflection and the concepts around what is required to build a therapeutic relationship. A useful book overall.
Meleis, A. Swyer, L. Im, E. Hilfinger, M. DeAnne, K. and Schumacher, K. (2000) Experiencing transitions: an emerging middle-range theory. *Advances in Nursing Science* 23(1): 12–28.
This seminal work on transitions is informative and good background reading for issues of transition.
Rogers, C. (1961) *On becoming a person*. Boston: Mifflin.
Rogers, C. (1980) *A way of being*. Boston: Mifflin.
Two old favourites to dip into and draw wisdom from. Rogers in the original has much to tell us about human nature, relationships and a way of being with others.
Sandgren, A. Thulesius, H. Fridlund, B and Peterson, K. (2006) Striving for emotional survival in palliative cancer nursing. *Qualitative Health Research* 16(1): 79–96.
This useful article provides a comprehensive framework for understanding how nurses deal with some of the emotional difficulties they face, in this instance in palliative care in hospital, but it is relevant in other settings too. It is a helpful tool for reflection and giving a language to the emotional experiences of nurses in their daily work.
Sellman, D. (2006) On being trustworthy. *Nursing Ethics* 13(2): 106–115.
This article looks at the concept of trust and discusses different perspectives evaluating its position in nursing – interesting and thought provoking.
Silverman, J. Kurtz, S. and Draper, J. (2005) *Skills for communicating with patients*. Oxford: Radcliffe Medical Press.
Although written from a medical perspective, this book gives a clear overview of many of the issues concerning consultations. It is practical in its approach to the topic, giving lots of useful examples as well as a helpful checklist to analyse the content and process of a consultation.
Walsh, M. Crumbie, A. and Reveley, S. (1999) *Nurse practitioners: clinical skills and professional issues*. Oxford: Butterworth-Heinemann.
A useful reference book encompassing a number of advanced skills as well as discussion on some of the topical issues facing nurse practitioners today.

DOMAIN 2: RESPECTING CULTURE AND DIVERSITY

AUDREY CALLUM

INTRODUCTION

> It is essential to know man it would seem, before attempting to do him good.
>
> Nathaniel Hawthorne (1850)

> There is no place for discrimination or harassment in the NHS on grounds of race or ethnicity, gender, sexual orientation, disability, religion or age.
>
> The Hon. John Reid, UK Department of Health

The context of health care is changing in response to changes in society and patterns of diseases, increasing patient expectations and challenging the new policy agenda for the NHS through its modernization programmes (DOH 1998a, 1999a, 2002).

The UK is rapidly becoming a multicultural, multilingual, multiethnic and pluralistic society as more and more people from ethnic minority groups have joined the UK population. The UK National Health Service (NHS) policies have clearly put the 'patient' at the centre of service provision (DoH 1998b, 1999a,b), which implies that nurses need to have an awareness of the demographic changes in the British population in order to implement these policies. There is also increasing evidence of inequalities in health linked to ethnicity (Townsend and Davidson 1982, Whitehead 1987, Nazroo 1997, Acheson 1998, DoH 1998a,b), which has created many challenges for health professionals, including those nurses working in advanced practice roles. This is important, as many of these professionals may lack cultural competence and may be unaware of how to meet the needs of culturally diverse clients. Nurses working in advanced nursing practice roles are in the frontline of care and must be skilled in providing culturally appropriate and competent care for their clients irrespective of their diverse clinical needs. Nurses need to have a sound cultural knowledge base as this will enable them to understand their own cultural values, biases, beliefs and prejudices. This should help to prevent biases, conflicting cultural encounters and unethical care. Having cultural knowledge can also help the advanced practitioner to articulate differences and accurately assess patients' individual needs through partnership in care planning.

This chapter focuses on two of the most challenging issues of contemporary health care for advanced nursing practice. In order fully to understand the concept of culture and spirituality within health care, other concepts need to be understood and applied. Once recognized, the advanced practitioner will be able to use this knowledge to inform areas of cultural and religious competence in advanced practice.

DEFINING CULTURE, ETHNICITY AND DIVERSITY

Culture

The terms culture, race and ethnicity are sometimes used interchangeably by health professionals and the public alike. However, these terms have differing meanings and interpretations.

There are many definitions of culture. According to Leininger (2001) culture can be defined as 'the values, beliefs, norms and practices of a particular group that are learned and shared and guide thinking, decisions and actions in a particular way'. However, culture is not static but is continually evolving, therefore, achieving cultural competence is ongoing (Henley and Schott 1999, Duffy 2001, Leininger 2001, Helman 2002). Consequently, as cultures evolve, health professionals need to keep abreast of changes to maintain cultural competence. Distinctions of race and ethnicity are socially constructed but they are not synonymous, and racial judgements are sometimes based on perceptions of physical appearance which are shaped by beliefs about the intrinsic, unchanging qualities of people of different races (Jenkins 1997, Macbeth and Shetty 2001). Conversely, in defining the nature of culture, Helman (2002: 2) believes that culture is 'a set of guidelines which an individual inherits as a member of a particular society and which tells him how to view the world and learn how to behave in it in relation to other people. It also provides him with a way of transmitting these guidelines to the next generation by use of symbols, language art and rituals' (Helman 2002: 2). Spector (1996), on the other hand, posits that it is a meta-communication system which is based on non-physical traits, such as beliefs, attitudes, customs, values, behaviour and language, that are shared by a group of people and passed down through generations. Despite the agreement in defining the term, the concept of culture remains problematic in the public domain. This fluidity of the cultural realm is evident during expressions of illness. Conversely, clinicians use cultural beliefs to understand particular illness behaviours, such as adherence to prescribed treatment modalities. During an encounter with the patient, nurses are said to be exposed to three cultures (De Santis 1994):

- the nurse's professional culture;
- the patient's culture;
- organizational culture.

All three cultures have their own sets of beliefs, values and practices and need to be considered when patient care is being planned. There is a universal need of all people to be treated with respect, which is predicated on the awareness of the interaction of these three cultures. This can also be experienced by patients as well as nurses, as patients are also confronted with these cultural phenomena which they, too, have to understand during the encounter with health professionals. The NMC (2008) requires that all nurses, including those working in advanced practice roles, respect the values, customs, spiritual beliefs and practices of all individuals and groups. A nurse who is culturally competent will be able to recognize and understand the impact their own culture and professional beliefs will have on workplace practices and will recognize that cultural differences occur across all levels of cultural diversity. Ignorance of any of these will create barriers to achieving a positive, productive and caring nurse–patient relationship. Consequently, the ability to give optimal, sensitive care will require knowing and owning feelings, beliefs and attitudes and recognizing their influence on patient care.

Ethnicity

Like culture, there are several definitions of ethnicity and its concept is also problematic as there does not seem to be a universally accepted definition of ethnicity.

Jones (1994: 292) believes ethnicity 'refers to cultural practices and attitudes that characterize a given group of people and distinguishes it from other groups', where the popular group is seen to be different by virtue of their religion, language, ancestry, common interests and other shared cultural practices, for example dietary habits or style of dress. There is an extensive body of anthropological and sociological literature relating to ethnicity, but the concept remains elusive as it is inextricably linked with concepts of race and racism (Jenkins 1997). This suggests that ethnic differences are wholly learned and are the result of socialization and acculturation (the process by which members of one culture or group adopt the beliefs and behaviours of another group) and not genetic inheritance. This needs to be considered when planning health care for clients from different ethnic groups and rests within the advanced practitioner's sphere of practice. All health professionals need to provide services that meet the needs of a multicultural society.

Diversity

Cultural diversity has become a very prominent feature in the British health care system and impacts significantly on the quality of nursing care. This poses a challenge for health care professionals, firstly because the British health care system is dominated by western values and secondly, because this population expects to receive a quality service that is culturally sensitive, and thirdly, because diversity is promoted as a fundament principle of nursing (Boyle 2000, Leininger 2001, NMC 2008). Cultural diversity is an inclusive concept that embraces not only ethnic groups but also other marginal or vulnerable people in society, for example those suffering from AIDS and drug abuse, because they too, may experience marginalization and discrimination based on their lifestyle choices.

Diversity, like health, means different things to different people. Leininger (2001) has argued that an understanding of cultural diversity is essential to the provision of effective and safe client care and that the knowledge of a client's cultural beliefs, values, and attitudes, is an integral part of providing health care. Nursing care and practice in the UK have undergone radical changes in recent years, as the population has become more culturally diverse. The demographic changes in the UK have meant that people from diverse groups and different cultural backgrounds will have health care needs requiring high-quality, effective needs-led services. Because of this, health care professionals working with these patients will need to keep abreast of the diversity of patients' cultures (Boyle 2000). The NMC (2008) also requires nurses to respect the values, customs, spiritual beliefs and practices of all individuals and groups. This means that nursing care needs to be delivered safely to patients, irrespective of their ethnicity and sexual orientation.

In any health care setting, the nurse who is culturally competent will recognize and understand the impact that his/her own cultural and professional beliefs will have on practices in the workplace and will be able to acknowledge that cultural differences will occur across all levels of diversity. Some researchers have suggested that cultural insensitivity can create barriers to accessing health care because of increased exposure to a multicultural and multilingual clientele and because of the patient-centred orientation of nursing, it is imperative that nurses are able to respond to the unique cultural needs of their client groups when challenged to provide effective caring and curing in varied cultural contexts. The role of advanced nurses is central to this, as they are strategically placed to provide culturally competent care through regular interaction with diverse cultural groups in their practice.

KEY POINTS

- The context of health care is changing as the UK continues to be a multiethnic, multicultural and multifaith society.
- The concepts of culture, race and ethnicity, although often used interchangeably, are problematic.
- Cultural insensitivity can create barriers to accessing health care.
- Advanced nurses are strategically placed to provide culturally congruent care for patients with diverse cultural needs.

LEGAL AND ETHICAL CONSIDERATIONS IN ADVANCED NURSING PRACTICE

Increasingly, nurses are being held accountable for providing care that is congruent for patients from cultural and linguistically diverse groups.

The United Nation's Universal Declaration of Human Rights (UNO, 1948) recognized access to adequate health care as a fundamental human right and imposed on all member states a moral obligation to attempt to provide health care to all its citizens without discrimination or regard to status. The International Council of Nurses Code (ICN 2000) with its relevance to nurses globally, stressed two areas of responsibility:

- promoting and restoring health;
- preventing and alleviating suffering.

This would, therefore, infer that nurses are deemed responsible for patients' human rights irrespective of their age, colour, ethnicity, culture, disability, gender, illness, politics, nationality, gender or their social status (ICN 2000) and reflects the accountability expected of all nurses.

The 2004 version of the Code of Professional Conduct stressed nurses' professional accountability, stating that as a registered nurse, midwife or specialist community public health nurse, you must:

- protect and support the health of individual patients and clients;
- protect and support the health of the wider community;
- act in such a way that justifies the trust and confidence the public have in you;
- uphold and enhance the good reputation of the profession.

It further stated that as nurses:

> you are personally accountable for ensuring that you promote and protect the interests and dignity of patients and clients, irrespective of gender, age, race, ability, sexuality, economic status, lifestyle, culture and religious or political beliefs.
>
> (NMC 2004: 2.2)

This clearly infers that nurses are personally and professionally accountable for ensuring that they have some knowledge of cultural competence with regards to race, culture and spirituality. Changes in demography internationally and nationally have meant that nurses at all levels who are caring for diverse client groups need to be able to demonstrate enhanced awareness of cultural differences in order to optimize health care delivery. Achievement of this is central to the role of advanced nursing practitioners who will be at the forefront of care delivery and provision. See also the 2008 version of the NMC Code (NMC, 2008).

Patient autonomy and choice

Involvement of patients, carers and the public in health care decision-making is at the heart of the NHS Modernization Agenda (DoH 1998b).

Autonomy refers to the right to act independently and respecting another person's autonomy involves respecting their human rights (Thompson, et al. 2006, Walsh 2006). The principle of respect for patient autonomy acknowledges the right of a patient to have control over his/her own life (Thompson et al. 2006). The respect for autonomy relates to the practitioner's duty of care to the patient/client and any breach of the NMC code (NMC 2008) would be deemed an act of negligence in a court of law. Advanced nurse practitioners (ANPs) need to have a working knowledge and understanding of the cultural beliefs and attitudes of patients that might influence their care and need to demonstrate that they can assist patients to become empowered. Patients and health professionals need to work collaboratively in the interest of the patient in order to achieve care that is optimum and culturally acceptable.

Scenario 4.1

A 48-year-old homeless man arrived at the practice to register with a doctor because he had rash on his leg which he had noticed for 2 weeks. The patient was seen as a temporary resident as he had not given a home address/abode. He was seen by the duty doctor who diagnosed an infected venous ulcer and requested that the man be admitted to hospital for a few days for treatment. However, he refused to be admitted, despite the GP advising him of the dangers of leaving the leg untreated. The GP asked the practice nurse to obtain a swab and gave the man a prescription for a week's course of antibiotics and asked him to return at the end of the week for a review. There was no reason to believe that he did not understand the consequences of his actions as it was not evident from his discussion with the GP that he had any mental health problems that would impair his judgement. Unfortunately, the patient did not return for follow-up of treatment.

Related cultural competencies

- Shows respect for the inherent dignity of every human being, whatever their age, gender, religion, socioeconomic class, sexual orientation, and ethnic or cultural group.
- Accepts the rights of individuals to choose their care provider, participate in care, and refuse care.
- Acknowledges their own personal biases and actively seeks to address them whilst ensuring the delivery of quality care.
- Actively promotes diversity and equality.
- Accesses culturally appropriate resources to deliver care.
- Assists patients from marginalized groups to access quality care.

Critical reflection

In considering this scenario, how would you manage a similar situation in your area of practice?

Feedback

This scenario reflects the importance of respecting patients' wishes. As suggested above, respect for the patient's autonomy acknowledges the right of patients to have control over their own life and is accepted as the practitioner's duty of care to the patient. It is therefore important for the advanced practitioner to treat every patient with respect and ensure every patient receives a high standard of care, irrespective of their culture or socioeconomic status.

KEY POINTS

- Nurses are personally and professionally accountable for providing culturally congruent care, for patients from culturally and linguistically diverse groups.
- ANPs should respect patients' autonomy and work collaboratively with patients in order to achieve optimum and culturally acceptable care.

CULTURAL COMPETENCE

As our society becomes more heterogeneous the need for cross-cultural competence becomes even more paramount.

In 1991, Leininger, the founder of transcultural nursing, said that practice needed to relate to cultural needs, and for it to be truly caring in the act of delivering culturally sensitive care, nurses need to be culturally competent. She argued that an understanding of cultural diversities is essential to the provision of effective and safe care for clients and that the knowledge of a client's cultural beliefs, values and attitudes is an integral part of providing health care (Leininger 2001).

Campinha-Bacote (1996) defines cultural competence as a process, not an endpoint. She describes a model of culturally competent care containing the components of cultural awareness, cultural knowledge, cultural skill and cultural encounter and desire. The model is a symbolic representation, in which cultural desire acts as a stimulus for the process of cultural competence, which requires nurses to visualize themselves as *becoming* rather than *being* culturally competent (Campinha-Bacote 2003). The Campinha-Bacote model of cultural competence (Figure 4.1), views cultural awareness, cultural knowledge, cultural skills and cultural encounters, as components of cultural competence in nursing care delivery. The model is a symbolic representation of a person's readiness and desire to engage in the process of cultural competence and the volcanic eruption stimulates the process of cultural competence (Campinha-Bacote and Munoz 2001).

Cultural awareness

According to Campinha-Bacote (1998), cultural awareness may be viewed as a deliberate, cognitive process in which health care providers appreciate and become sensitive to the values, beliefs, practices and problem-solving strategies of their patients' culture. Cultural awareness ultimately involves recognition and

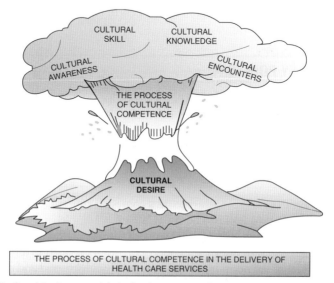

FIGURE 4.1 *The Campinha-Bacote model of cultural competence. Reprinted with permission from the author and publisher, Campinha-Bacote, J. (2003). 'Many faces: addressing diversity in healthcare'. Online Journal of Issues in Nursing 8 (1).*

examination of one's own prejudices and biases and an exploration of one's own cultural background, in order to avoid ethnocentricity. Self-awareness is necessary for the advanced practitioner in order to enable him/her to start the process of becoming culturally competent.

Cultural knowledge

This involves obtaining knowledge about patients with regard to specific physical, biological and physiological differences among ethnic groups (Purnell and Paulanka 1998). Caring for people in a multicultural and multiethnic society will require an understanding of the differences within that group as well as an understanding of the inequalities in health to which the group may be exposed. Therefore, an understanding of the group's cultural values and beliefs will go a long way towards helping to improve their health. Cultural knowledge and an understanding of patients' cultural beliefs can enable enhanced understanding of the barriers to health behaviours.

Cultural skills

This is defined as the ability to collect cultural data that are relevant to the patient's presentation of illness and to perform a culturally competent physical examination (Campinha-Bacote 1999) which can be carried out on patients from differing ethnic backgrounds.

Cultural encounter

This is defined as the process that encourages the nurse to engage directly with patients from culturally diverse backgrounds and involves assessing linguistic needs of clients (Campinha-Bacote 1998). This helps to increase cultural competence, which is an ongoing process and provides nurses with the opportunity to learn and appreciate the norms and uniqueness of patients from diverse cultures (Campinha-Bacote and Munoz 2001).

KEY POINTS

- Cultural awareness, cultural knowledge, cultural skills and cultural encounters are important for ANPs in understanding patients' cultural beliefs and can enable enhanced understanding of the barriers to health behaviours.

HEALTH

Health is, and continues to be, a contested concept. The World Health Organization (WHO 1986) defined health as 'a state of complete physical, mental and social well-being and not merely the absence of disease'. Although this definition provides a broad view of health, the concept of 'health' is open to differing interpretations because the meaning of health is socially constructed and means different things to different people. Perceptions of the determinants of health are socially constructed (Davey et al. 2005) and this has implications for advanced practitioner practice in the delivery of health promotion messages and treatment of illness. The social model of health sees the health of the individual as the outcome of socioeconomic and political determinants as well as medical care (Townsend and Davidson 1982, Whitehead 1987). The concepts of health and illness are embodied in the everyday life of people of all cultures and religions, making it difficult to establish universal consensus. In 1974, the Canadian Minister of Health, Lalonde, argued that health and illness are dependent not only on medical conditions but also on environmental and living conditions. The WHO (1986) definition of health had been intended to have universality but this concept of health is unattainable and sets aspirational targets for its achievement. Health also has a negative connotation of 'illness and disease', which are attributes of the medical model of health. This overlooks the important elements of well-being, psychosocial and economic factors embedded within cultures, which should be reflected in any meaningful definition of health for it to reflect cultural aspects. Health care practitioners, including advanced practitioners, are both providers of services as well as agents of change, who will facilitate the empowerment of clients and the wider community in increasing their control over and improvement of their health. Therefore, a universal definition of health has implications for health, health care, health promotion and nursing practice. In an attempt to reduce inequalities in health and provide holistic care for patients, ANPs need to understand the impact that culture has on the health of the individual, as well as the biopsychosocial, religious, environmental and economic impact, as this will go a long way towards achieving care that is holistic and culturally congruent.

Concepts of health and illness experience

In western thinking health and illness are said to coexist, whereas other cultures employ the notion that harmony and balance exist between various parts of the body in health, and illness is regarded as a state of disharmony and imbalance (Helman 2002). Because health and illness cannot coexist in this cultural realm, it has implications for the ways in which people conceptualize illness and its treatment. This provides a challenge for health care professionals to provide treatment and care that is meaningful to patients. Government policies have emphasized the importance of improving and increasing access to services for all users, including black and ethnic minorities (DOH 1998b); therefore, health professionals are required to consider the physical as well as emotional and psychological dimensions of care. This puts the onus on health professionals to consider how care will be experienced by patients from different cultures, depending on their cultural values, attitudes and beliefs about health and the ways in which the experience of health and illness are defined, together with expectations of treatment modalities. Medical pluralism (a multiplicity of choices of healers and medical practices from which patients can seek or choose medical or traditional treatment or therapy) exists (Holland and Hogg 2001, Helman 2002); therefore, nurses need to have the time to listen and question people about their individual beliefs as this will help to progress beyond superficial knowledge of cultural patterns. Health professionals need to learn about an individual's personal interpretation of a presenting illness and be able to manage and negotiate with patients within the context of the particular interaction. Patients will not attain a sense of complete health unless their cultural needs are fully met.

Importantly, the way we care for patients and their response to this care is greatly influenced by their cultural beliefs and attitudes. Health professionals must possess the ability and knowledge to communicate and understand health behaviours and recognize how these are influenced by culture. Having this ability and knowledge can eliminate barriers to the delivery of health care. It is also important that health professionals recognize clinical differences among people of different ethnic and racial groups (e.g. the propensity for hypertension in Afro-Caribbeans) and that they respect an individual's belief system, and the effects of those beliefs on their well-being, as this is of critical importance in achieving culturally competent care.

Ethnocentrism

Ethnocentrism is the belief that the ethnic group with which an individual identifies is superior to all other ethnic groups (Giger and Davidhizar 2004, Marks et al. 2004, Papadopoulos 2006). Consequently, the individual persistently uses membership of the ethnic group as the primary criterion when forming relationships with others and when evaluating and making judgements about other individuals. The tendency towards ethnocentrism makes health care environments challenging. This belief exists in all people and affects the provider and recipient of health care services. Professionally, nursing is influenced by a western middle-class ideology, which permeates the health care system and affects many aspects of the care processes. A paternalistic attitude is evident and may consequently affect the way care is delivered, resulting in a conflicting relationship between nurses and patients.

THE HEALTH BELIEF MODEL AND EXPLANATION OF HEALTH BEHAVIOURS

The health belief model (HBM) is a psychological model that attempts to explain and predict health behaviours. This is done by focusing on the attitudes and beliefs of individuals (Rosenstock 1966, Becker 1984).

The HBM was explained in terms of four constructs representing perceived threat and net benefits: perceived susceptibility, perceived severity, perceived benefits and perceived barriers. These concepts were proposed as accounting for people's 'readiness to act'. An added concept, cues to action, would activate that readiness and stimulate overt behaviours. A recent addition to the HBM is the concept of self-efficacy, or one's confidence in the ability successfully to perform an action. However, the HBM has been widely criticized, as it does not take age or ethnicity into account, which has implications for practice as people have their own lay beliefs about health and illness that differ from those referred to in the HBM.

Lay health beliefs

Health beliefs are inherent in every ethnic group. A patient's culture influences health beliefs. These diverse beliefs are embedded in practices and lifestyles in accordance with peoples' worldviews and values. This results in wide discrepancies in practice between patients and health care practitioners and the medical belief system, and helps to explain the difficulties which occur between patient and health care practitioners. The beliefs individuals hold about their illness will determine how they cope (Henley and Schott 1999, Holland and Hogg 2001).

In working towards a reduction in equalities in whatever context, freedom from illness is everyone's responsibility (McClachlan 1997, Gerrish 1998). There are wide variations in health beliefs between and within different cultures. Health care professionals need to consider that patients will experience care in different ways, depending on their cultural values, attitudes and beliefs about health, which will influence the ways in which they define and experience health and illness and their expectations of treatment. Therefore, having the ability and knowledge to understand health behaviours that are influenced by culture can eliminate barriers to health care delivery.

Explanatory models of illness

Kleinman (1980) described explanatory models (EMs) as the conceptions of causation of illness and appropriate treatment held by individuals experiencing illness. Explanatory models are defined as 'the notions about episodes of sickness and its treatment that are employed by all those engaged in the clinical process'. Explanatory models are held by both health professionals and patients and provide an explanations of an illness. Kleinman (1980) asserts that lay EMs tend to be 'idiosyncratic and changeable' and influenced by personality and cultural factors. They are used by individuals to explain, organize and manage episodes of impaired well-being (Helman 2002). Kleinman's (1980) view of EMs is focused on illness and uses five constructs to elicit EMs of illness:

*   aetiology of illness;
*   symptoms onset;
*   pathophysiology;
*   course of the illness;
*   recommended treatment.

The understanding of illness helps patients to make sense of an illness experience. This understanding is not formalized consciously but tends to change over time and is influenced by the individual's social environment, ethnicity and culture (Kleinman 1980, Spector 1996, Pool and Geissler 2005), as well as past experiences and tacit knowledge. Respect for others' belief systems and the resultant effects of those beliefs on patient well-being is of critical importance to competent care. Lack of understanding, tolerance and respect for other peoples' beliefs will cause conflict in any interaction with patients from differing cultural backgrounds.

KEY POINTS

*   Health is a contested concept, which is open to differing interpretations.
*   The concept of health and illness is embodied in the life of people from different cultures and religions, making it difficult for universality of meaning.
*   ANPs need to understand the impact of culture on health to enable them to provide holistic and culturally congruent care.
*   ANPs need to be able to communicate with patients and understand how their culture influences health behaviours.
*   EMs are held by practitioners and patients and used to explain, organize and manage episodes of illness.
*   Lack of understanding, tolerance and respect for peoples' beliefs will cause conflict when interacting with patients from differing cultural backgrounds.

Scenario 4.2

Mr Abraham is a 60-year-old Afro-Caribbean gentleman who was recently diagnosed with hypertension by his GP and was prescribed an anti-hypertensive drug to control his blood pressure. At the review 3 months later, his blood pressure remained high and the doctor decided to increase his medication because he assumed that the drug prescribed wasn't strong enough to reduce Mr Abraham's blood pressure; another appointment was given in 3 months' time. Mr Abraham's blood pressure was even higher than the previous reading. The GP decided to add another drug and another appointment was arranged in a further 3 months. The blood pressure reading remained high despite a further increase in both drugs. A month after his last appointment Mr Abrahams visited the surgery for an appointment with the nurse practitioner for lifestyle advice. His blood pressure was taken by the nurse practitioner, who after assessing his notes saw that his blood pressure had remained high despite the medication. On further questioning, Mr Abrahams revealed to the nurse practitioner that he had not taken his tablets as he feared that they would harm him; thus, the reason for the non-reduction in his blood pressure.

Related cultural competencies

- Shows respect for the inherent dignity of every human being, whatever their age, gender, religion, socioeconomic class, sexual orientation and ethnic or cultural group.
- Accepts the rights of individuals to choose their care provider, participate in care, and refuse care.
- Acknowledges their own personal biases and actively seeks to address them whilst ensuring the delivery of quality care.
- Actively promotes diversity and equality.
- Incorporates cultural preferences, health beliefs and behaviours and traditional practices into management plans as appropriate.
- Accesses culturally appropriate resources to deliver care.
- Assists patients from marginalized groups to access quality care.

Critical reflection

What implications do these beliefs have for your practice?
How would you manage this presentation?

Scenario 4.3

Mrs Thomas is a 79-year-old woman who migrated to the UK from Jamaica in 1964. Since the death of her husband 15 years ago, she has lived with her 34-year-old unmarried son. She has nine other children, some of whom live locally and the others live overseas. She was diagnosed with type 2 diabetes and hypertension 10 years ago but does not adhere to any of the advice given to her by health professionals from the hospital or from the primary health care team. As a consequence, she is now living with resultant chronic complications from both diseases.

Related cultural competencies

- Shows respect for the inherent dignity of every human being, whatever their age, gender, religion, socioeconomic class, sexual orientation, and ethnic or cultural group.
- Accepts the rights of individuals to choose their care provider, participate in care, and refuse care.
- Acknowledges their own personal biases and actively seeks to address them whilst ensuring the delivery of quality care.
- Actively promotes diversity and equality.
- Incorporates cultural preferences, health beliefs and behaviours and traditional practices into management plans as appropriate.
- Provides patient-appropriate educational materials that address the language and cultural beliefs of the patient.
- Assists patients from marginalized groups to access quality care.

Critical reflection

When caring for Mrs Thomas what action would you take in this situation? How would you elicit this lady's beliefs about her health?

Feedback for Scenarios 4.2 and 4.3

It is evident from these two presentations that both patients had different beliefs about their health/illness from those of the health professionals they had encountered. Peoples' beliefs about health and illness are individual and are influenced by their culture and worldviews. Misunderstanding how a patient defines health can ultimately lead to cross-cultural conflict. These beliefs are powerful and strongly held and people cannot always be dissuaded from practising them by the arguments of health professionals.

It is important to explore health and illness beliefs and negotiate care with respect and communication, for this may help the nurse practitioner and patient mutually to agree plans of care delivery which may lead to adherence. Understanding peoples' health beliefs is fundamental to nursing practice and will allow the ANP to care for patients holistically and deliver culturally safe and effective care.

SPIRITUAL COMPETENCE

There have been many definitions of spirituality and there is conclusive evidence to suggest that spirituality enhances health. However, defining the concept of spirituality is elusive, making it problematic. One reason for this elusiveness is that spirituality is considered by many to be an individual, personal and subjective concept (McSherry et al. 2004). Another reason is that one aspect of the meaning of spirituality is inextricably bounded up with religion (McSherry 2000) in relation to the patterns of worship and prayer, such as past religious observance. Respect for beliefs is an important part of practice for nurses and allied health professionals (NMC 2008). Human spirituality is not homogeneous and ANPs need to acknowledge the importance of adopting an individualistic and non-judgemental approach to care delivery, and they need to explore issues of spirituality with their patients. Spiritual care is person-centred, and the best use of personal and spiritual resources helps patients cope with suffering and ill health, as well as the experience of a new and unfamiliar health care system. Spirituality can also be of particular significance in end-of-life care, enabling patients to find meaning and purpose in death as in life.

Some researchers have suggested that spirituality and religion provide health benefits in terms of prevention, improved health status, recovery from illness or enabling people to cope with illness and diversity (Dein and Stygall 1997). Spirituality can also benefit health by providing meaning and purpose in life. However, illness can also bring meaning and purpose and can promote spiritual healing (Hall 1998), which helps people deal with death and gain some control over the fear of dying.

Scenario 4.4

Mrs Baktari, a 36-year-old mother of two, was found collapsed at the side of the road by a passer-by and was taken to the A&E department by ambulance. On arrival in the unit she was resuscitated, but this was unsuccessful. Her documents revealed that she was of the Hindu faith, but the nurse who was allocated to her had no experience of the religious rituals or customs regarding the death of a Hindu person. She sought advice from a colleague who told her to 'make the body presentable' for the relatives, who had been contacted and were on their way to the hospital. On arrival at the ward, the relatives were escorted to the cubicle but were annoyed that the body had been touched and asked that the body be released immediately to their care.

Related cultural competencies

- Shows respect for the inherent dignity of every human being, whatever their age, gender, religion, socioeconomic class, sexual orientation, and ethnic or cultural group.
- Actively promotes diversity and equality.

Related spiritual competencies

- Assists patients and families to meet their spiritual needs in the context of health and illness experiences, including referral for pastoral services.
- Provides appropriate information and opportunity for patients, carers and families to discuss their wishes for end-of-life decision-making and care.
- Respects wishes of patients and families regarding expression of spiritual beliefs.

Critical reflection

In considering this scenario, how would you ensure that religious rituals are adhered to for patients in the future?

Where do you access religious resources in your area of practice and how could you enhance your knowledge of end-of-life care for patients with diverse religious beliefs?

Feedback

In considering this scenario it is important for the ANP to understand the religious beliefs and practices of the Hindu faith pertaining to end-of-life care and death and dying. It may be useful also to explore general cultural beliefs and attitudes about Hinduism and offer support to the family as necessary.

Scenario 4.5

Mr Patel is a 52-year-old with type 2 diabetes, which is managed by diet and oral hypoglycaemic tablets. He was driven to the A&E department by his son because he had complained of feeling sweaty and drowsy. On examination and further investigation, it was found that he was hypoglycaemic. On questioning, it was revealed that Mr Patel had been taking his tablets at regular times but had not eaten because he had been fasting for Ramadan and had refused to eat, despite having discussed this with the diabetes specialist nurse at the clinic. Strong religious beliefs had prevented adherence to health care advice.

Related cultural competencies

* Shows respect for the inherent dignity of every human being, whatever their age, gender, religion, socioeconomic class, sexual orientation, and ethnic or cultural group.
* Accepts the rights of individuals to choose their care provider, participate in care, and refuse care.
* Acknowledges their own personal biases and actively seeks to address them whilst ensuring the delivery of quality care.
* Actively promotes diversity and equality.
* Incorporates cultural preferences, health beliefs and behaviours into management plans as appropriate.
* Provides patient-appropriate educational materials that address the language and cultural beliefs of the patient.
* Accesses culturally appropriate resources to deliver care.
* Assists patients from marginalized groups to access quality care.

Related spiritual competencies

* Respects the inherent worth and dignity of each person and the right to express spiritual beliefs.
* Assists patients and families to meet their spiritual needs in the context of health and illness experiences, including referral for pastoral services.
* Assesses the influence of patients' spirituality on their health care behaviours and practices.
* Incorporates patients' spiritual beliefs in the care plan.
* Respects wishes of patients and families regarding expression of spiritual beliefs.

Critical reflection

How do you care for patients during religious festivals?

Feedback

During Ramadan, Muslim patients fast between sunrise and sunset. Those who are sick, although not expected to fast, do so regardless of discussions about their illnesses with health professionals. If a hospitalized patient wishes to fast during Ramadan, food should be available before sunrise and after sunset. Essential medicines can also be administered during this period. It is thus important for the ANP to understand the patient's spiritual beliefs and the impact these may have on care delivery and the ANP must be able successfully to negotiate culturally congruent care that respects the wishes of the patient. For further information, please see Kemp and Bhungalia (2002) and the National Association of Health Authorities and Trusts (1996).

DEFINITION OF SPIRITUALITY AND RELIGION AND MEETING THE NEEDS OF PATIENTS

Because the UK is a multifaith society, it is important for providers of care to take the cultural and spiritual needs of patients into account in order to enable the NHS to continue to provide culturally congruent care of the highest standard to patients.

Spirituality is often used to refer to an individual's personal beliefs, experiences and principles (Markham 1998, McSherry 2000). Religious beliefs may help people focus on spirituality and can lead to positive effects. This may be because the meaning of spirituality is inextricably tied up with religion (Narayanasamy 1999b, Davidhizar and Bechtel 2000). Spiritual needs may be experienced by anyone, not just those who have faith. Therefore, the acknowledgement of language, culture, dietary habits, customs, fears and anxieties are some of the components of spiritual care.

Addressing the spiritual needs of patients is a fundamental part of holistic care and may be the most neglected area of care. However, there have been changes in the way people describe their religion or spirituality. In the recent population census (ONS 2004), 76% of the UK population answered positively regarding religion. There is also growing research evidence to support the notion that a large percentage of the UK population within the health care system has strong spiritual beliefs, even in the absence of a specific religious affiliation. The NICE (2004) guidance for palliative care states that spiritual care concerns all staff who have contact with patients, and if they cannot respond to such needs or if it is inappropriate for them to do so, they should make these needs known to other members of the multidisciplinary team. Narayansamy (2001) suggests that nursing care must explore the language of spirituality to ensure that an aspect of holistic care is not dismissed, as this may be crucial to patients' well-being and the integrity of nursing. It is, therefore, of crucial importance that ANPs acquire the skills and knowledge needed to prepare them to meet these needs.

KEY POINTS

- A large percentage of the population within the UK health care system holds strong spiritual beliefs.
- Spirituality enhances health but defining the concept is problematic because spirituality is inextricably linked with religion.

- Human spirituality is not homogeneous and needs to be fully explored with patients.
- It is important for ANPs to take the cultural and spiritual needs of patients into account.
- Cross-cultural communication skills are important for successful nurse–patient relationships.

BARRIERS TO ACHIEVING CULTURAL, LINGUISTIC AND RELIGIOUS COMPETENCE

Barriers exist because most organizations have not been designed to facilitate cultural diversity for the following reasons:

- there may be a lack of facilities to accommodate certain cultural or religious needs;
- staff shortages may limit time spent to attend to patients' specific religious/spiritual needs;
- in hospital, some practices relating to religious preparation for or after death are not possible due to organizational barriers and restrictions on the number of visitors to the bedside, which may hinder communication between families in respect of religious preferences;
- communication barriers between staff and patients;
- lack of time and funding for staff training and education;
- concerns about projecting own beliefs and attitudes to patients;
- uncertainties and concerns over managing some issues relating to death.

Critical reflection

When considering the above barriers to communication consider the following questions:

- How are patients/religious/spiritual needs assessed in your area of practice?
- What would suggest to you that a patient has religious needs?
- How would you ensure that a patient's religious needs are met?

Feedback

It is important for ANPs to have some understanding of the basic concepts and principles underpinning other religious and spiritual beliefs. It may be helpful in this context to find out what religious services, facilities and resources are available for patients in the area of practice, and local community knowledge gained can be shared and disseminated to other health care professionals through on-site training, induction or hospital intranet services within the area of practice. There should be wide access to specific information concerning death and dying, and the contact numbers of local religious and community outreach workers should be available in the practice. These could include booklets, leaflets and other written information, which should be available for all health care staff and patients from different cultures. Access to NHS trust guidelines with regards to good practice in addressing the spiritual and religious needs of patients should be available to all involved in caring for patients from diverse cultural backgrounds. Collaboration between the multidisciplinary team is important to successfully achieve culturally congruent religious care.

CULTURAL LINGUISTICS

Shifting demographic trends offer challenges both to those delivering services and government organizations in providing care that is culturally and linguistically competent. Communication across cultures and faiths can have a profound effect on individuals collaborating in care delivery. Therefore, successful relationships will be dependent on cross-cultural communication skills and capabilities. Linguistic competence adheres to the principle that patients who have limited English proficiency have the right to medically trained interpreter services (Luckman 1999). If health professionals are unable to understand or be understood, this will contribute to poor health outcomes for the patient, irrespective of gender, culture, ethnicity or social class, as culture is not just about ethnic minorities.

Scenario 4.6

Mrs Ali is an Ethiopian Muslim woman who was invited for a cervical smear by the local primary care trust. She arrived at the clinic accompanied by her husband who spoke 'little English'. He handed the letter to the practice nurse saying his wife did not speak any English. The nurse took the letter and told the couple that the letter was an invitation for Mrs Ali to have a smear test. The nurse tried to explain the reasons why she should have the smear and assumed that this was understood by the couple. The nurse then proceeded to take Mrs Ali to the treatment room to perform the test. Her husband refused to have his wife's clothes removed as this was against his religion and they left the surgery.

Related cultural competencies

- Shows respect for the inherent dignity of every human being, whatever their age, gender, religion, socioeconomic class, sexual orientation, and ethnic or cultural group.
- Accepts the rights of individuals to choose their care provider, participate in care, and refuse care.
- Acknowledges their own personal biases and actively seeks to address them whilst ensuring the delivery of quality care.
- Actively promotes diversity and equality.
- Provides patient-appropriate educational materials that address the language and cultural beliefs of the patient.
- Accesses culturally appropriate resources to deliver care.

Related spiritual competencies

- Respects the inherent worth and dignity of each person and the right to express spiritual beliefs.
- Assesses the influence of patients' spirituality on their health care behaviours and practices.
- Provides appropriate information and opportunity for patients, carers and families to discuss their wishes for end-of-life decision-making and care.
- Respects wishes of patients and families regarding expression of spiritual beliefs.

Critical reflection

Consider this scenario, how would you ensure that Mrs Ali's dignity, privacy and respect for her religion were addressed? How would you have acted on this occasion?

Feedback

In order for culturally appropriate care to take place, the ANP needs to know and understand how health behaviours are influenced by culture and religion. It is important to remember that perceptions of health, illness, disease and their causes will vary culturally. Therefore, ANPs must possess the ability and knowledge to communicate and understand patients' spiritual and religious needs. Showing respect for people from different cultures and their religious and cultural beliefs and being able to listen and communicate with patients from diverse cultural backgrounds is very important.

CONCLUSION

The UK is a multicultural, multiethnic and multifaith society which has a major impact on the demographic discourse of the British population. As Britain embraces its demographic challenges, so do health care environments, service provision and care delivery in an attempt to manage these changes. There are numerous challenges for health care practitioners who are required to become competent and creative in their delivery and provision of services. It is evident that the concepts of health, ethnicity, diversity, religion and spirituality remain problematic, for there is no universal consensus about these concepts. The traditional approach to focus care on the indigenous population is no longer enough in a multiethnic society. Individuals from other cultures have different beliefs and concepts about health and illness that conflict with western beliefs about medicine and treatment. This requires nurses, as well as ANPs, to have the knowledge and skills to become culturally competent in order to deliver culturally congruent care.

PRACTICAL STEPS IN ACHIEVING DOMAIN 2: CULTURAL AND RELIGIOUS COMPETENCIES

The scenarios and examples provided in the text will help you to demonstrate how the NMC competencies relating to Domain 2 can be achieved. This section provides information that will help you to reflect critically on the scenarios presented in the text and will help you to consider the context in which a patient's culture is addressed within your own area of practice and the steps you would take as an advanced practitioner to achieve the competencies.

Suggestions for achieving cultural and religious competencies

- Written critical reflective accounts of a significant event or critical incidence reviews (identifying the key elements of cultural, religious and spiritual care and personal knowledge, skills and develop action plans to achieve competence).
- Portfolio of evidence for achieving competencies (Appendix 3)
- Learning contracts to identify strengths and weaknesses in relation to each cultural and religious competence (see Appendices 4 and 5).

Tools for developing competencies

- Job description – identify, select and critically reflect on appropriate elements of your roles and responsibilities within your job description that relate to the appropriate competence, to demonstrate how the competence would be achieved.
- Study days, seminars, workshops – attendance at any event relating any of the competencies could be achieved by critical reflection, showing how appropriate competence has been achieved.
- Induction training – any element of your induction training that relates to caring for patients with diverse cultural and religious needs could be used to reflect achievement of the related competence and evidence of this supplied in your portfolio.
- Training courses, e.g. first contact, continuing professional education and continuing personal development courses, courses for nurse practitioners, etc., could be used to demonstrate achievement of any of the competencies, through critical reflection.
- Case or critical incidence reviews.
- Discussions at multidisciplinary and interdisciplinary and professional meetings.
- Personal and professional development reviews, such as, appraisals and personal and professional development plans.
- Research and dissemination.
- Attendance at conferences.
- Publications in journals.

A written critical, reflective analysis of each of these could be used to support learning and be mapped against each competence to demonstrate achievement.

ELIMINATING LINGUISTIC BARRIERS

ANPs can help to eliminate linguistic barriers through collaboration and partnership with other members of the multidisciplinary team and with the wider community in the following ways:

- developing religious diversity initiatives in practice that will promote respect and inclusive care;
- developing strategies to integrate religious diversity into patient care plans;
- identifying obstacles to communication between self and people from other cultures and identifying ways to build relationships with people from different cultures;
- understanding the racial, ethnic and cultural demographics of the community in which you practice;
- ensuring access to trained interpreters is available for translation;
- ensuring linguistically appropriate resources/literature are available in identified languages;
- liaising with religious and spiritual organizations to help facilitate care;
- being aware that clients/patients from different cultures may hold conflicting beliefs about the causes and treatment of their illness;
- identifying training needs of self and others;
- adapting educational materials for the appropriate ethnic group, because literal translation of health information will not be culturally specific and will not be able to address lay beliefs (Gerrish 1998) and could be viewed as ethnocentric because they fail to acknowledge the patient's own cultural perspectives;
- developing health education materials that are culturally specific;

- providing culturally congruent resources, e.g. forms, leaflets, videos and audiovisual aids;
- incorporating cultural awareness into assessment and treatment, e.g. diabetes in Asian people;
- offering training to staff in communication skills.

Examples for achieving religious and spiritual competencies

- incorporate spiritual care into patients' care plans in partnership with patients and carers/families;
- foster a multidisciplinary approach to assessment of spiritual health and care needs of patients;
- communicate with spiritual bodies (e.g. local temples and elders, etc.) of different faiths for spiritual support;
- provide access to a private and suitable place for prayer and religious observance;
- document patients' spiritual needs in patients' records;
- develop and broaden knowledge base for spirituality in multifaith religions;
- identify training needs in relation to bereavement care, and communication and interpersonal skills, and find ways of achieving them;
- respect patients' choices for religious preferences/rituals through communication, negotiation and respect;
- preserve patients' autonomy for as long as possible;
- access chaplaincy services in order to provide and facilitate spiritual care of patients;
- regularly review patients' spiritual issues and care as necessary;
- help patients/carers/staff articulate their spiritual and religious needs and identify sources to address them;
- act as a resource for knowledge, support, training and education of other staff members;
- identify and develop resources to aid spiritual care within the unit/department;
- participate and influence development of local and national initiatives to facilitate spiritual care through collaboration with public, private and voluntary organizations.

REFERENCES

Acheson, D. (1998) *An independent inquiry into inequalities in health*. London: Stationery Office.

Becker, M.H. (1984) Compliance with medical care. In *Health care and human behaviour*, Steptoe, A. and Matthews, A. (eds). London: Academic Press.

Boyle, P. (2000) Multicultural health care. *The World of Irish Nursing* 8(7): 14–15.

Campinha-Bacote, J. (1996) The challenge of cultural diversity for nurse educators. *Journal of Continuing Education in Nursing* 27: 59–64.

Campinha-Bacote, J. (1999) A model and instrument for addressing cultural competence in health care. *Journal of Continuing Nursing Education* 38(5): 203–207.

Campinha-Bacote, J. (2003) Cultural desire: The key to unlocking cultural competence. *Journal of Nursing Education* 42(6): 239–240.

Campinha-Bacote, J. (2003) Many faces: addressing diversity in health care. *Journal of Issues in Nursing* 8(1): manuscript 2.

Campinha-Bacote, J. and Munoz, C. (2001) A guiding framework for delivering culturally competent services in case management. *Case Manager* 12: 48–52.

Davey, B. Gray, A. Seale, C. (2005) *Health and disease: A reader*, 3rd edn. Berkshire, UK: OUP.

Davidhizar, R. and Bechtel, G. (2000) The spiritual needs of hospitalised patients. *American Journal of Nursing.* 100(7): 1–4.

Dein, S. and Stygall, J. (1997) Does being religious help or hinder coping with chronic illness? A critical literature review. *Palliative Medicine* 11: 291–298.

Department of Health (1998a) *Saving lives: our healthier nation.* London: HMSO.

Department of Health (1998b) *The new NHS, modern, dependable.* London: HMSO.

Department of Health (1999a) *Reducing inequalities: an action report.* London: The Stationery Office.

Department of Health (1999b) *Making a difference: strengthening the nursing, midwifery and health visiting contribution to health and health care.* London: NHS.

Department of Health (2002) *The NHS plan: a plan for investment, a plan for reform.* London: The Stationery Office.

De Santis, L. (1994) Making anthropology clinically relevant to nursing care. *Journal of Advanced Nursing* 20: 707–715.

Duffy, M. (2001) A critique of cultural education in nursing. *Journal of Advanced Nursing* 36(4): 487–495.

Gerrish, K. (1998) Preparing nurses to care for minority ethnic communities. *International Nursing Review* 45: 115–127.

Giger, J. and Davidhizar, R. (2004) *Transcultural nursing: assessment and intervention,* 4th edn. Missouri: Mosby.

Hall, B.A. (1998) Patterns of spirituality in persons with advanced HIV disease. *Research in Nursing and Health.* 21: 143–152.

Hawthorne, N. (1850) *The scarlet letter.* Boston, MA: Ticknor, Reed and Field.

Helman, C.G. (2002) *Culture health and illness,* 4th edn, Chs 1 and 5. London: Arnold Publishers.

Henley, A. and Schott, A. (1999) *Culture, religion and patient care.* London: Age Concern.

Holland, K. and Hogg, C. (2001) *Cultural awareness in nursing and health care: an introductory text.* London: Arnold.

International Council of Nursing (2000) *Code of ethics.* Geneva: ICN.

Jenkins, R. (1997) *Rethinking ethnicity.* London: Sage.

Jones, L.J. (1994) *The social context of health and healthwork.* Basingstoke: MacMillan Press.

Kemp, C. and Bhungalia, S. (2002) Culture and the end of life: A review of major world religions. *Journal of Hospice and Palliative Nursing* 4(4): 235–242.

Kleinman, A. (1980) *Patients and healers in the context of culture.* CA: University of California Press.

Lalonde, M. (1974) *A new perspective on health of Canadians: a working document.* Ottowa: Govenment of Canada.

Leininger, M.M. (2001) *Culture, care, diversity and universality: a theory of nursing.* Sudbury, MA: Jones and Bartlett.

Luckman, J. (1999) *Transcultural communication in nursing.* Albany, NY: Demar Publications.

Macbeth, H. and Shetty, P. (2001) *Health and ethnicity.* London: Taylor & Francis.

MacLachlan, M. (1997) *Culture and health.* Chichester: John Wiley & Sons.

McSherry, W. (2000a) *Making sense of spirituality in nursing practice: an interactive approach.* Edinburgh: Churchill Livingstone.

McSherry, W. Cash, K. Ross, L. (2004) Meaning of spirituality: implications for nursing practice. *Journal of Clinical Nursing* 13(8): 934–941.

Markham, I. (1998) Spirituality and the world of faiths. In *The spiritual challenge of health care,* Cobb, M. and Bradshaw, V. (eds), pp. 73–88. Edinburgh: Churchill Livingstone.

Marks, D. Murray, M. Evans, B. Willig, C. Woodhall, C. Sykes, C. (2004) *Health psychology: theory, research and practice,* 2nd edn. London: Sage Publications.

Narayanasamy, A. (1999b) Learning spiritual dimensions of care from a historical perspective. *Nurse Education Today* 19(3): 386–395.

Narayanasamy, A. (2001) *Spiritual care: a practical guide for nurses and health care practitioners,* 2nd edn. Wiltshire: Quay Publishing.

National Association of Health Authorities and Trusts (1996) *Spiritual care in the NHS: a guide for purchasers and providers.* Birmingham: NAHAT.

Nazroo, J. (1997) *The health of Britain's ethnic minorities.* London: Policy Studies Institute.

Nursing and Midwifery Council (2004) *The code of professional conduct: protecting the public through professional standards.* London: NMC.

Nursing and Midwifery Council (2008) *The Code. Standards of conduct, performance and ethics for nurses and midwives.* London: NMC.

National Institute of Clinical Excellence (2004) *Improving supportive and palliative care for adults with cancer: Manu*al. London: NICE.

Office for National Statistics (2004) *Population trends.* London: The Stationery Office.

Papadopoulos, I. (2006) *Transcultural health and social care: development of culturally competent practitioners*, Chs 3 and 5. Edinburgh: Churchill Livingstone.

Pool, R. and Geissler, W. (2005) *Medical anthropology.* Berkshire: OUP.

Purnell, L.D. and Paulanka, B.J. (1998) *Transcultural health care: a culturally competent approach.* Philadelphia: F.A. Davis.

Rosenstock, I.M. (1966) Why people use health services. *Milbank Memorial Fund Quarterly.* 44: 94–124.

Royal College of Nursing (RCN) (2007) *Competencies for NPs.* RCN: London.

Spector, R.E. (1996) *Cultural diversity in health and illness*, 5th edn. Upper Saddle River, NJ: Prentice Hall.

Thompson, I. Melia, K. Boyd, K. Horsburgh, D. (2006) *Nursing ethics*, 5th edn. London: Churchill Livingstone.

Townsend, P. and Davidson, N. (1982) *Inequalities in health: the Black report.* Harmondsworth: Penguin Books.

UNO (1948) *Universal declaration of human rights.* New York: United Nations Organization.

Walsh, M. (2006) *Nurse practitioners: clinical skills and professional issues*, 2nd edn. Philadelphia PA: Butterworth Heinemann, Elsevier.

Whitehead, M. (1987) *The health divide.* London: Health Education Council.

WHO (1986) *The Ottawa charter.* Geneva: World Health Organization.

FURTHER READING AND RESOURCES

American Nurses Association's Statement on Cultural Diversity: http://www.nursing world.org

CRE (2002) *Towards racial equality: an evaluation of the public duty to promote race equality and good race relations in England and Wales.*

CRE (2004) *The strategic health authority race equality guide: a performance framework.* London: NHS.

Cultural diversity in the workplace: http://www.diversityinc.com

Cultural issues that influence the health of the individual and families: http://www.xculture.org

Diversity Rx. http://www.diversityrx.org

Ethnicity online: http://www.ethnicityonline.net

HARP (health for asylum seekers and refugees portal): http://www.harpweb.org.uk

http://www.minorityhealth.gov.uk/docs/stepbystep.pdf

National Institute of Clinical Excellence (2004) *Improving supportive and palliative care for adults with cancer.* London: NICE.

London Health Observatory: http://www.lho.org.uk

Research Centre for Transcultural Studies in Health (2004) Middlesex University Homepage. http://www.mdx.ac.uk/www/rctsh/homepage.htm (accessed 26/7/06.)

Scottish Refugee Council (2003) Briefing: asylum seekers and refugees in Scotland. http://www.scotlandrefugeecouncil.org.uk (accessed 26/7/06.)

Transcultural Nursing Society: http://www.tcns.org

http://www.statistics.gov.uk/focuson

http://www.statistics.gov.uk

http://www.adherents.com (Religion)

5 DOMAIN 3: MANAGEMENT OF PATIENT HEALTH/ILLNESS STATUS

ANNALIESE WILLIS

INTRODUCTION

The third domain of the Nursing and Midwifery Council (NMC) Standards of Proficiency for Advanced Nurse Practitioners (NMC 2005) is concerned with the skills and competencies required for the clinical assessment and management of patients. It requires advanced nurse practitioners (ANPs) to demonstrate:

- health promotion strategies;
- a holistic health assessment approach, which includes diagnosis and management of acute, chronic, urgent and complex patient problems;
- evidence-based practice;
- autonomous/independent practice within a multidisciplinary team context;
- self-awareness of competency level.

This chapter will illustrate the type of evidence that can be used in the assessment and accreditation process to gain NMC recognition for the competencies in Domain 3. It is designed to provide guidance and support to ANPs on how to recognize and evaluate their practice experience and knowledge and how this can be collected and used.

Background

The development of advanced practice roles in the UK over the last 15 years has been influenced by a range of factors including health care policy (DoH 1999a, 2000a, 2006a), health care restructuring (NHSME 1991, Bryant-Lukosius et al. 2004), the international experience of advanced nursing roles (Mantzoukas and Watkinson 2006) and recognition of the unique and valuable role of nursing (DoH 1999b, UKCC 1999, NMC 2005). In addition, nurses themselves are key drivers for these role and service developments, with a large percentage involved in direct patient care and undertaking role functions such as patient assessment/referral, autonomous decision-making and offering specialist advice (RCN 2005). Assessment and management of patients during health and illness episodes has always been a core component of nursing practice, but in the context of advanced practice these activities can be seen to involve new role functions for nurses. These new skills include physical examination of body systems, clinical reasoning, diagnosing and prescribing, which have traditionally been associated with medical practice. Role development for advanced practice, therefore, tends to be diverse, with significant blurring of interprofessional role boundaries (Daly and Carnwell 2003). The effectiveness of advanced nursing roles has been assessed in relation to patient assessment skills (history-taking and physical examination of body systems), patient diagnosis and management, and the overall clinical role and found to be equivalent to the level of care provided by medical practitioners (Horrocks et al. 2002) at no extra cost but with increased patient satisfaction (Venning et al. 2000). In addition, Mantzoukas and Watkinson (2006) identified seven generic features of an ANP, including the use of knowledge in practice, critical thinking and analytical skills, along with clinical judgement and decision-making skills. These particular features are evident within Domain 3.

The competencies for Domain 3 are listed in Appendix 1 and this chapter recommends the types of evidence you might use to demonstrate that you have met these competencies (see Table 5.1). It outlines how to ensure that the evidence you use is robust (see the section *Collecting evidence for Domain 3*) and provides four case studies (scenarios) illustrating application of evidence to the competencies. The aim of this chapter is to familiarize you with the competencies for Domain 3 and to help you understand what evidence to choose and how to apply it to this domain.

TABLE 5.1   *Types of evidence suitable for Domain 3*

Evidence	Requirements
Critical reflective review to demonstrate achievement of a competency, i.e. reflect and cite evidence on how each competency is met	Verified by a peer or other colleague to confirm that this is representative of your normal practice
OSCA/OSCE station that you have successfully completed	Verified by university
Video/dvd/audio-recording of a patient consultation with reflection on elements of the consultation	Submit recording with completed self-assessment tool or reflective account
Consultation assessed using Calgary Cambridge (Silverman et al. 2005) (or similar) framework	Self-assessment and/or peer/university assessment
Assignment from an assessed course	Mark sheet and comments, qualification certificate or university transcript of units, course information
Testimonial	Signed by a patient, peer/colleague or university lecturer
University transcript of modules or qualification certificate	Course information or university mapping of course content to NMC competencies
Learning objectives from clinical placements	Verified as achieved by appropriate assessor
Guidelines, strategies, reports, profiles, patient information related to clinical area that you have developed or implemented	Verify your role as author/implementer, accompanied by case history to illustrate how patient benefits, or use patient testimonial
Letters, minutes of meetings	Permission from author of letters, chair of meetings to present data in your portfolio
Copies of patient's notes/files that you have completed including investigation results	Permission from patient to use (essential to ensure patient anonymity), permission from employer to use

OSCA/OSCE, objective structured clinical assessment/examination.

The scenarios presented demonstrate a range of exemplars and evidence and you will find that each one is mapped against specific competencies. All the competencies for this domain have been addressed and some have been met by more than one scenario. This is desirable in that it demonstrates triangulation which supports the robustness of the evidence and is necessary to ensure that some competencies are fully met (e.g. competency 24 requires you to demonstrate knowledge of pathophysiology of conditions commonly seen in practice and Scenarios 5.1 and 5.2 illustrate knowledge about two different commonly presenting pathologies, i.e. sore throat and peptic ulcer disease). However, you will notice that the breadth of evidence chosen for these scenarios does not demonstrate that all competencies have been fully met and this is something that you would need to do when you submit your portfolio of evidence. (For example, the diagnoses and management of acute and long-term conditions has not been fully met by the scenarios presented.) It is your responsibility to ensure that all the competencies have been fully met by the evidence you present before submitting your portfolio. Although this may seem a daunting task, it is worth noting that the exemplars provided in this chapter may be used as evidence against competencies in the other domains.

The scenarios presented in this chapter are representative of the author's practice setting and should not be considered as the ideal or correct form of exemplar for you; every practitioner will present different cases or evidence which should reflect their individual clinical setting/role. You should be able to use these cases to understand what is needed in order for each competency to be met fully and how to apply evidence to them. This allows you to reflect on your practice and to apply your knowledge and skills to the competencies.

So how do you get started? First, familiarize yourself with the domain and the competencies; you may find it helpful to list all the competencies in a table so you can start brainstorming ideas on what evidence you might use to meet each competency. Refer to Table 5.1 for help on the types of evidence that may be useful and consider whether you have similar evidence that you can use. Once you have identified some evidence, cross-match it against the competencies and think about whether the evidence partially or fully meets the competencies you are considering (e.g. the competency demonstrating critical thinking is fully met by Scenario 5.1). Then assess the evidence itself against the key criteria detailed in the section entitled *Collecting evidence for Domain 3* (e.g. find the mark sheet and comments for the assignment, Scenario 5.2). Finally, start collecting and organizing your evidence into a portfolio.

COLLECTING EVIDENCE FOR DOMAIN 3

Much of the evidence you collect for this domain should be readily available to you as a consequence of any relevant study that you may have undertaken, including independent learning, or will be evident/collectable from within your normal clinical practice. The types of evidence that could be used for Domain 3 are suggested in Table 5.1.

The material that you use to demonstrate that you have fully met the competencies for Domain 3 must meet some key criteria; it should be:

- verifiable (by someone relevant, e.g. a colleague testimonial, which must be signed by your colleague and their contact details must be available so the examiner can contact them if required);

- applied to specific competencies (so that it is clear that every competency has been met);
- diverse (a wide range of evidence is more robust and aids triangulation and credibility of the evidence);
- of high quality (you should show analysis of the evidence to ensure its relevance to any given competency is clear and to demonstrate higher or master's level thinking);
- signposted (to create a logical flow through the work and to facilitate clarity of what is being claimed).

For more advice on collecting evidence for your portfolio, please refer to Chapter 10.

Type of evidence

This section describes the evidence needed for your portfolio and four scenarios are considered. The first is a critical reflective review of a patient presenting in practice.

Scenario 5.1

Diana (pseudonym) was a 22-year-old student who came to the walk-in centre complaining of a sore throat for the previous 3 days. She reported recent coryzal symptoms, fever but no headache, vomiting, photophobia or a rash. She was drinking well and had a fair appetite. She had no difficulty swallowing but this was painful. She had no cough. She admitted to finding her course quite stressful and didn't want to miss any time from studying so having had symptoms for 3 days she was feeling worried.

Past medical history: fit and well; previous tonsillitis episodes ×2 treated with antibiotics by her GP.

Medication: Microgynon; over the counter Beechams Hot Lemon; echinacea drops daily.

Allergies: nil.

On examination: looks well; temperature 37.3°C; ears: tympanic membrane visualized, no signs of infection, throat red, tonsils slightly enlarged – no exudates; minimal cervical lymphadenopathy; no neck stiffness, no rash.

The issues that I wish to consider in relation to Scenario 5.1 and would discuss during the consultation are: diagnosis; use of investigations; patient expectations, beliefs and concerns; management – clinical decision-making and ethical considerations; use of antibiotics; self-care advice and treatment.

Diagnosis

Sore throat is a very common presentation in primary care and can be caused by bacterial and viral infections. It is generally a self-limiting illness with most patients recovering within 8 days (Lindbaek et al. 2006). Clinically, viral and bacterial signs can be similar. The most common bacterial organism is Group A beta-haemolytic streptococcus and this can be isolated from up to 30% of patients presenting with sore throat (Drugs and Therapeutics Bulletin 1995).

After history-taking and examination I took the following into account before making a diagnosis:

- recent coryzal symptoms are suggestive of viral cause;
- low-grade fever, lack of exudates, minimal cervical lymphadenopathy, no photophobia, no neck stiffness or rash all reassure me that the illness is mild in nature and serious pathology at this time (e.g. meningitis) is ruled out;
- the patient's age is relevant, as an alternative diagnosis in this age group is infectious mononucleosis (glandular fever); however, at present I was able to put this to one side as she was feeling able to carry out normal activities of daily living, and the symptoms were mild and of short duration. I would consider a blood test for glandular fever if the sore throat persists longer than 7–10 days or in patients who do not respond when treated with antibiotics;
- clinically there were no exudates and minimal cervical lymphadenopathy;
- she was taking no other drugs except for the oral contraceptive pill. In decision-making around differential diagnoses it is important to recognize the effects of drugs such as carbimazole, which can cause bone marrow suppression, one of the signs being a sore throat.

Use of investigations

Throat swabs are not thought to be useful routinely in sore throats as they cannot differentiate between infection and carriage (MeReC 1999). They have poor sensitivity, with results taking up to 48 hours to be reported, and the test is relatively expensive (Little and Williamson 1996). However, I do take swabs in patients whose symptoms are prolonged or in high-risk groups.

Other tests available are rapid antigen tests which give almost immediate results (not thought to be cost-effective) and anti-streptolysin O (ASO) titres, which can identify whether a person has recently been infected with streptococcus, and may be useful for people who remain unwell or who develop complications. A further test is an anti-DNAse B test, which, when combined with ASO titres, gives more useful results.

In the walk-in centre the clientele generally have acute presentations and patients are encouraged to return to their own GP if symptoms do not resolve, so there is little need for these tests in my current practice, although it is useful to have knowledge of them.

Patient expectations, beliefs and concerns

An important part of the consultation is to understand the reason that patients attend. Many patients attend for a seemingly obvious reason but often the presenting complaint is not the only complaint. Presentation with a sore throat may be part of a wider agenda (Scottish Intercollegiate Guidelines Network 1999). Several authors on communication skills teaching recognize the importance of this element in a consultation (Byrne and Long 1976, Neighbour 2004, Silverman et al. 2005).

In exploring the patient's expectations I considered the fact that she has had antibiotics on previous occasions for sore throat presentations and may well have attended expecting to receive them again. A third of patients attending want or expect an antibiotic (Butler et al. 1998). She had also been taking echinacea drops daily for the last month hoping that this would stop her getting colds this winter and so it was possible that she perceived a need for conventional medicine because the complementary therapy appeared to have been unsuccessful.

Diana's main reason for attendance was that she wondered if she needed antibiotics because the pain was not being controlled by the over-the-counter measures she had tried. Patients' expectations are known to influence prescribing decisions (McFarlane et al. 2002) and as a nurse prescriber I must be alert to this request.

Clinical decision-making

In coming to any decision, ethical considerations are an important part of the thought process. I have a duty of care to the patient to ensure that she receives safe competent care and I must act within my NMC code of professional conduct (NMC 2008). I have a responsibility to patients who expect to receive a diagnosis, advice and treatment for their presenting problem.

Seedhouse (1998) has designed a grid to help formulate ethical considerations used in decision-making. I wanted the most beneficial outcome for the patient and in this consultation I was aware of my professional responsibilities and the need to respect patients as partners in their care.

Part of any consultation includes 'safety netting' (Neighbour 2004). This requires an understanding of the likely cause of the disease and possible complications so that information can be given to the patient to seek further help if any deviation from anticipated natural progress occurs.

It is known that sore throat symptoms resolve within 7 days whether or not they are treated with antibiotics (Del Mar et al. 2007), and I used this knowledge to explain to Diana that antibiotics are not thought to be necessary in treating most causes of tonsillitis. There was nothing in her past medical history that would make me more likely to treat with antibiotics, for example rheumatic fever or being immunocompromised.

More common complications I thought of were otitis media and sinusitis, with more serious complications being a quinsy, rheumatic fever or glomerulonephritis. In clinical practice, however, it is not practical to go through all possible scenarios with the patient. It would be too time-consuming and too worrying, so I generally explain the normal signs and symptoms, expected length of illness and ask them to return if they feel more unwell or any new signs or symptoms appear. I discussed when to seek further help with Diana so that she would feel confident in managing her illness. Obviously, I must work within my scope of professional practice (NMC 2008). Should there be any clinical signs that could suggest a more serious illness I would refer on to a medical colleague – either to an ENT specialist (e.g. if I had diagnosed a quinsy) or to a GP (e.g. if the patient presented with more severe or unusual symptoms or had a complex medical history that could mean complications were more likely to develop).

I also use the walk-in centre written guidelines on the management of sore throat presentations as a guide to my clinical care. This information is provided by the Prodigy web site (www.prodigy.co.uk) Patient Information Leaflet service.

Use of antibiotics

Diana had no risk factors or signs/symptoms to suggest antibiotics would be appropriate in managing this episode of illness. She was generally well and, as I discussed earlier, had symptoms of a coryzal illness suggesting a viral origin. I discussed with her my thought that it was more likely to be a viral sore throat and would not improve with the use of antibiotics. To encourage acceptance of this decision I discussed possible side-effects of antibiotics, for example vaginal thrush, interaction with oral contraception and risk of developing an allergy to the drug. However, it is useful to re-look at antibiotic therapy in the management of sore throats to demonstrate my knowledge and understanding, should the clinical indications be different.

In writing clinical care guidelines for the walk-in centre I researched the use of antibiotics for the treatment of acute sore throat. This involved speaking and writing to experts in the field of sore throat management, for example the local microbiologist, and appraising clinical guidance from respected organizations.

The National Institute for Health and Clinical Excellence (NICE 2001) recommends antibiotics in the following situations:

- features of marked systemic upset secondary to acute sore throat;
- unilateral peritonsillitis (quinsy);
- a history of rheumatic fever;
- an increased risk from acute infection (such as a child with diabetes mellitus or immunodeficiency).

The antibiotic of choice in treating tonsillitis is Penicillin V unless there is a known allergy to penicillin in which case erythromycin should be used instead. A 10-day course is recommended to eradicate possible streptococcal infection (Drug and Therapeutics Bulletin 1995, Scottish Intercollegiate Guidelines Network 1999). Shorter courses are sometimes given because there is no good correlation between microbiological and clinical cure for relief of symptoms. The Public Health Laboratory Service (PHLS) recommends either twice or four times daily dosing for 7–10 days for penicillin and 5–10 days for erythromycin (PHLS 2000).

It is known that the prescription of an antibiotic increases re-attendance rates for further episodes of sore throat (Little et al. 1997). There is also the risk of adverse reactions, and there is a concern that indiscriminate prescribing increases bacterial resistance in the community (Standing Medical Advisory Committee 1999, Drug and Therapeutics Bulletin 2007).

Self-care advice and treatment

Having explained to Diana the nature and likely course of the illness, I offered reassurance, and gave advice on symptomatic treatment.

I recommended paracetamol or ibuprofen as analgesics for sore throats. As she was already taking Beechams Hot Lemon with little effect, I mentioned that she might like to try ibuprofen as an alternative or in addition. Beechams Hot Lemon contains paracetamol and I was careful to remind her that she should not take both together because they contain the same drug and could result in overdose. An alternative analgesic to Ibuprofen is soluble aspirin gargles but there is little evidence to demonstrate the efficacy of this method.

I discussed her use of echinacea drops and explained that there was conflicting evidence surrounding the benefits. Some studies found no evidence to support that echinacea prevents colds and flu or shortens the duration of the illness (Barrett et al. 2002), whereas others suggested some benefits (Fugh-Berman 2003). On reviewing the safety of echinacea, the Medicines Control Agency state that the main risks appear to be of allergy, particularly for people suffering from hayfever (Medicines Control Agency 2002).

As well as addressing her physical symptoms I attempted to explore Diana's feelings of stress related to her studying. I gave her some practical advice on stress management including relaxation techniques.

Where possible I follow up verbal advice with a patient information leaflet to reinforce the advice given. This helps patients to manage their illness confidently. Diana agreed to follow a self-management strategy and I re-emphasized the need to seek further help should she develop other signs or symptoms that made her feel worse.

Conclusion

Writing this scenario has demonstrated the thought processes I used to underpin the clinical decisions during my consultation with Diana. I have been surprised at the breadth of knowledge I draw upon in my clinical practice. It provides evidence demonstrating that I am a safe, competent nurse practitioner in the assessment, diagnosis and management of a patient presenting with an acute illness.

In order to reach this decision I have shown that I have an understanding of sore throat presentations, the natural progression of the illness and how to assess for the severity of the disease. I understand the pharmacological and non-pharmacological approaches to modifying disease and promoting health and can link theory to practice. I can take a comprehensive medical history and undertake an appropriate physical examination in order to make a diagnosis, which also considers various other differential possibilities. Although I rarely take swabs for sore throats I have knowledge of what tests are available to aid patient management and when it is appropriate to request tests.

Scenario 5.1 enables you to demonstrate a range of competencies within this domain that will be discussed below. Some of these competencies can be seen to be met fully, for example formulating an action plan, and others will only be met partially, for example diagnosing and managing acute and long-term conditions.

Obtains, analyses and interprets history, presenting symptoms, physical findings and diagnostic information to develop the appropriate differential diagnoses

A brief patient history is provided in this Scenario 5.1 and, importantly, the history and physical findings are interpreted and analysed. For example, the diagnosis of viral sore throat is explicitly informed by key information gained from the history (recent coryzal symptoms, lack of marked systemic upset); the physical examination (looks well, no exudates visible on tonsils, minimal cervical lymphadenopathy); and the potential use of investigations (throat swab). Differential diagnoses are also considered based on information from the history (patient's age makes infectious mononucleosis a possibility) and the physical examination (absence of photophobia, neck stiffness or body rash eliminate meningitis as a diagnosis).

Diagnoses and manages acute and long-term conditions while attending to the patient's response to the illness experience

The scenario clearly discusses management of an acute condition (sore throat) and describes the awareness of the patient's feelings and potential response to the illness. However, in order to meet this competence fully you need to offer further evidence demonstrating how you have diagnosed and managed a long-term condition while attending to the patient's response.

Prioritizes health problems and intervenes appropriately, including initiation of effective emergency care

This scenario demonstrates how you have been able to discriminate between serious (meningitis) and minor (viral sore throat) pathology and that you have appropriately intervened to manage a minor health problem. You would need to demonstrate how you prioritize and initiate effective emergency care. This could be achieved by using other types of evidence (see Table 5.1); for example, by providing evidence of successful completion of an OSCE/OSCA (objective structured clinical examination/assessment) station of a patient who presents requiring urgent care (i.e. patient having an asthma attack or an epileptic fit).

Employs appropriate diagnostic and therapeutic interventions and regimens with attention to safety, cost, invasiveness, simplicity, acceptability, adherence and efficacy

The use of a throat swab in this scenario has been considered, taking into account cost, simplicity and efficacy. By reflecting on the patient's perception of having a throat swab and any risks to the patient as a consequence of this investigation, the remaining descriptors (safety, invasiveness, acceptability) will have been met. Likewise, this scenario effectively analyses the use of antibiotics as a therapeutic intervention incorporating all the descriptors except cost and adherence.

Formulates an action-plan based on scientific rationale, evidence-based standards of care, and practice guidelines

The scenario describes the use of clinical guidelines (NICE) as well as reference to local experts who will be aware of local guidance (microbiologist) to underpin the decision on whether or not to prescribe antibiotics. In addition, the evidence to support the use of relevant investigations (throat swab) is reviewed.

Provides guidance, counselling, advice and support regarding management of the health/illness condition

Within this scenario it has been demonstrated that the patient is provided with guidance (under what circumstances they must return for review), counselling (self-management strategy), advice (on medications to relieve sore throat symptom) and support (recognizing that the patient may have other concerns but uses the sore throat symptom as an excuse to access help). To meet this competency fully you would also need to demonstrate this for a patient who does not have an illness, but perhaps requires help with management of a general health issue, for example healthy eating.

Demonstrates critical thinking and diagnostic reasoning skills in clinical decision-making

This competency is fully met by the scenario. Diagnostic reasoning was evidenced via the identification of a range of differential diagnoses and final choice of diagnosis.

Critical thinking was evidenced by the appraisal of the value of a throat swab, safety-netting and the clinical decisions related to treatment and use of medications.

Analyses the data collected to determine the health status

Analysis of the patient's history and physical examination findings (i.e. when you discuss how you make a diagnosis) enables the health status of the patient to be determined within this scenario.

Demonstrates knowledge of the pathophysiology of acute or chronic diseases or conditions commonly seen in practice

For this competency, it is important that evidence is provided demonstrating your knowledge of pathophysiology relating to a range of clinical conditions that present in your normal working environment. The scenario illustrates your knowledge in relation to one commonly presenting condition only.

Applies theories and evidence-based practice pertinent to guide practice

Within this scenario, the discussion about the use of throat swabs, and whether or not to prescribe an antibiotic, demonstrate that you apply an evidence-based approach to practice.

Evaluates the use of complementary/alternative therapies used by patients for safety and potential interaction

This competency is partially met, in that you have commented on the safety of echinacea, but you do not explicitly mention whether you investigated if Diana had a past medical history of hayfever. You would also need to comment on the potential for drug/complementary therapy interaction to meet this competency fully.

Integrates appropriate non-drug-based treatment methods into a plan of management

The management plan incorporates a non-drug-based method (relaxation techniques) of treatment for Diana's stress-related problems.

Orders, may perform, and interprets common screening and diagnostic tests

The discussion about the value of throat swabs in the scenario illustrates competency in appropriately ordering/performing and interpreting a diagnostic test. Further evidence would be required to demonstrate that you have achieved this with regard to screening tests, in order to meet this competency fully (For X-ray referral guidance, see Appendix 2.).

The next exemplar and scenario is a direct extract from an assignment done whilst studying on the Nurse Independent and Supplementary Prescribing course, 2006.

Introduction

Tobacco smoking is associated with high levels of morbidity and mortality in a range of disease processes. This recognition is reflected in recent health policy documents (DoH 1999c,d, 2000b, 2004). The national smoking cessation strategy involves a three-tiered approach: health care practitioners to provide smoking cessation advice to patients opportunistically; intermediate support via dedicated appointments or clinics in both primary and secondary care; and referral pathways to specialist services. Currently, there are two pharmacological interventions available for patients to assist with smoking cessation: nicotine replacement therapy (NRT) or Bupropion (British Medical Association and Royal Pharmaceutical Society of Great Britain 2007).

Nurse prescribing has a long history in theory (DHSS 1986, DOH 1989) but has only recently become a reality (DoH 1999a, 2006b). In the last decade there has been a paradigm shift in nursing, with recognition of different levels of practice resulting in an explosion of new nursing roles in both primary and secondary care (Daly and Carnwell 2003). This has been influenced by some key policy changes, including reduction in junior doctors' working hours (NHSME 1991), introduction of the *Scope of Professional Practice* and its subsequent development (UKCC 1992, NMC 2004), recognition of the unique nursing role (DoH 1999b, 2000a, 2006a) and a drive to encourage greater multiprofessional working (NHSME 1999). Nurses are therefore well placed in a number of arenas to support patients with smoking cessation, for example in general practice, walk-in centres, cardiac rehabilitation, diabetes care and others.

Scenario 5.2 presents a case study of a patient who presented for smoking cessation advice in a general practice setting. It highlights the importance of providing patient information and support, as well as pharmacological interventions. The complexities of prescribing, including weighing up the risks and benefits of NRT for this patient, will be debated.

Scenario 5.2

Harry (pseudonym) is a 75-year-old retired office worker who smokes approximately 25 g of tobacco a day via a pipe. He has smoked continuously since the age of 18 years. He stopped smoking cigarettes about 30 years ago and started to use a pipe and tobacco. He has never attempted to stop smoking. He lives alone and socializes with friends, who are all smokers, three times a week. He has a high alcohol consumption, averaging about 35 units per week. He is normally fit and well.

He has a past medical history of hiatus hernia, peptic ulcer, hypertension and recently atrial fibrillation. His current medications include ramipril 2.5 mg once daily and aspirin 75 mg once daily. He does not take any over-the-counter medication other than paracetamol occasionally for headaches.

Harry had presented for advice because his GP had told him that his recent experience of atrial fibrillation and his hypertension were probably a result of his smoking habit. He was shocked by this and felt motivated to attempt to stop smoking in order to maintain and prevent deterioration of his health. Becker (1984) suggests that a patient's belief about their susceptibility to a serious disease directly affects their motivation and the likely success of behaviour modification to reduce their risk.

A patient-centred consultation style was adopted in order to facilitate a catalytic and supportive environment (Heron 2001) and which would allow exploration of Harry's health beliefs and motivation and encourage a partnership approach to care. This is important because Harry was going to have to do all the hard work in order to be successful in his attempt to quit. This approach reflects the philosophy of the social-psychological consultation model, which focuses on human behaviour within a therapeutic relationship. Pendleton et al. (2003) state that establishing a relationship and promoting collaboration and partnership with the patient are key aims of a consultation. Additionally, the quality of the interaction between a patient and a health care practitioner has been found to affect patient concordance with treatment (Crumbie 1999a).

Harry expressed some concern that he had left it too late to stop smoking; however, age should not be a barrier to smoking cessation intervention (Rigotti 2005, Davidhizar et al. 2002). Ageism has a significant effect on the motivation of older people to concord with treatment (Resnick 1991) as does lack of choice or coercion (Sherwood 1995), i.e. if a patient believes they must alter their behaviour in order to prevent further ill-health. It was therefore important to reinforce the potential health gains associated with smoking cessation to Harry, as well as offering him choices in all aspects of the quit attempt.

The key components of the consultation were patient assessment and information giving. Assessment centred around ascertaining Harry's smoking history and factors that influenced his smoking, judging whether he was addicted to nicotine, investigating how he felt about giving up smoking as well as clarifying his current health status. This information would help inform the decision-making in relation to whether pharmacological treatment was an option for this quit attempt.

Local guidelines on the assessment and management of smoking cessation interactions were utilized (Manchester, Salford and Trafford Health Promotion Department 2002). Guidelines that synthesize evidence into clear recommenda-tions for practice are valuable to practitioners who may experience practical difficulties accessing, assessing and assimilating health information and can lead to improvements in both the process and outcomes of care (Rycroft-Malone 2002).

Harry required information relating to the harmful effects of smoking, difficulties associated with trying to stop smoking and strategies that may help him overcome problems he may experience, for example NRT to reduce craving. Heron (2001) emphasizes the importance of ensuring that the information is relevant to the individual patient's needs and is delivered in such a way that it encourages the patient's active involvement in the learning process. Harry expressed an interest in trying NRT, which has been found to be effective in aiding smoking cessation (West et al. 2000), and felt that the patches would be easiest to manage.

The prescribing dilemma

In weighing up the risk/benefit of treatment with NRT, Harry's past medical history of peptic ulcers, his current health status of hypertension and the recent episode of atrial fibrillation needed to be considered. Smoking is associated with the pathogenesis of gastric ulcers by causing gastric hypersecretion and compromising the mucosal defence mechanisms (Crumbie 1999b) and consequently contributes to delayed ulcer healing and relapse of peptic ulcer disease. Additionally, smoking is considered a causative factor in the development of heart disease, lung disease and various cancers (DoH 2004). The British Medical Association and Royal Pharmaceutical Society of Great Britain (BNF 2007) advise that NRT should be used with caution in patients with cardiovascular disease or a history of gastritis and peptic ulcers and it should not be used in patients with severe cardiovascular disease, including severe arrhythmias. Review of the evidence supporting the use of NRT in patients with these conditions suggests that nicotine medication is not a significant risk factor for cardiovascular events (Murray et al. 1996, McRobbie and Hajek 2000, West et al. 2000), including atrial fibrillation (Tobacco Advisory Group of the Royal College of Physicians 2000), and is not likely to cause peptic ulcer disease (Murray et al. 1996).

Therefore, NRT appeared to be a suitable option for Harry. However, it has been established that Harry has a high alcohol intake, which predisposes him to further peptic ulcer disease (Cabrera and Groer 2001) and his anxiety about his current health problems could result in a rise in his blood pressure and cause palpitations. It was necessary to address these issues with Harry in order to prevent any resulting symptoms being falsely perceived as attributable to the NRT.

NRT patches are available in either 16- or 24-hour doses and in a range of strengths (BNF 2007). Harry preferred the 16-hour dose because he was anxious not to experience sleep disturbances. He did not usually start smoking within the first hour of rising in the morning so was used to low circulating nicotine levels as a result of smoking abstinence overnight. He did not have any skin problems that would make using a patch difficult. In order to reduce the likelihood of recognized side-effects such as palpitations, chest pain and dyspepsia, which might worry Harry, and to improve concordance with the treatment, I recommended trying a medium dose 10-g Nicorette patch, which releases 10 mg of nicotine over 16 hours. Additionally, I was anxious about his recent episode of atrial fibrillation and this contributed to my decision to prescribe cautiously. Following a brief case review, the prescription was signed by the GP mentor.

Having agreed on a treatment and management plan, Harry was issued with a prescription and a further appointment for 1 week to review his progress. It was important to be positive and to encourage Harry but also to be realistic: the quitting process may be difficult and may not be achieved on first attempt. Relapse is common and should not be viewed as failure but as part of the learning process (Clarke 1999).

Reflection

On further discussion of this case, the GP mentor proposed that I might have been overcautious in my prescribing decision. Having decided that the benefits of smoking cessation to Harry were significant and the use of NRT was safe and acceptable, he questioned whether I might have jeopardized the quit attempt by issuing a subtherapeutic treatment dose. There is some evidence that in patients who are medium to heavy smokers, lower strength patches are not as effective as higher strength patches (West et al. 2000). However, I did not want to cause iatrogenesis, which may be more likely in older people because of altered pharmacokinetics (Downie et al. 2003) and polypharmacy (DoH 2001). Guidelines for prescribing for elderly people suggest that drug dosages should be reduced in order to account for these factors (British Medical Association and Royal Pharmaceutical Society of Great Britain 2007). Therefore, I felt it was reasonable to start at a lower dose. There was also the option of using another form of NRT, for example gum, alongside the patches if the patches were insufficient in reducing symptoms of nicotine withdrawal. Combining the patch with other forms of NRT is safe and may be more effective than the patch alone (West et al. 2000).

Conclusion

The risks to health resulting from smoking are well established and a smoking cessation strategy is part of the current health agenda. The development of a prescribing role for nurses could have a significant beneficial impact on patient care, particularly in relation to health promotion activities such as smoking cessation. Nurses need to be cognisant of their underpinning knowledge base in relation to pharmacology, utilize local and national guidance, provide a rationale for decision-making processes and regularly reflect on practice in order to be effective and safe prescribers.

Scenario 5.2 demonstrates how to provide evidence relating to health promotion/health protection and disease prevention as well as therapeutic interventions (e.g. safe prescribing practice) within Domain 3. The competencies covered by this scenario are described below.

Provides health promotion and disease-prevention services to patients who are healthy or who have acute and/or chronic conditions

A thorough assessment of the patient's health education and health promotion needs relating to smoking cessation is provided in this case study, including knowledge requirements and consideration of readiness to change behaviour. The evidence would fully meet the requirements for this competency.

Evidence of a smoking cessation programme offered to individual patients is provided, including your role in planning, developing and implementing care for a particular patient. You have made explicit your attempts to promote health and well-being (benefits of stopping smoking at any age, reducing iatrogenesis) and addressing individual needs (consideration given to patient's existing health problems, patient's smoking habits).

Provides health education through anticipatory guidance and counselling to promote health, reduce risk factors, and prevent disease and disability

In undertaking a thorough assessment of this patient you have demonstrated effective guidance and counselling that supports health promotion (benefits of smoking cessation being explicitly linked to the patient's health concerns), and reduction of risk factors (preventing iatrogenesis as well as reducing the patient's risk of health ill associated with continuing smoking). In addition, you have recognized potential disease and disability (heart disease, peptic ulcer disease) that the patient is at risk from if he continues smoking and used this knowledge effectively within your health education strategy.

Develops and uses a follow-up system within the practice workplace to ensure that patients receive appropriate services

It is clear that the patient management plan incorporates patient review within this clinical setting. To meet this competency fully, evidence of a comprehensive follow-up system which demonstrates a range of services that may be beneficial for the patient, for example smoking cessation support groups, repeat prescriptions policy for patients taking NRT, recall of patients who miss review appointments, would need to be provided.

Employs appropriate diagnostic and therapeutic interventions and regimens with attention to safety, cost, invasiveness, simplicity, acceptability, adherence, and efficacy

The decision-making process associated with the therapeutic intervention for this patient clearly demonstrates that you have considered safety (risks of adverse effects), invasiveness (giving the patient a choice of therapeutic intervention), simplicity (one patch a day which can be supplemented by nicotine gum if required), adherence and acceptability (rationale for choice of 16-hour patch) and efficacy (reference to appropriate literature). You would need to consider cost issues, and all of the above for a diagnostic intervention or regimen, in order to meet this competency fully.

Formulates an action plan based on scientific rationale, evidence-based standards of care, and practice guidelines

A scientific rationale has been utilized (reference to appropriate published literature), evidence-based standards of care (guidelines for prescribing for older people, Tobacco Advisory Group of the Royal College of Physicians) and practice guidelines (Manchester, Salford and Trafford Health Promotion Department guidelines) in the formulation of an action-plan for this patient and so have fully met the competency.

Provides guidance, counselling, advice and support regarding management of the health/illness condition

This scenario demonstrates that this competency has been fully met in relation to management of a patient's health problem, i.e. management of smoking cessation. You would need to do the same with respect to management of an ill patient.

Demonstrates critical thinking and diagnostic reasoning skills in clinical decision-making

Critical thinking has been demonstrated when reflecting on the prescribing decision in this case, as well as sound clinical decision-making. This would need to be evidenced with regard to diagnostic reasoning in order fully to meet this competency.

Formulates a problem list and prioritized management plan

A problem list has been formulated (investigation of the patient's smoking history, assessing if he was addicted to nicotine, discovering his thoughts and feelings about smoking cessation and clarifying his health status) and a prioritized management plan (discussing alcohol intake and anxiety levels, use of NRT patch, positive encouragement with quit attempt and a follow-up appointment) presented in this scenario. Therefore this competency is fully met.

Demonstrates knowledge of the pathophysiology of acute or chronic diseases or conditions commonly seen in practice

Pathophysiological knowledge of peptic ulcer disease is clearly demonstrated within this case study. Additional evidence demonstrating pathophysiological knowledge relating to some other common conditions is necessary to show the range of knowledge required to meet this competency fully.

Applies principles of epidemiology and demography in clinical practice by recognizing populations at risk, patterns of disease, and effectiveness of prevention and intervention

Understanding of the epidemiology of smoking-related illnesses has been utilized to provide a potentially effective intervention (smoking cessation) and illness prevention strategy (prevent progression of potential cardiovascular disease while being cognisant of iatrogenesis) for a particular patient. Knowledge of populations that are at risk (smokers with co-morbidity such as diabetes or peptic ulcer disease, as well as smokers generally) and that patterns of smoking-related disease may be more likely to present in the older adult has been demonstrated.

Provides information and advice to patients and carers concerning drug regimens, side-effects and interaction, in an appropriate form

A patient-centred approach has been taken to provision of information and advice for this patient. The patient was helped to choose an appropriate form of NRT and consideration was given as to whether a 24-hour or 16-hour regime should be recommended. Analysis of risk to the patient relating to side-effects (reactivation of peptic ulcer disease, deterioration of cardiovascular status) and potential interactions relating to use of NRT (skin condition of patient) is evident. No mention is made of providing information via another format (e.g. written leaflets), and this would be required to meet this competency fully.

If legally authorized, prescribes medications based on efficacy, safety, and cost from the formulary

This case study was undertaken as part of the Nurse Independent and Supplementary Prescribing course and so the nurse was not legally authorized to prescribe the treatment. However, it has been demonstrated that the nurse has made an appropriate prescribing decision, and has clarified that the actual prescription was signed by the GP mentor. The prescribing decision demonstrates due consideration has been given to efficacy (literature that supports NRT patches and gum as a combined therapy, as well as the value of smoking cessation interventions to older adults), safety (lower dose for an older adult, taking a thorough past medical history) and cost (if patient is concordant with the regime then medication will not be wasted).

Schedules follow-up visits appropriately to monitor patients and evaluate health/illness care

This competency has only been partially met with respect to planning a follow-up visit for this patient. You would need to evidence how you have appropriately monitored a patient (how the patient was reviewed, by whom and when, the use of investigations or tools to determine the efficacy of the intervention) and evaluated the prescribed care for patients you have to see, for both health promotion and illness-related health issues.

Scenario 5.3 consists of a testimonial from Mr Candy, consultant gynaecologist, at North Kent Foundation Trust; a referral letter for patient x; and the reply following her gynaecological treatment.

Scenario 5.3

Dear Alice   17th November 2006

RE: Your referrals to the gynaecology services at North Kent NHS Foundation Trust

In the last 18 months you have appropriately referred patients with a range of gynaecological problems to the gynaecological services at North Kent NHS Trust. These referrals have included urgent presentations including post-menopausal bleeding and suspected ectopic pregnancy as well as more routine problems such as cervical dyskaryosis and menorrhagia. Your referral letters have been comprehensive and inclusive of all relevant information.

Yours sincerely
Mr J. Candy

Dear Mr Candy   1st July 2006

RE: X, DOB 4.4.80

I would be grateful if you would urgently review X who presented with a 24-hour history of increasing left iliac fossa pain and vaginal bleeding. She had a positive pregnancy test on 29.5.06 and her LMP was on 27.4.06. She complains of constant pain in the left iliac fossa region, which started yesterday morning, has been getting worse and is unrelieved by oral analgesia. The pain is now more generalized over her lower abdomen and she also feels nauseous but has not vomited. There have been no bowel changes and she has not opened her bowels in the last 24 hours. She describes the vaginal bleeding as 'spotting' only.

She is normally fit and well and has a past medical history of asthma, which is currently well controlled. Her last cervical smear was negative in August 2005. She discontinued the oral contraceptive pill, Marvelon, in December 2005, and since then her menstrual cycle has been a regular 28-day cycle with approximately 5 days of bleeding.

Medication: salbutamol inhaler prn; becodtide inhaler qds; folic acid 400 μg od; No known allergies.

She is married and this pregnancy was planned. She works as a shop assistant. Her husband will be accompanying her to A&E. They are both distressed and very concerned about the implications of an ectopic pregnancy.

On examination, she is pale and obviously in pain. Her BP is 100/70 mmHg, P 86, RR 20. She demonstrates mild guarding of her abdomen on palpation and she is acutely tender in the left iliac fossa. No organomegaly. Quiet bowel sounds were heard on auscultation. On vaginal examination the cervical os was slightly open and she had a small amount of bright red blood in the vagina. She was very tender in the left adnexa and demonstrated cervical excitation. PR exam was not performed.

I am concerned that she is presenting with an ectopic pregnancy and so would appreciate an urgent review.

Yours sincerely
Alice White

Dear Alice   19th July 2006
RE: X DOB 4.4.80

Thank you for your prompt referral of X, who unfortunately did have an ectopic pregnancy. She was admitted from A&E on 1.7.06 and underwent a left salpingectomy. The procedure was uncomplicated and she was discharged on 3.7.06.

I have advised her to avoid getting pregnant for the next 3 months and she is planning to use condoms for contraception. I will review her in the outpatient clinic in 3 months' time to discuss fertility issues.

Yours sincerely
Mr J. Candy

The testimonial and referral letters enable you to demonstrate the competencies Domain 3 described below.

Diagnoses and manages acute and long-term conditions while attending to the patient's response to the illness experience

In the evidence the appropriate management of an acute condition (ectopic pregnancy) is discussed and highlights awareness of the patient's (and her husband's) feelings and potential response to the health problem. However, in order to meet this competence fully you would need to offer further evidence demonstrating how you have diagnosed and managed a long-term condition while attending to the patient's response.

Prioritizes health problems and intervenes appropriately, including initiation of effective emergency care

The action taken with this patient (immediate referral to A&E) demonstrates the seriousness and urgency of this patient presentation and appropriate intervention has been prioritized, thereby meeting this competence fully in relation to emergency care. You would need to demonstrate that that you can perform in the same way for other health problems, other than those requiring emergency care, in order to provide breadth of evidence for this competency.

Initiates appropriate and timely consultation and/or referral when the problem exceeds the nurse's scope of practice and/or expertise

This competency has been fully met with respect to appropriate and timely referral. You would need to consider presenting evidence that demonstrates how you would seek help with a patient presentation that exceeds your scope of practice or expertise, other than via referral, for example discussing the case with a colleague in your workplace.

Assesses and intervenes to assist the patient in complex, urgent or emergency situations

The appropriate assessment (history and physical examination) and management of this patient (urgent referral to A&E) demonstrates the ability to assess and intervene in urgent and emergency situations. You would need to provide evidence on assessment and intervention of a complex patient situation in order fully to meet this competency. Clarification of what you believe made the situation complex would be helpful.

Rapidly assesses the patient's unstable and complex health care problems through synthesis and prioritization of historical and immediately derived data

This competency is fully met with respect to patients presenting with unstable health care problems but would need more evidence to demonstrate a complex health care problem. Once again, clarification of what you believe made the situation complex would be helpful.

Diagnoses unstable and complex health care problems using collaboration and consultation with the multiprofessional health care team as indicated by setting, speciality, and individual knowledge and experience

The evidence presented confirms that a correct diagnosis has been made of a potentially unstable health care problem via appropriate referral and consultation with a consultant gynaecologist. You would need to present some additional examples which outline a range of health care problems (including complex ones) to demonstrate the required breadth of evidence for this competency.

Obtains a comprehensive problem-focused health history from the patient or carer

This competency has been fully met by this evidence. Please note it is important that the evidence details the history fully.

Performs a comprehensive problem-focused, age-appropriate physical examination

This competency has been partially met by this evidence. A comprehensive (includes general inspection, baseline observations) problem-focused (abdominal and pelvic examination) age-appropriate (i.e. pelvic examination for a woman who is sexually active) physical examination has been undertaken. Further examples of patients with different health problems and in different age groups is needed to cover the breadth of evidence for this competency. Please note that you would need to have evidence of formal assessment of your physical examination techniques (i.e. via an OSCE/OSCA or a colleague testimonial) in order to demonstrate competence in physical examination skills.

Analyses the data collected to determine health status of the patient

Clear evidence of clinical reasoning and analysis of the available evidence is not presented in this evidence. A reflective account that details the differential diagnoses that were considered for this patient presentation and what elements of the history and/or physical examination were required in order to accept or refute the differentials is needed to meet this competency.

Assesses, diagnoses, monitors, coordinates, and manages the health/illness status of patients during acute and enduring episodes

This competency has been met in relation to assessment, diagnosis and coordination of the health/illness status of a patient during an acute episode. Details on monitoring a patient are needed for an acute episode, for example for this patient, description of the care provided before the patient attended A&E (regular observations, advising patient to be nil-by-mouth, providing analgesia) is required. All of the above needs to be evidenced for a patient experiencing an enduring episode, for example description of the assessment, diagnosis, monitoring and management of a patient with a long-term health condition.

Communicates the patient's health status using appropriate terminology, format and technology

This competency has been clearly met with regard to a referral situation. Providing evidence of your communication of a patient's health status in electronic and/or written patient notes and/or verbally (e.g. a colleague testimonial of a verbal handover) would provide the breadth of evidence required.

Works collaboratively with other health professionals and agencies as appropriate

Evidence of collaborative working is provided in the consultant's letter about the referrals. Further evidence of how you work collaboratively with health agencies, for example social care, would help you to meet this competency fully.

The final scenario comprises an extract of your documentation in a patient's medical notes.

Scenario 5.4

Mr N; DOB, 11.8.40;
4.3.07; 10.30 am

Mr N is a 67-year-old Asian man who has recently come to England from India to live with his son. He complains of feeling generally unwell for the last 2 weeks and has developed chest pain and mild shortness of breath in the last 2 days. Today he coughed up some blood, which worried him so he self-referred to the A&E department.

Symptoms of lethargy, malaise, night sweats and a mild cough for the last 2 weeks. Wakes at night feeling hot and sweaty most nights, denies sweats during the day, has not taken his temperature. Has 'no energy' and does not feel rested after sleep, sleep disturbed by sweats and cough. Has been unable to help out in his son's shop in the last week because of fatigue. Dry cough with no sputum until this morning when expectorated purulent sputum, which was blood stained. No relieving or aggravating factors for cough. Has been self-medicating with paracetamol 1 g tds for last 2 days. No one else in the family is unwell. Patient worried he may have cancer.

Previous medical history

1952 appendicectomy
December 2006 diabetes mellitus (diet controlled)
No regular medications
No known allergies
Vaccinations: tetanus 2005; does not recall TB vaccination, no scar on arm

Family history

Father died at age 35 in a road traffic accident, mother died at age 80 from a CVA, brother age 59 years fit and well, sister age 62 years diabetes mellitus.

No FH of heart disease, jaundice, thyroid disease, renal disease, cancer, asthma or mental illness.

Social history

Widower – wife died last year (brain haemorrhage). Lives with his son and family in a two-bedroom flat; it is very cramped, with a total of three adults and three children sharing the accommodation. No other children. Moved to England from India in November 2006 following the death of his wife. Speaks English well, planning to stay in England.

Non-smoker, drinks alcohol rarely (less than 1 unit per week), does not exercise but usually helps out in his son's shop, which involves lifting boxes.

Review of systems

General: unintentional weight loss in last few months, approximately 3.18 kg (7 lbs), but pleased about this because advised he needed to lose weight when he was diagnosed with diabetes.

Skin: no rashes, no skin changes.

Neck: no lumps or swollen glands.

Respiratory: never had a chest radiograph, no wheezing, no recent infection, cough noted with productive sputum, haemoptysis one today, none previously, has noticed SOB on exertion in last 2 days, relieved by rest. No dyspnoea at rest.

Cardiovascular: no known heart disease, BP normal when last checked approximately 2 months ago, no palpitations, no orthopnoea. Intermittent, dull chest pain for last week on right side of anterior chest, no radiation of pain, no aggravating or relieving factors.

Gastrointestinal: poor appetite in last few weeks, has been trying to lose weight since diagnosed with diabetes, avoids sugar and high carbohydrate foods. No nausea/vomiting or indigestion symptoms. Opens bowels daily, no constipation, diarrhoea or rectal bleeding. No abdominal pain, no jaundice.

Urinary: no frequency, dysuria or nocturia.

Musculoskeletal: no joint pain but muscles feel 'weak'.

Neurological: recently bereaved but feels he is coping, denies low mood. No fainting, seizures or memory loss. No sensation loss.

Endocrine: diet-controlled diabetes mellitus, no thyroid problems.

Physical examination

Mr N is fully mobile and is not experiencing acute chest pain or SOB. He is alert and orientated. He looks tired and his clothes look loose suggesting recent weight loss.

Vital signs

Height 1.7 m, weight 87 kg.

BP 142/88 mmHg, pulse 92 regular, respiratory rate 22, temperature 38.6°C, oxygen saturation 98% on air.

Respiratory

Symmetrical chest, dull percussion note and crackles heard in apex of right lung, resonant percussion note and vesicular breath sounds heard over rest of lung fields. No pleural rub. No cervical lymphadenopathy.

Cardiovascular

JVP 2 cm, S1 and S2, no adventitious sounds. No bruits, no ankle or sacral oedema.

Impression: ? TB, ? pneumonia.

Plan: for chest radiograph, sputum for M,C&S ×3, bloods (FBC, ESR, CRP, U+Es, LFTs, RBS, HbAIC).

Refer to respiratory physician

Mark Jenning
Nurse practitioner

11.15 am

Patient developed a sudden onset of SOB at rest and worsening sharp chest pain located in upper right chest. Patient distressed, fully conscious. Respiratory rate 30, pulse 110, oxygen saturation 91% on air. On respiratory exam, trachea deviated to left, hyper-resonant percussion note and absent breath sounds in right upper chest.

Patient reassured and moved into a resuscitation bay, high flow oxygen 100% administered via a non-rebreathing mask, refer to casualty officer and for urgent chest radiograph.

Pneumothorax in apex of right lung seen on chest radiograph, for chest drain insertion.

> *Mark Jenning*
> *Nurse practitioner*
>
> 12.15 pm
>
> Patient stable, intercostals chest drain inserted without difficulty or further trauma, patient remains on high flow oxygen, analgesia given.
> BP 145/88 mmHg, pulse 96 regular, respiratory rate 22, temperature 38.6°C, oxygen saturation 97%.
> Diagnosis – pneumothorax secondary to probable erosion of TB lesion
> No suspicion of multidrug resistant TB in this patient so patient does not need to be transferred to a negative pressure room at this point (NICE 2006), refer to TB specialist nurse. Discussion with Mr N and his son regarding the possible diagnosis of TB. Explained that all family members will need screening for TB and possibly vaccination or treatment. In addition, advice will need to be sought on whether contact tracing of customers who were served in the shop or co-workers will be needed. The immediate care plan was explained, including admission to hospital to manage the pneumothorax and the subsequent drug treatment regime. The importance of concordance with the treatment regime was emphasized.
>
> *Mark Jenning*
> *Nurse practitioner*

Scenario 5.4 enables you to demonstrate the competencies within Domain 3 described below.

Recognizes environmental health problems affecting patients and provides health protection interventions that promote healthy environments for individuals, families and communities

Consideration of the potential impact of environmental factors (Mr N's cramped home circumstances) is demonstrated in this scenario. In addition, referral to the TB specialist nurse will ensure that relevant health protection interventions are addressed for this family and potentially for the local community. In order to fully meet this competency you would need to provide further evidence of your role in providing health protection interventions for individuals, families and communities (i.e. other than via referral to another practitioner).

Analyses and interprets history, presenting symptoms, physical findings, and diagnostic information to develop the appropriate differential diagnoses

A comprehensive history and physical examination has been documented and two differential diagnoses identified for this patient. So whilst it is clear that the history and physical examination findings have been obtained and interpreted, the information has not been analysed and so clinical decision-making is not explicit. In addition, the range of differential diagnoses is limited (more could have been considered but there is no evidence of this documented). This evidence could be supplemented by a critical reflection of the clinical reasoning process.

Diagnoses and manages acute and long-term conditions while attending to the patient's response to the illness experience

This competency has been met with respect to diagnosing and managing an acute condition (chest pain and dyspnoea) while attending to the patient's response to the illness experience (recognition of the patient's distress and provision of support and reassurance). This would need to be repeated with a patient who has a long-term condition in order to meet this competency fully.

Prioritizes health problems and intervenes appropriately, including initiation of effective emergency care

Evidence has been presented to demonstrate prioritization of a health problem (deterioration in the patient's breathing) and appropriate intervention by providing effective emergency care (commencing oxygen therapy, transfer to resuscitation bay for close monitoring) so this competency has been fully met.

Formulates an action plan based on scientific rationale, evidence-based standards of care, and practice guidelines

Within this case study a plan of care making explicit reference to NICE guidance on diagnosis and management of TB has been outlined, demonstrating that practice has been informed by scientific rationale and evidence-based standards of care.

Provides guidance, counselling, advice and support regarding management of the health/illness condition

The final entry in the patient's notes details how both the patient and his son have been supported by providing advice and guidance on the diagnosis and immediate management plan. Evidence would need to be provided to illustrate how counselling has been provided to the patient in order to meet fully this competency. Patient feedback would be a useful form of evidence here.

Initiates appropriate and timely consultation and/or referral when the problem exceeds the nurse's scope of practice and/or expertise

The referral to the casualty officer on clinical deterioration of the patient's condition demonstrates appropriate and timely consultation/referral. This, in addition to referral to the TB specialist nurse, conveys clearly the boundaries with regard to your professional knowledge and expertise.

Plans and implements diagnostic strategies and therapeutic interventions to help patients with unstable and complex health care problems regain stability and restore health, in collaboration with the patient and multiprofessional health care team

The request for sputum sample examination and chest radiograph (routine and urgent) demonstrate an ability to plan and implement relevant diagnostic interventions for a patient with a complex and unstable health care problem. Initiation of emergency care (commencing oxygen therapy, moving to the resuscitation bay for closer observation) and prompt referral to other multi-professional team members (casualty officer, TB specialist nurse) demonstrates effective planning and implementation of therapeutic interventions that restore stability but not full health, for this patient. You need to make explicit how you worked in collaboration with both the patient and the multiprofessional team in order to meet fully this competency.

Rapidly and continuously evaluates the patient's changing condition and response to therapeutic interventions and modifies the plan of care for optimal patient outcome

Within this case study there is evidence of a rapid response (initiation of oxygen therapy, removal to resuscitation bay) and continuous evaluation (regular review of patient) of the patient's changing condition, and appropriate changes to the care plan have been documented.

Obtains a comprehensive problem-focused health history from the patient or carer

This has been fully evidenced within this case study.

Performs a comprehensive problem-focused, age-appropriate physical examination

This scenario contains a comprehensive problem-focused physical examination. You would need to illustrate how it was age-appropriate or choose another example to illustrate effectively this aspect of the competency. Please note that you would need to provide evidence of formal assessment of physical examination techniques (i.e. via an OSCE/OSCA or a colleague testimonial) in order to demonstrate competence in physical examination skills.

Analyses the data collected to determine health status of the patient

This is implicit within the case study. It would be helpful to provide a reflective commentary on your clinical reasoning with regard to the differential diagnoses which would enable you to demonstrate explicit analysis of the data and how it informed your reasoning.

Assesses, diagnoses, monitors, coordinates and manages the health/illness status of patients during acute and enduring episodes

Assessment (history and physical examination), diagnosis, monitoring (observation of patient's deterioration) and management (action taken on patient's deterioration) of a patient during an acute episode of ill health has been demonstrated. You would need to do the same for a patient with an enduring episode of ill health in order to meet fully this competency.

Communicates the patient's health status using appropriate terminology, format and technology

This competency has been fully met by the case study. In order to demonstrate breadth in this competency it would be helpful to provide evidence on how you have done this via other media, for example electronically, verbally.

Uses community/public health assessment information in evaluating patient needs, initiating referrals, coordinating care and programme planning

The reference to TB guidelines to inform your clinical decision-making provides evidence of how public health assessment information has been utilized to make an appropriate referral. In order to meet fully this competency evidence in relation to evaluating patient needs, coordinating care and programme planning is required.

Applies principles of evidence-based practice pertinent to their area of practice

This competency has been fully met (use of NICE guidance).

Provides information and advice to patients and carers concerning drug regimens, side-effects and interaction, in an appropriate form

Provision of information about the drug treatment regime to both the patient and his son has been illustrated; however, the exact regimen or discussion of side-effects and interactions have not been detailed. This would need to be evidenced – as would provision of information in another format, for example use of a leaflet or website.

Orders, may perform, and interprets common screening and diagnostic tests

Within this case study diagnostic tests (chest radiograph, sputum and blood tests) have been ordered but have not been interpreted. Evidence of interpretation of these tests, as well as ordering and interpreting common screening tests is needed in order to meet this competency fully.

Evaluates results of interventions using accepted outcome criteria, revises the plan accordingly, and consults/refers when needed

This competency could have been met by evaluating the intervention of providing oxygen therapy to the patient in response to his dropping oxygen saturation rate. This would best be achieved by a short reflective account, making reference to guidance on management of a patient showing deteriorating oxygen saturation and clarifying the decision to commence oxygen therapy, as well as outlining when this therapy would be discontinued, and when, and to whom, referral would be made if the patient continued to deteriorate.

CONCLUSION

Domain 3 of the NMC Standards of Proficiency for ANPs (NMC 2005) is concerned with the work of ANPs relating to direct patient care. Therefore, the evidence likely to be used by practitioners to demonstrate achievement of the competencies will be specific to the clinical area for the individual nurse and derived from clinical practice. This chapter has shown how a range of clinical practice data can be applied to the competencies in order to evidence the ANP role within this domain.

REFERENCES

Barrett, B.P. Brown, R.L. Locken, K. Maberry, R. Bobula, J.A. and D'Alessio, D. (2002) Treatment of the common cold with unrefined echinacea: a randomized, double-blind, placebo-controlled trial. *Annals of Internal Medicine* 137(12): 939–946.

Becker, M.H. (ed.) (1984) *The health belief model and personal behaviour.* Thorofare, NJ: Charles B. Sack.

British Medical Association and Royal Pharmaceutical Society of Great Britain (2007) *BNF 53.* London: British Medical Association and Royal Pharmaceutical Society of Great Britain.

Bryant-Lukosius, D. DiCenso, A. Browne, G. and Pinelli, J. (2004) Advanced practice nursing roles: development, implementation and evaluation. *Nursing and Health Care Management and Policy* 48(5): 519–529.

Butler, C.C. Rollnick, S. Pill, R. Maggs-Rapport, F. and Stott, N. (1998) Understanding the culture of prescribing: qualitative study of general practitioners' and patients' perceptions of antibiotics for sore throats. *British Medical Journal* 317: 637–642.

Byrne, P.S. and Long, B.E.Z. (1976) *Doctors talking with patients.* London: HMSO.

Cabrera, M. and Groer, M. (2001) Gastrointestinal and hepatic disorders. In *Advanced pathophysiology: application to clinical practice,* Groer, M. (ed.), pp. 308–329. Philadelphia: Lippincott.

Clarke, C. (1999) The respiratory system. In *Nurse practitioners: clinical skills and professional issues,* Walsh, M. Crumbie, A. and Reveley, S. (eds), pp. 105–121. Oxford: Butterworth-Heinemann.

Crumbie, A. (1999a) Assessment and management of the patient with chronic health problems. In *Nurse practitioners: clinical skills and professional issues,* Walsh, M. Crumbie, A. and Reveley, S. (eds), pp. 227–238. Oxford: Butterworth-Heinemann.

Crumbie, A. (1999b) The abdomen. In *Nurse practitioners: clinical skills and professional issues,* Walsh, M. Crumbie, A. and Reveley, S. (eds), pp. 122–137. Oxford: Butterworth-Heinemann.

Daly, W.M. and Carnwell, R. (2003) Nursing roles and levels of practice: a framework for differentiating between elementary, specialist and advancing nursing practice. *Journal of Clinical Nursing* 12: 158–167.

Davidhizar, R., Eshlerman, J. and Moody, M. (2002) Health promotion for ageing adults *Geriatric Nursing* 23(1) 29–35.

Del Mar ,C.B. Glasziou, P.P. and Spinks, A.B. (2007) *Antibiotics for sore throats.* Cochrane database systematic review 3 (CD000023).

Department of Health (1989) *Report of the advisory group on nurse prescribing,* 1st Crown Report. London: HMSO.

Department of Health (1999a) *Review of the prescribing, supply and administration of medicines*, 2nd Crown Report. London: The Stationery Office.

Department of Health (1999b) *Making a difference: strengthening the nursing, midwifery and health visiting contribution to health and healthcare.* London: The Stationery Office.

Department of Health (1999c) *Smoking kills: a white paper on tobacco.* London: The Stationery Office.

Department of Health (1999d) *Saving lives.* London: The Stationery Office.

Department of Health (2000a) *The NHS plan: a plan for investment, a plan for reform.* London: The Stationery Office.

Department of Health (2000b) *National service framework for coronary heart.* London: The Stationery Office.

Department of Health (2001) *National service framework for older people* The Stationery Office: London.

Department of Health (2004) *Choosing Health: making healthy choices easier.* London: The Stationery Office.

Department of Health (2006a) *Modernising nursing careers: setting the direction.* London: The Stationery Office.

Department of Health (2006b) *Medicines matters.* London: The Stationery Office.

Department of Health and Social Security (DHSS) (1986) *Neighbourhood nursing – a focus for care* (Cumberlege Report). London: HMSO.

Downie, G. Mackenzie, J. and Williams, A. (2003) *Pharmacology and medicines management for nurses* Edinburgh: Churchill Livingstone.

Drug and Therapeutics Bulletin (1995) Diagnosis and treatment of streptococcal sore throat. *Drug and Therapeutics Bulletin* 33: 9–12.

Drug and Therapeutics Bulletin (2007) Avoiding antibacterial over-use in primary care. *Drug and Therapeutics Bulletin* 45: 25–28.

Fugh-Berman, A. (2003) Echinacea for the prevention and treatment of upper respiratory infections. *Seminars in Integrative Medicine* 1(2): 106–111.

Heron, J. (2001) *Helping the client: a creative practical guide,* 5th edn. London: Sage.

Horrocks, S. Anderson, E. and Salisbury, C. (2002) Systematic review of whether nurse practitioners working in primary care can provide equivalent care to doctors. *British Medical Journal* 324(7341): 819–823.

Lindbaek, M. Francis, N. Canings-John, R. Butler, C.C. and Hjortdahl, P. (2006) Clinical course of suspected viral sore throat in young adults: cohort study. *Scandinavian Journal of Primary Health Care* 24(2): 93–97.

Little, P. and Williamson, I. (1996) Sore throat management in general practice. *Family Practice* 13: 317–321.

Little, P. Williamson, I. Warner, G. Gould, C. Gantley, M. and Kinmonth, A.L. (1997) Open randomised trial of prescribing strategies in managing sore throat. *British Medical Journal* 314: 722–727.

Manchester, Salford and Trafford Health Promotion Department (2002) *Smoking cessation guidelines.* Manchester: Manchester, Salford and Trafford Health Promotion Department.

Mantzoukas, S. and Watkinson, S. (2006) Review of advanced nursing practice: the international literature and developing the generic features. *Journal of Clinical Nursing* 16: 28–37.

McFarlane, J. Holmes, W. Gard, P. Thornhill, D. McFarlane, R. and Hubbard, R. (2002) Reducing antibiotic use for acute bronchitis in primary care: blinded, randomised controlled trial of patient information leaflet. *British Medical Journal* 324(7329): 91–94.

McRobbie, H. and Hajek, P. (2000) *Nicotine replacement therapy in patients with cardiovascular disease*. London: Royal London Hospital.

Medicines Control Agency (2002) *Safety of Herbal Medicinal Products*. London: Department of Health.

MeReC (1999) Managing sore throats. *MeReC Bulletin* 10: 41–44.

Murray, R.P. Bailey, W.C. Daniels, K. and Bjornson, W.M. (1996) Safety of nicotine polacrilex gum used by 3,094 participants in the Lung Health Study. *Chest* 109: 438–445.

National Institute for Clinical Excellence (2001) Recurrent episodes of acute sore throat in children aged up to 15 years. In *Referral advice: a guide to appropriate referral from general to specialist services*. London: National Institute for Clinical Excellence.

National Institute for Health and Clinical Excellent (NIHCE) (2006) *Tuberculosis: clinical diagnosis and management of tuberculosis, and measures for its prevention and control.* London: NICE.

Neighbour, R. (2004) *The inner consultation: how to develop an effective and intuitive consulting style*. Abingdon: Radcliffe.

NHS Management Executive (NHSME) (1991) *Junior doctors: the new deal.* London: NHSME.

NHS Management Executive (1999) *Working together: securing a quality workforce for the NHS.* Health Service Circular 79.

Nursing and Midwifery Council (2004) *The NMC code of professional practice: standards for conduct, performance and ethics*. London: Nursing and Midwifery Council.

Nursing and Midwifery Council (2005) *The proposed framework for the standard for post-registration nursing*. online http://www.nmc-uk.org/aArticle.aspx?ArticleID=82 (accessed on 01/09/07).

Nursing and Midwifery Council (2008) *The code. Standards of conduct, performance and ethics for nurses and midwives*. London: Nursing and Midwifery Council.

Pendleton, D. Schofield, T. Tate, P. and Havelock, P. (2003) *The new consultation: developing doctor–patient communication*. Oxford: Oxford University Press.

Public Health Laboratory Service (PHLS) (2000) *Management of infection guidance for primary care: draft for consultation and local adaptation*. London: Department of Health.

Resnick, B. (1991) Geriatric motivation: clinically helping the elderly to comply. *Journal of Gerontological Nursing* 17(5): 17–21.

Rigotti, N. (2005) *Smoking cessation*. In *Primary care medicine*, 5th edn, Goroll, A.H. and Mulley, A.G. (eds), pp. 405–512. Philadelphia: JB Lippincott.

Royal College of Nursing (2005) *Maxi nurses: advanced and specialist nursing roles*. London: Royal College of Nursing.

Rycroft-Malone, J. (2002) *Clinical guidelines*. In *Clinical decision making and judgement in nursing*, Thompson, C. and Dowding, D. (eds), pp. 147–164. London: Churchill-Livingstone.

Scottish Intercollegiate Guidelines Network (1999) *Management of sore throat and indications for tonsillectomy: a national clinical guideline*. Edinburgh: Scottish Intercollegiate Guidelines Network.

Seedhouse, D. (1998) *Ethics: the heart of health care*. Chichester: John Wiley and Sons.

Sherwood, A. (1995) Kicking the habit of a lifetime. *Care of the Elderly* 7(1): 28–29.

Silverman, J. Kurtz, S. and Draper, J. (2005) *Skills for communicating with patients*, 2nd edn. Oxford: Radcliffe Publishing.

Standing Medical Advisory Committee (1999) *The path of least resistance*. London: Department of Health.

Tobacco Advisory Group of the Royal College of Physicians (2000) *Nicotine addiction in Britain*. Royal College of Physicians: London http://www.rcplondon.ac.uk/pubs/books/nicotine/contributors.htm (accessed on 01/09/07).

United Kingdom Central Council for Nursing, Midwifery and Health Visiting (1999) *A higher level of practice.* London: United Kingdom Central Council for Nursing, Midwifery and Health Visiting.

United Kingdom Central Council for Nursing, Midwifery and Health Visiting (1992) *Scope of professional practice.* London: United Kingdom Central Council for Nursing, Midwifery and Health Visiting.

Venning, P. Durie, A. Roland, M. Roberts, C. and Leese, B. (2000) Randomised controlled trial comparing cost effectiveness of general practitioners and nurse practitioners in primary care. *British Medical Journal* 320: 1048–1052.

West, R. McNeill, A, and Raw, M, (2000) Smoking cessation guidelines for health professionals: an update. *Thorax* 55: 987–999.

6

DOMAIN 4: THE EDUCATION FUNCTION

FIONA SMART

INTRODUCTION

This chapter examines the role of the advanced nurse practitioner (ANP) within the domains of practice identified by the Royal College of Nursing (2002) as the teaching and coaching function. (Note that this is referred to by the NMC as the education function.) It approaches the analysis against the backdrop of three policy documents: *The expert patient: a new approach to chronic disease management for the 21st century* (DoH 2001), *Choosing health: making healthy choices easier* (DoH 2004) and *Our health, our care, our say* (DoH 2006). It draws into the frame the experiences of ANP students as they work with patients, clients and carers, with the intention of enabling health and managing illness. It uses examples from a range of everyday practice settings to illustrate the inherent challenges of the teaching and coaching function of the ANP, at the same time as recognizing its significance if patients, clients and carers are to be enabled to make choices that might optimize their well-being. Before this, however, some statistics are presented to focus thinking on why education is an invaluable component of advanced nursing practice.

THE HEALTH OF THE POPULATION

As the DoH (2006b) acknowledges, we are faced with a number of challenges that need to be accounted for and worked with if nursing is to be responsive in its role. Although society is increasingly complex in respect of its social, cultural and ethnic composition, health inequalities persist, a fact evidenced in the statistic which notes that infant mortality rates vary from 1.6 per 1000 live births in Eastleigh, Hampshire to 9.8 per 1000 live births in Birmingham. The consequence of disadvantage cannot be underestimated, not least its potential to create a sense of disengagement which risks damage both to the individual and to society as a whole. Alongside the reality and impact of health inequalities within some sections of society, expectations of health care and its providers continue to rise, as evidenced by the determination of individuals to be treated as partners and equals while they engage with the different elements of the service, and to have choices and options made available to them.

If health and its protection is the priority of some members of society, it is also the case that 15 million individuals live with long-term conditions which either do, or will, limit and shape their lives. This equates to approximately 25% of the population, a proportion of society which clearly cannot afford to be ignored. Embedded within this statistic are others; for example, obesity rates have doubled over the last 10 years. If the trend continues, it is estimated that by 2010, 1 in 4 individuals will be clinically obese, and, as a consequence, will be at an increased risk of cardiovascular disease, notably strokes and heart attacks, and the onset of type 2 diabetes. Smoking is still the single greatest cause of illness and premature death in the UK, killing at least 86 500 people a year and accounting for a third of all cancers and a seventh of all instances of cardiovascular disease. Its significance as a problem to society has been targeted via the smoking bans in public places across the UK. Yet without understanding smoking as a behaviour and its addictive components, health care providers cannot hope to work positively with individuals who smoke and who at this point in time may, or may not, wish to stop (Rollnick et al. 1999).

In this context it is noted that health care spending continues to increase. Figures from the Department of Health record that the NHS budget has doubled since the Labour party took office in 1997. Predictions estimate that it will have trebled by 2008 when it reaches £93.6 billion. Intentions to modernize the way in which monies are spent is evidenced by the plethora of National Service Frameworks (NSFs) issued since the Labour Government took up office in 1997. Although NSFs centre attention on specific groups or health problems, for example, the older person and diabetes mellitus, collectively they can be seen as frameworks with the potential to drive policy forwards.

PERSPECTIVES FROM POLICY

The expert patient: a new approach to chronic disease management for the 21st century

The premise upon which the expert patient policy rests is the acknowledgement that an individual living with a chronic disease commonly understands his or her illness better than the health care providers responsible for its management (DoH 2001). As a result, individuals with chronic diseases cannot simply be the passive recipients of care but, instead, can and should be key players in the decision-making that is central to the maintenance of their well-being and the moderation of the impact of the disease on their life:

> … by ensuring that knowledge of their condition is developed to a point where they are empowered to take some responsibility for its management and work in partnership with their health and social care providers, patients can be given greater control over their lives.
>
> DoH (2001)

Clearly the view is that if chronic disease, earlier acknowledged as impacting directly on the lives of 25% of the population, is to be better managed, then the knowledge-base of individuals living with long-term conditions needs to be enabled so that they can take control of the diseases affecting their lives. However, two points provoke reflection. First, there is the assumption that all individuals with a chronic disease want to assume the role of expert patient in the way the policy describes. Secondly, there is the issue of 'control-surrender' on the part of health care providers to the patient, an exchange of power which may not be as easy to make happen as the above quotation suggests. Thinking both points through it seems important to remember that in seeking to drive forward the intentions of the expert patient agenda, patient choice should not be ignored. In the event that this is the direction that patients want to travel, it is suggested that concurrent with the need for health care providers to fashion opportunities for patients to learn about their illness, it will be necessary to create the space for the emergence of a new relationship between the two parties.

The government has added further detail to its vision of the expert patient via its long-term conditions model (DoH 2005). Underpinned by a determination to secure effective joint working of all providers operating in health and social care settings, the model identifies three categories of patients (Figure 6.1).

Despite the argument that it is important to enable all individuals living with a long-term condition to acquire knowledge and understanding, the model depicted in Figure 6.1 suggests that efforts need to be targeted at the 70–80% of individuals at Level 1 so that disease progression either in terms of its complexity or co-morbidity might be delayed.

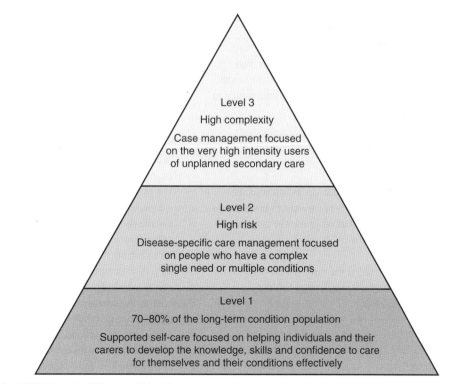

FIGURE 6.1 *The NHS and social care long term.*

One particular strategy is in place to facilitate the government's vision: the Expert Patient Programme. Described as a 'lay-led self-management programme', it seeks to support people so that their confidence is increased, their quality of life improved and their condition better managed (DoH 2006). Made available through primary care trusts and partner organizations, data generated from an evaluation of its impact on 1000 participants who completed the programme between January 2003 and January 2005 indicate its effectiveness in improving health outcomes for patients and provide evidence of a reduction in the extent to which they used health care services (DoH 2007).

Choosing health: making healthy choices easier

Described as a new approach to the health of the public that is 'more down to earth' and practical in its orientation *Choosing health* seeks to support people in making better choices for their health and the health of their families. Its perspective is wide-ranging, paying attention to key themes and areas of activity, including health inequalities, consumerism, community-based action, health at work and a health-promoting NHS. It is underpinned by three core principles (Table 6.1) and a number of priorities identified as reducing the numbers of people who smoke; reducing obesity and improving diet and nutrition; increasing exercise; encouraging and supporting sensible drinking; improving sexual health and improving mental health.

TABLE 6.1 *The principles underpinning* Choosing health

The principle	A footnote to the principle
Informed choice	Qualification of the principle
Recognizes that people want to make their own decisions about choices impacting on their health and to have credible and trustworthy information to help them do so	Noted that society needs to exercise a special responsibility for children who are too young to make their own informed choices Noted that special arrangements need to be in place where one person's choice causes nuisance or harm to another individual, e.g. second-hand smoke
Personalization	The intention
Recognizes that deprived groups and communities are not always in receipt of services that meet their needs. Understands that services may be available, but difficult to access	The provision of support tailored to the realities of individual lives, with services and support sensitively personalized and provided flexibly and conveniently
Working together	The expectation
Recognizes that neither the government nor individuals can make progress on healthy choices in isolation	The public looks to the government to lead, coordinate and promote partnerships across communities including local government, the NHS, business, retailers, the voluntary sector, the media and faith organizations. The public looks to individuals to take their health seriously, and that of their families, and expects constructive engagement in the process of health protection

An analysis of the substance of *Choosing health* highlights the importance of the role of the nurse, whether working with individuals, groups or in communities in comparative isolation or operating collaboratively with other agencies and providers. Thinking particularly, but not exclusively, about the role of the ANP and its potential to create a climate for positive change, *Choosing health* notes the need to build a 'comprehensive and integrated prevention framework' that maximizes the opportunities afforded by the 'millions of encounters that the NHS has with people every week' (DoH 2004). In so doing, it acknowledges the importance of embedding the opportunities for health improvement in everyday work with patients. In other words, the policy is arguing that health improvement is not something separate that only some health care providers engage with, rather it is everyone's business. Thinking then about the role of the ANP whose work commonly centres on gathering information from patients, clients and carers in a range of settings, *Choosing health* would invite every conversation to be inclusive in its focus, rather than exclusively centred on the presenting problem. Clearly there are implications for practitioners, not least the need for them to be prepared to open up discussions in ways that value the priorities of the patient and which appreciate the limitations of the health care provider's knowledge base. At this point, readers are invited to reflect on how the incorporation of the ideals and intentions of the policy into their everyday practice might work to challenge health inequalities and to facilitate what can be a difficult decision for some patients, i.e. to choose health.

Our health, our care, our say: a new direction for community services

Our health, our care, our say (DoH 2006)sets out a vision which looks to provide people with good-quality social care and NHS services in the communities where they live. As such, its goals can be seen to be consistent with the Labour government's 10-year plan to promote health, to be more responsive and to facilitate independence, choice and control across the field of health and social care provision.

Although debatable, it is possible to argue that the outcome focus of the goals as presented in Table 6.2 sets outline targets that can be used to create opportunities for health and social care providers to progress the government's agenda and to challenge current systems and processes which disable the policy's vision.

Although the ease with which at least some of the anticipated outcomes can be readily audited is an issue, a review of the policy's success over a 9-month period suggests that positive change is under way. For example, the NHS Life Check is being piloted as a two-part service: a self-assessment followed by personalized advice and support for those shown to be at risk. It aims to help people to assess the risk of ill-health created by their own lifestyles (DoH 2006). Of course, the initiative depends on a number of factors, not least its ability to reach the people most in need of teaching/coaching to facilitate their health and well-being. This said, by focusing on three key life stages – the first year of life, adolescence and mid-life (age 50–60 years), NHS Life Checks can be understood as targeting three specific groups: parents, who can create a positive environment in the home which supports the health and well-being of children; young people, who are widely recognized to be among the most healthy members of society, but may be at risk of harm by virtue of self-selected lifestyle choices; and individuals at mid-life, who could maximize their well-being and reduce unnecessary risks to their health.

TABLE 6.2 *The goals and anticipated outcomes of* Our health, our care, our say

The goals	Anticipated outcomes
Better prevention and early intervention for improved health, independence and well-being	Reduction in the prevalence of damaging underlying determinants of health, e.g. smoking and obesity and associated service usage Reduction in the number of people out of work or unable to work due to ill health or dependency Shift in resources and in planning emphasis to prevention and early intervention, supported by robust cost–benefit analysis Increased self-care and condition management among service-users
More choice and a stronger voice for individuals and communities	Service users and carers have more say over where, how and by whom their support is delivered and better access to information that informs their choices. Individuals and communities are able to influence the shape and delivery of local services and to trigger action to look at problems Service-users are more satisfied with their overall experience of care
Tackling inequalities and improving access to services	More services provided in the community Improved range of services for urgent care Streamlined GP registration and appointments processes to improve access and convenience Partnership working across health and social care communities to understand and address inequalities
More support for people with long-term needs	Service-users with long-term needs and their carers receive supportive services that respond to their preferences and choices, in a location convenient to them More support for self-care including increased participation and take-up of the expert patient/carer programme Ongoing reduction in avoidable hospital admissions Better coordination of health and social care services to meet the needs and wishes of individuals with long-term needs

THE DEVELOPING ROLES AND FUNCTIONS OF THE NURSE

The recent move towards to enhancing the health of the nation and minimizing the impact of illness has been evidenced in the host of consultation documents and White Papers produced since 1997. Expectations of nursing are also clear. Although differently expressed and variously focused, all of the government's policies and papers that centre on the reform of health care look, in some way, for nurses to drive forward change; witness, for example, *Liberating the talents* (DoH 2002). However, it is worth noting that the development of nursing pre-dates the late 1990s. Particularly significant to its evolution and the resultant diversification of the traditional role of the nurse was the United Kingdom Central Council's (UKCC) (1992) *Scope of professional practice*, which sanctioned the expansion of the individual nurse's role as defined by his/her own analysis of the boundaries to their competence.

Perhaps unsurprisingly, the UKCC's (1992) decision to place responsibility for the decision to undertake an aspect of practice, or indeed not, with the individual nurse did attract controversy. Not least among the questions that it invited was the possibility that practitioners may not be the best judges of the boundaries to their own professional competence. It was a concern that focused attention on the unconsciously incompetent and the potential for the safety of the patient to be compromised. Even so, *Scope* provided a framework for a new way of working for all nurses, and as a consequence breathed life into an emergent area of practice that was already challenging traditional roles. This area of practice was the role of nurse practitioner.

Analysis of the role of ANP and its functions helps to explain the negativity with which it is sometimes, but not always, associated (Horrocks et al. 2002, Wilson and Bunnell 2007). The fact that its area of work butts up to and extends over the boundary of medical practice was always going to be both an enabler and a constraint to its ongoing development and acceptance by fellow nurses, medical practitioners and allied health professionals. As noted by Beattie (1995), territorial protectionism of roles and responsibilities is a feature of the health care system.

Although the role of the ANP, as it is currently described by the Royal College of Nursing (2005), continues to attract debate and divide opinion, some of its elements are less contentious, for example the aspects of practice captured within the education domain. Unlike, for example, the skill set that centres on health assessment, diagnostic reasoning and clinical decision-making, there is an expectation that the work of any nurse will, in some way, involve the process of enabling learning. It is an expectation that finds form in the standards of proficiency for nursing which define the benchmark for the registrant at the point when they first are admitted to the professional register (Nursing and Midwifery Council 2004). Specifically, at this point in their career, initial registrants are required to demonstrate the ability to 'create and utilise opportunities to promote the health and well being of patients, clients and groups' (NMC 2004). As such, even novice registered nurses can be understood to be capable of contributing to the strategic vision set out in *The expert patient: a new approach to chronic disease management for the 21st century* (DoH 2001), *Choosing health: making healthy choices easier* (DoH 2004) and *Our health, our care, our say* (DoH 2006).

Expectations of the ANP build on those required of the initial registrant and find life in the standards set out by the Royal College of Nursing and adopted by the NMC (2005) with the intention of regulating the role (Appendix 1). However, careful consideration of the substance of the education domain invites comment. Conversations with nurses who have developed into a range of roles, notably, but not exclusively, that of the clinical nurse specialist, suggest that the expectations of the ANP in relation to education are not dissimilar to the work undertaken by nurses operating in other roles. Inevitably this raises the question whether this particular aspect of advanced nursing practice is any different for nurses working in different roles. In pursuing this argument there is a risk of seeking to argue that ANPs somehow 'do it better', but that is not the intention. Rather, the aim is to consider that perhaps, because of their role, ANPs may get to 'do it differently'. In order to pursue this possibility and to illustrate the scope of the domain, specific examples are drawn from information provided by ANP students. As the detail unfolds it will become apparent that the strength of the ANP role lies, in part, in its capacity to complement the work of fellow health care providers so that health opportunities can be maximized as envisaged by the government in its plans for the nation's health. However, first, in order to facilitate the analysis some theoretical perspectives are introduced.

PROMOTING HEALTH: MODELS AND THEORETICAL PERSPECTIVES

Whether the individual is fit and well or living with a long-term condition that already is, or will in time shape their lives, the intention to promote health can be argued to be an appropriate goal because it maximizes health opportunities. However, different approaches to the promotion of health are available for use. Situated within the options that are available to practitioners are subtleties which centre on the explicitness, or not, of the approach as it concerns the intention to influence, and perhaps even change the patient's, client's or carer's behaviour. Rather than seeing these differences in approach negatively, or perceiving some to be better than others, it may be the case that the most effective practitioner is the one who can alter their approach dependent on the person/people and the accompanying contextual factors which need to be taken into account. Although this may be so, it is the case that nurses generally and ANPs specifically tend to have preferred ways of working in their teaching and coaching roles.

Reviewing the literature, it is clear that the contrast between the different models and theoretical perspectives available for use reflects something more than a variance in the words used to describe an approach. For example, the knowledge, attitude, behaviour (KAB) model appears soft in its stance, in that it appears to rely on the potential of information to transform behaviour. In effect, the message is that an increase in knowledge will facilitate attitudinal and then behavioural change. It is a premise that appears naïve and invites criticism because of an evidence base which makes it clear that knowledge of itself, although necessary to the promotion of health, is insufficient. In other words, factors other than knowledge are powerful in their potential to influence attitudes and behaviours.

In contrast, Becker's (1974) health belief model operates with a premise which maintains that behavioural change depends on a cost–benefit analysis undertaken by the individual whose health might be promoted. It recognizes that for behavioural change to take place, the individual must:

- have an incentive to change;
- feel threatened by their current behaviour;
- feel a change would be beneficial with few adverse consequences;
- feel competent to carry out the change.

Different again is Ajzen's (1991) theory of planned change, which suggests the need to consider three particular variables if behaviour is to be understood, influenced and altered:

- *Attitudes*: because they present as the outward manifestation of beliefs focused on the consequences of behaviour and the ensuing appraisal of potential positive and negative outcomes.
- *Subjective norms*: because they connect to ideas about what 'significant others' do and expect and to the degree to which the individual wants to conform to prevailing norms.
- *Perceptions of control*: because of the recognition that behavioural change will depend on the extent to which the individual perceives that they are in control of the situation as it relates to the health issue in focus.

Tones' (1995) Health Action Model offers a contrasting perspective because it emphasizes the influence of self-esteem on the behaviour of the individual and indicates that life skill education may be a prerequisite for change. It is an approach

TABLE 6.3 *Factors influencing behavioural change*

Importance Why?	Confidence How? What?	Readiness When?
Is it worthwhile?	Can I?	Should I do it now?
Why should I?	How will I do it?	What about other priorities?
How will I benefit?	How will I cope with x, y and z?	
What will change?	Will I succeed if ?	
At what cost?	What change ?	
Do I really want to?		
Will it make a difference?		

that contexualizes health choices within a range of environmental, social and psychological determinants and seeks empowerment for the individual by helping them to value themselves and to invest in the skills necessary to the change process.

Reflecting on the approaches presented, their similarities and differences, and the evidence which indicates that education, of itself, will not necessary influence behaviour, it seems important to consider factors that might make a difference to the individual with whom the ANP works. This thinking finds life in Rollnick et al.'s (1999) analysis of behavioural change. Specifically they argue that three factors could make a difference: the importance of the message to the individual, the confidence of the individual and readiness of the individual (Table 6.3). To elaborate their thinking, Rollnick et al. (1999: 21) suggest the kind of questions people might ask themselves or voice in their interactions with others about readiness, importance and confidence.

It seems that Rollnick et al.'s (1999) thinking offers an orientation to the person which accepts that health behaviour change can provoke a multitude of questions for the individual which might overlap and could well compete. What Rollnick et al. (1999) argue is that by recognizing the possibility that all, or some, or just one of these questions could be featuring in the individual's mind has the potential to open up a conversation which might enable change. Put another way, the failure to recognize that these questions, or others like them, might exist, risks closing down the opportunities for discussions that could help the individual to make decisions with the potential to support and enhance their health and well-being.

If it is important to promote the opportunity for conversations with the intention of promoting health, at the same time as bolstering the individual's confidence and supporting their readiness for behavioural change, Rollnick et al. (1999) urge practitioners to recognize the risk of resistance and to consider the impact of a lack of motivation. They go on to suggest that resistance, although not inevitable, can be a common factor in a health-focused conversation introduced either because of what the individual brings to the consulting room, or because of what the practitioner elicits. Sometimes they see that potentially negative outcomes are the outcomes of the interaction between the two individuals (Rollnick et al. 1999). Clearly the need to minimize resistance in individuals matters, as does the importance of avoiding traps likely to induce it. With a view to supporting practitioners committed to promoting health and well-being, Rollnick et al. (1999) isolate three traps and suggest three strategies to address them (Table 6.4).

If resistance suggests active disengagement with the process of behavioural change, a lack of motivation on the part of the individual suggests passivity. However, Rollnick et al. (1999) caution against simplistic thinking with regards to motivation,

TABLE 6.4 *Resistance: traps and strategies to avoid them*

Trap	What not to do	Strategy
Take control away	Ignore the resistance and proceed with advice-giving to tick the box	Leave control with the individual, respecting where they are at the moment and their right to choose
Misjudge importance, confidence or readiness	Assume that it doesn't matter how ready the individual is or what his/her feelings are about importance or confidence	Review where the individual is regarding the importance of the message, their confidence and readiness for change. Stay aligned with their reality
Meet force with force	Attack or defend	Back off and come alongside the individual

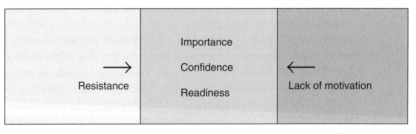

FIGURE 6.2 *Isolating key factors influencing health behaviour change using Rollnick et al. (1999).*

or rather the lack of it, and, in particular, advise practitioners not to fall into the belief that motivation will be enhanced if the individual can be helped to understand the importance of the health message. As such, it is a view that supports evidence arguing that knowledge is a necessary, but insufficient condition for behavioural change. Just because something is understood to be important, does not mean that individuals will alter what they do. As Rollnick et al. (1999) appreciate, the importance of the message, combines with the confidence of the individual to support their readiness for change and so boosts their motivation.

Taking Rollnick et al.'s (1999) ideas as a whole it is possible to present them diagrammatically in a way which illustrates how resistance and a lack of motivation can impact negatively on the individual's appreciation of importance of the message, their confidence and/or their readiness for change (Figure 6.2).

Rollnick et al.'s (1999) thinking, as it concerns health behaviour change, is as capable of critique as any other. This said, its overt patient-centredness is congruent with the aspirations of the role of the ANP (RCN 2002). Moreover, its recognition that conversations with patients can be one-off, time-limited exchanges, as well as developed over a period of time, suggests its flexibility. As such it has the potential to progress the intentions embedded in *The expert patient*, the potential of *Choosing health* and the hopes of *Our health, our care, our say*. As the chapter moves to introduce the reality of working within the education domain of practice using the lived accounts and reflections of ANP students, Rollnick et al.'s (1999) propositions will be drawn upon together with other models and theoretical perspectives. The material shared will serve to illustrate the challenges inherent within this area of practice and its potential. As the analysis unfolds, it will become evident that despite the expectation that all nurses have an education function, the enhanced knowledge and skill base of the ANP can be seen to create different opportunities for health promotion and health protection focused on the interests of individuals and communities.

INTRODUCING THE ANP STUDENTS

In total, eight ANP students agreed to provide reflections on their education function and examples to illustrate their practice. Names and any other details likely to risk a breach of confidentiality have been altered in order to protect the identity of the individual, their place of work and the patients/clients with whom they work.

- Isabel's background is in acute care, mainly in the environment of A&E. She is now in a developmental post in a primary care setting where she is employed by the local primary care trust.
- Gloria also works in the primary care setting, but with the armed forces. Although her patients are defined as being fit and well, maintaining their health and well-being in a culture which can invite risk through lifestyle choices is a factor that Gloria needs to account for.
- Kate is a lone worker in the community setting. A children's nurse by background, much of her work involves supporting parents so that they can manage the care of their children who are living with life-limiting illnesses.
- Ruby works in a district general hospital in a role bridging two environments: A&E and a surgical assessment unit (SAU). She openly acknowledges feeling more at home in the SAU.
- Beth also works in an acute setting, where her role is that of a critical care outreach sister. It is a role that involves facilitating discharge from critical care units to the wards, preventing the deterioration of patients on the wards and, where necessary, enabling the timely transfer of patients from the wards to the critical care areas.
- Wendy works in a minor injuries unit in an isolated setting within which access to services necessary to the management of serious health care problems is complicated by distance. It is also an environment within which the patients who attend frequently are well known.
- Jackie's role is new and centres on female street workers.
- And finally, there is Allison, who works in a primary care setting for two partners. The population she works with is by definition 'deprived' and unemployment is high.

REFLECTIONS ON THE EDUCATION FUNCTION OF THE ROLE

Different as individuals and varied in terms of the focus on their work, each of the students share something in common, namely their positive orientation to the education function of their roles. In a variety of ways they speak of the fact that it is intrinsic to their work. As Kate explains:

> teaching families nursing care procedures, enabling them to manage their child's health care needs within the home environment and to act as a specialist resource for health and social care workers is a key component of my role.

Isabel agrees, but, as she does so, considers the change in emphasis from an acute to primary care setting that she has experienced:

> In my previous role in A&E, health promotion was specifically related to the short-term goals of accident prevention and improving recovery. There was

not the emphasis placed on coaching and health promotion that there is in primary care and so this was a steep learning curve, particular in relation to the coaching that relates to long-term conditions.

Gloria's perspective on the importance of the education function of the role connects with her work with the armed forces, where, as she observes:

> The primary task of the Forces Medical Services is the preservation of the health of the troops; therefore, disease prevention, health promotion and health education must be part of the remit of every health care provider in the military.

If the students agree on the significance of this domain of practice, they also share a common understanding that effectiveness within its parameters depends on well-refined communication skills. As Beth puts it, without them 'teaching patients about their health and guiding them to understand their illness' becomes very difficult. She goes on to consider that the way in which the ANP communicates may be key in supporting motivation that will support lifestyle change. It is a point which connects back to Rollnick et al.'s (1999) thinking.

Interestingly, Allison's experience highlights the willingness of patients experiencing significant challenges to their health and well-being to listen to positive health messages, providing they are offered in a way which respects them as individuals. Ruby also subscribes to a belief in the significance of communication skills reflecting that they have the potential to:

> promote an alliance with the patient that creates a belief in themselves and their ability to handle situations effectively from their strengths and personal power.

Ruby continues, insisting that simply telling people what to do is not enough. Citing Benner (1984), she argues that ANPs need to become:

> experts in coaching patients through an illness so that … they take what is foreign and fearful to the patient and make it less frightening.

Importantly, she then adds a comment which suggests an understanding of what has changed for her since commencing her ANP studies:

> I feel my expanding clinical knowledge base, coupled with my increasing ability to perform an extensive physical examination and a comprehensive assessment at a more advanced level, is enabling me to provide more information which reflects my patients' needs.

Ruby's reflection on what has changed for her in her practice is important for another reason, because it begins the process of connecting together the different domains of the advanced practitioner role. Yes, communication skills matter, but that could be argued to be the case for all nurses. In this particular context with this particular role in focus, Ruby is indicating that the conversation with the patient alters because of the knowledge and skill base she has been enabled to develop.

PRACTICE, POLICY, THEORETICAL PERSPECTIVES AND ROLE DEVELOPMENT

The experiences of three student ANPs are used to clarify the education function in relation to the role of the ANP. The first connects with the strategic vision embodied in *The expert patient*, the second links to the aims of *Choosing health* and the third focuses on the intent of *Our health, our care, our say*. Each example is offered because of the dimension it offers and its potential to facilitate understanding of how the education function of the ANP can take shape. Readers are invited to consider what is shared and to reflect on which theoretical perspectives and models might have been influencing the practice of the three students. It may be that alternatives present which could be used to inform future practice.

The expert patient

Wendy offers the account of her work with Bob, described as a regular attendee in the Minor Injuries Unit, with whom she developed a positive working relationship. Bob first attended the unit in 2004 with a graze to his leg sustained in the garden 6 weeks previously. The graze had not healed and had deteriorated to such an extent that Bob attended the hospital to see his GP at the insistence of his wife. He was reviewed by his GP, commenced on a course of flucloxacillin and referred to the Wound Management Clinic (WMC). He was subsequently referred back to our department for a dressing change at the weekend because the WMC was closed.

> Bob was 72 years old when I first met him. He lived with his wife in a bungalow in the centre of town. He had two children, both of whom had left home. Bob had been retired from his profession in the local town for over 10 years and identified his hobbies as walking, cycling and meeting his friends once a week in their local pub.

> Bob was on medication for hypertension and had a medical history of osteoarthritis and a previous DVT in his left leg – the leg that had developed the ulcer. His GP had noted at the time that signs of venous hypertension had been observed bilaterally, with an oedematous left lower leg. The WMC had carried out a Doppler reading on his leg with an ABPI of 0.5; it was decided that the ulcer was arterial in origin and that he was unsuitable for any form of compression therapy. Investigations had been undertaken on his referral to WMC to eliminate any other contributing untreated medical condition such as diabetes mellitus.

> On initial examination the ulcer was very superficial in depth, measuring $10 \times 5 \times 0.3$ cm. Because of the good state of the ulcer when Bob first began visiting us for weekend dressings, staff believed that it would heal well. However, it soon became apparent that Bob's views were quite different from ours. The first inkling that we had of this was during one of the early dressings, when we were talking about the wound and I was asked how long it would take to heal. Knowing the complexity of wounds and the chance of it regressing, I mentioned that I thought that it would take some months for it to heal. I remember seeing the look of surprise on Bob's face. Observing this I asked him how long he thought it would take, and was surprised when he told me his time-frame was measured in weeks rather then months. I decided at this point to ascertain his knowledge of his ulcer.

> Bob believed that his wound was like any other and would heal quickly enough. At this early stage I didn't want to overburden him with information, especially as it was probable that we would see a lot of each

other. Information, therefore, was provided on what Bob wanted to know and what I thought was important with the intention of building on it. I pointed out that ulcers were unlike normal wounds and because of a number of factors were slower to heal than other wounds. Although at the time I thought that Bob had understood what I had told him, with hindsight I realized that he had not. Throughout the consultations, advice and suggestion were given on factors that can help/hinder healing, such as nutrition, age, medication, infection, smoking, chronic diseases such as diabetes, sleeping and psychosocial aspects (Russell 2000, Dealey 2005).

Kolb (1984 cited by Oliver and Endersby 1994) identified four types of learning competencies: feeling, perceiving, thinking and behaving. A person's life and past experiences will affect the way in which he learns, for Bob it was found that he preferred actively to seek and experiment, leading me to see him as an accommodator (Oliver and Endersby 1994).

Because of the nature of my shifts it was over a month later when I saw Bob again. I realized that he was having some problems with his wound. When he arrived for his dressing, Bob appeared less talkative then usual. On asking how he was and how he was getting on, he informed me that he was feeling a bit down. He'd had the ulcer for a number of months now and had seen no improvement; in fact, he thought that it was getting worse. He commented that it appeared slightly bigger and was producing more 'stuff'. He also confessed that it was beginning to bother him. When I asked him to elaborate on this, using listening skills that I had begun to learn, Bob told me that it was becoming sore and this, along with everything else, was beginning to get him down. Normally I would have provided him with advice on what he needed or could do. But I somehow knew that this was not what he needed. Instead I invited Bob to talk and I listened. I noted that Bob appeared to be in a brighter mood when he left and seemed determined to try some of the suggestions that had been mentioned to him in previous consultations.

Nevertheless, the ulcer continued to deteriorate and with it came a change in Bob's attitude, general demeanour and appearance. As the wound steadily broke down, Bob became more withdrawn and began to banter less and less with myself and the other staff. He had always given the appearance of being younger than his years, so it was a shock to see him almost visibly age in front of the staff. It was also observed that his clothing was stained and badly fitting, whereas his appearance at the initial contact had been smart and clean.

Investigations were undertaken by me, my colleagues and the staff of the WMC, with whom we closely liaised. An infection of the wound had previously been identified on more that one occasion via clinical signs and through results of wound swabs. Although prescribed medication had appeared to halt the progression of the infection, the wound continued to deteriorate.

In October 2005, a routine blood test revealed that Bob had a high alcohol content in his blood. A study by Stephens et al. (1996) found that alcohol delays the healing process through its effect on fibroblast function and collagen synthesis. When dressing his wound, I mentioned the blood test and the result. Bob made it clear that he was unhappy to receive any advice on this subject. His notes indicated that staff in the WMC had also strongly advised him to cut back on his drinking. I began to wonder whether it had increased in response to the poor healing of his ulcer.

Using the CAGE questionnaire I enquired about his alcohol intake (Mayfield et al. 1974 cited by Bickley 2003). Bob told me that as well as going out once a week at the weekend, he was now drinking most nights at home. He appeared to be rather defensive about his alcohol intake and I did not enquire any further. Although I would have liked to have given him advice and for him to follow it, through constant contact I had discerned that Bob was a person who would change his behaviour when he decided he was ready to and would not be pressured or told. On reflection, Bob was at the pre-contemplation stage of the stages of change model regarding his alcohol intake (Prochanska et al. 1992 cited by Rutter and Quine 2002). I decided that at this stage the relationship between us was more important than his alcohol intake. Although I was worried by the increase, his self-assessment indicated that he was within recommended limits.

However, Bob's alcohol intake was not his only problem. Colleagues were extremely concerned about his emotional well-being. Depression has been categorized by the American Psychiatric Association (1994) as the patient showing or complaining of five or more symptoms over a period of 2 weeks, from a symptom list of nine. Depression, anxiety and hostility have been reported in the literature by patients with chronic wounds such as ulcers (Franks et al. 1994, Gould 1999). I approached Bob's GP to express my concerns. Patients who develop low self-esteem can lose the motivation to persevere with treatment, believing that their ulcer will never heal and thus fulfil their own prophecy. The steady deterioration in the ulcer may have accounted for the state that Bob was in.

Bob still complained occasionally of pain in his ulcer and although he had been prescribed analgesia, the team was not aware whether he was using it or not.

There is a perceived cultural difference in the response to pain, which can lead to stereotyping. The young person is believed to be more vocal and demanding regarding pain relief, whereas the older population appear to 'make do', not wanting to cause a fuss (Gould 1999). The effect of ulcers on patients' quality of life can include pain, reduced mobility, disfigurement, lack of energy and affect their work and social life (Callam et al. 1985, Franks and Moffatt 1998). This effect can be more pronounced on men than women and can engender negative feelings and emotions in the patient (Frank and Moffatt 1998). Patients reported feeling unclean because of the smell of the exudate from the wound, which led to them withdrawing from people and isolating themselves (Douglas 2001).

The condition of Bob's ulcer had deteriorated until it was almost circumferential and covered most of the anterior leg, with satellite ulcers to the posterior of the leg. The wound, especially at its distal aspect, had become much deeper. The amount of exudate had increased so that daily dressings were required for its management. The distal aspect of his foot had become swollen and blue in colour, and there was an offensive smell and deterioration in the surrounding skin.

The nursing staff at the WMC decided to refer Bob to the hyperbaric chamber for treatment in late 2005. However, Bob's attendance was sporadic. He found that the procedure was uncomfortable and increased the amount of pain and exudate to his ulcer. He decided to stop going, but was persuaded on a number of occasions to try the therapy again. By November 2005, Bob had decided that he would not attend the chamber anymore despite the risks, which included the need for amputation.

At this point, there appeared to be a positive turn around in Bob's emotional state. Throughout the period mentioned, I had consistently supported Bob and offered suggestions for improving the healing progress. After making the decision regarding the treatment via hyperbaric oxygen and being supported in this, Bob decided to visit France with his wife in March 2006. Dressings and referral notes were taken with him and the weekend proved to be a success. Bob felt happier in going out and more confident. He did not feel so self-conscious regarding the smell of the wound. After a few visits to France, Bob returned home with a few new treatments that he wanted to try out. One was the use of magnet therapy, which he had read about on the Internet. Electromagnetic therapy supposedly works by promoting healing through fields of electricity. Its benefit has been debated in the literature with no conclusive evidence established (Ravaghi et al. 2006). Another was a cream to be applied to the skin surrounding the ulcer. The composition of the cream was: 40 g of cérat de Galien, which was made up of 53.5% sweet almond oil, 33% rose water, 13% beeswax and 0.5 sodium borate; 30 g of fucidine; and 30 g of diprobase.

The use and effectiveness of alternative and complementary medication has been debated in the literature, with moves towards the need for professional regulation being highlighted (Mills 2001, Simpson and Roman 2001, Barnes 2003, Shang et al. 2005). After deciding on the basis of the evidence that neither of these 'treatments' would inhibit skin healing nor have a detrimental effect, Bob was supported in his decision-making. The importance of listening and involving the patient in their treatment has been highlighted by Ebbeskog and Emami (2005) and in policies such as *The NHS improvement plan* (DoH 2004b).

The change in mood also coincided with a change in the ulcer itself. The exudate became much lighter so that Bob was able to return to alternate-day dressings. Most remarkably, the skin surrounding the ulcer made a huge improvement and no longer looked macerated. Health-promoting advice continued to be offered in small amounts. Bob has made changes to his diet, which had been very calorific. He has reduced his alcohol intake to normal levels. He now only drinks socially, but is unwilling to give up alcohol at the moment. His expectations of healing are now more realistic as he realizes that it is a long process. According to Morse's (1991) work on nurse–patient relationships, my relationship with Bob is a connected relationship. Our relationship has build into a therapeutic one over a period of time. Talking and listening is at the heart of the relationship, which accounts for much of Bob's attendance at the department, without it becoming over-involved.

Poulton (1991) wrote that individuals modify their health behaviours when they can see a clear and obvious benefit. Bob has since given up alcohol and has lost approximately 9 kg. Although he misses drinking and finds it hard at times, he believes that the benefits are worth the effort.

Choosing health

Gloria offers this account of a one-off interaction that took place in a military medical reception station (MRS), using de Bono's (1985) *Six thinking hats* as an organizing framework.

> A 22-year-old male soldier (Mr Z) arrived 'on spec' one evening for the treatment of heel blisters. There are set times for attending the MRS and only emergencies should be seen outwith these times. Most staff, especially military combat medical technicians (CMTs), turn soldiers away to return at the appropriate time (07.30 at sick parade). As an Ministry of Defence nurse I totally understand the military culture of following orders, but nonetheless I also understand the pressure cadets are under to perform. The ethos of not letting the side down and the fear of the wrath of their training officers if they want to attend 'sick' in the morning puts the cadets under tremendous pressure. As a student ANP, I know that there could well be a rampant, infective, cellulitic blister lurking in Mr Z's socks! I make sure cadets know the MRS rules so they don't end up being told off by others, but I never turn them away.

The combination of soldiers traditionally having a 'macho' stereotype (Dawson 1994 and Goldstein 2001) and the stereotype of men as healthy, strong and self-sufficient (Robertson and Williams 1998) means that many feel that they need to live up to this image, although it may prevent them from seeking advice. Once Mr Z was reassured that I would not be 'telling him off' for attending out of hours and by not trivializing his concerns, I felt he relaxed and we built up a good rapport.

Red hat: my feelings

> While treating his blisters Mr Z asked if I could help him stop smoking. I'd just returned from training as a smoking cessation (SC) advisor, and was more than keen to put my newfound knowledge into practice and was full of the most up-to-date evidence about smoking cessation advice, although I explained that I was a novice in the field. Consequently, I asked if he would object to my sitting in on his first session with a more experienced advisor and to follow his progress. We spent some time discussing his motivation for stopping and what help we could offer at the MRS. We discussed in detail where he could foresee problems and talked about coping strategies for these; basically I worked through the Four A system (ask, advise, assist and arrange). He explained that he had tried to stop smoking in the past using patches but 'they gave him nightmares'. He was a 20+ a day smoker and lit his first cigarette before he got out of bed in the morning; he thus scored highest in the Fagerstrom test for nicotine dependence (Heatherton 1991), thus he was a perfect candidate for intense intervention therapy. Although the latest NICE (2006) guidelines say that there is no evidence

that the transtheoretical (stages of change) model is more effective than any other approach, I deduced that Mr Z was in the contemplation stage (Prochaska and DiClemente 1982). An appointment was made for a couple of days later when I looked forward to helping Mr Z on his journey to becoming a non-smoker. I was excited at his determination and felt positive that we would be able to help him.

Black hat: negative side

Presently the only smoking cessation services offered in this practice are 30-minute appointments at the medical centre, which inevitably restricts access. During the consultation, I sat quietly to one side. My colleague took Mr Z's smoking history and told him 'jokingly' that he had to succeed because she needed a success! She prescribed 16-hour nicotine replacement patches (as opposed to 24-hour ones). After I tentatively mentioned nicotine gum to supplement the patches, she said he could have gum to take in the evenings as he couldn't chew gum in uniform. I had to bite my tongue, as I couldn't believe that she was giving suboptimal advice (Hajek 2006), but it would have been unprofessional to start a discussion within the consultation, despite the fact that the evidence indicated that my colleague was not working to recent guidelines and was almost setting this soldier up for failure. Unsurprisingly, Mr Z didn't come back after the second week.

Yellow hat: positive side

I was deeply disappointed that a good opportunity had been missed and became determined to improve soldiers' access to SC clinics and up-to-date practice, so affording them the optimal chance of success. Nicotine replacement therapy, in whatever form, is an established pharmacological aid to help smokers quit and has consistently been shown to almost double the abstinence rate, irrespective of the level of additional interventions (Stead and Lancaster 2005). NRT and SC Clinic availability in medical centres offer the best chance of quitting for soldiers (Mahony-Zahe 2002). Some barriers to successful quitting include the military hierarchical rank structure, military duties and training exercises that take soldiers away from camp regularly, and peer pressure, especially among the young recruits who don't want to 'lose face'. Nevertheless, there are also enablers. NRT is free to serving soldiers, and the discipline within the military could provide a positive influence if more people, not just nurses, were involved in smoking cessation.

Research has shown that the more a soldier smokes, the poorer his or her fitness performance, with a resultant increase in injuries (Jones et al. 1993). It is also the case that following surgery, smokers' wounds take longer to heal (Bahrke et al. 1988). Historical evidence suggests that military efficacy could be compromised because a smoker is to some extent visually challenged in darkness, requiring some 20% more time to readapt following a 'flash' (von Restorf and Hebisch 1988) and logistically, the frequency with which smoker's cough, the lighting of a cigarette or the smell of tobacco can give away the soldier's location (Adam and Ladell 1953). Bearing all these factors in mind it is not only the physical health of the soldier that needs to be considered when planning smoking cessation within the army, but also the battlefield implications.

Green hat: application to practice

Initially I spoke to my mentor about how to handle this sensitive situation and we decided that instead of a teaching session on the latest evidence-based practice, which we knew would provoke the same antagonistic reaction, it would be better to start by inviting the drug representative from our NRT supplier to come and give us the most up-to-date information about the products. Meanwhile, I prepared handouts from my recent course to distribute at the meeting. I don't believe that direct confrontation is always the answer. Letting people think something is their own idea often leaves them in their own 'space'. Nevertheless, I would like to work on my people skills so that I can handle situations like this without feeling uncomfortable.

Blue hat: application to other situations

Nurses need to understand the requirements of their target population while implementing public health policy during clinical practice, and advice about smoking in the military may be a component of primary (discourage from starting), secondary (encouraging otherwise healthy smokers to stop) and, although less common in this setting, tertiary health promotion (encourage to stop after disease is established) (Donaldson and Donaldson 2000).

Within the army, the Maudsley Model is considered to be the most suitable base for an effective programme. I envisage that the establishment of group sessions could utilize the camaraderie and support that is inherent between soldiers. Drop-in clinics in the messes or gym, or even IT solutions, such as text-messaging communications of encouragement could be beneficial. The government White Paper *Choosing health* (DoH 2004) advocates that people need to make informed choices so, perhaps, physical training instructors (PTIs) (in charge of soldiers' fitness) and the combat medical technicians (CMTs) (who accompany the soldiers in training), both of whom understand the culture and ethos of the military lifestyle, are the ideal 'message bearers' between the health care providers and the soldiers. They could become the 'heath trainers', as envisaged in the White Paper. Army dental services could also play a vital role in smoking health education (Barnfather et al. 2005).

Although the implementation of these solutions would involve extra cost both in training and man-hours, the long-term benefits could far outweigh the costs. Discussions are now under way between the GPs, smoking advisors, practice manager, PTIs, CMTs and platoon commanders to negotiate the most appropriate way forward so that this vital public health issue can be addressed.

Our health, our care, our say

In contrast to the two previous examples, which illustrate the potential of the ANP role on a one-to-one basis, Jackie's emergent role embraces a specific population focus and brings to life particular elements of the education function within the context of

Our health, our care, our say. It highlights the work of an outreach worker whose role centres on substance abuse in a population of street workers.

The role was specifically developed in recognition of the particular health needs of the substance-misusing, female street worker population and the belief that an outreach ANP could encourage clients into mainstream services via the delivery of locally based services. In order to focus what might risk becoming a diffuse service, Jackie's role centred on massage parlours and the need for health input concentrated on hepatitis B and contraceptive advice. As such, it sought to work collaboratively with prostitution as an activity, defined by the Home Office (2004) as the exchange of sexual services in return for a payment, be it money or drugs, and with prostitutes as individuals. Importantly, Jackie's role recognized the risk to female street workers that comes from their reluctance to disclose their area of work, whilst at the same time understanding that the locally based Centre for Sexual Health is currently overstretched, with excessive waiting times. Furthermore, Jackie notes that despite the fact that services provide free condoms, support and educational advice, evidence suggests that female street workers remain reluctant to access them. Jackie questions why this is the case in the context of *Paying the price* (Home Office 2004), which acknowledges that individuals involved in prostitution require specialist support by means of outreach services.

Jackie goes on to describe a growing understanding of the target population.

> The age range of the sex workers is between eighteen and fifty-three. Contact with the parlour girls is quite regular … and they appear happy to disclose personal information. Some workers are married, some have long-term relationships but it appears that very few of the girls disclose their occupation to their partners. Many appear to use the occupation of care home workers to cover up the shift patterns, or state they are receptionists at the parlours. All use pseudonyms. Some of the women are mothers who state they work to give their children things they would otherwise not be able to afford. Locally in the parlours the cost appears to be forty pounds with the parlours taking a cut of this; however, more can be earned in negotiation with the customer. The busiest periods were stated as the summer months, when the holidaymakers were about and the slackest period after Christmas. All the girls stated they use condoms all the time whilst at work; however, split condoms do occur. It also appears that outside of work, in their own personal relationships, the girls do not use condoms.

Determined to develop an evidenced-based service, Jackie recounts her analysis of the literature and the identification of key themes, specifically the correlation between sex workers and drug use; inconsistencies in use of condoms by sex workers; understanding of sexually transmitted infections (STIs) among sex workers; and the provision of outreach services for marginalized groups.

Jackie concludes that evidence from Britain and abroad highlights that sex workers find it difficult to access mainstream service provision. The reasons for this include the fact they are perceived as undesirable or difficult (Weiner 1996). In addition, the work itself promotes social exclusion along with illegal aspects involved in it. Jackie argues that to be a sex worker brings with it discrimination and hostility and so argues the need to provide an outreach service provision for sex workers which has an in-built educational perspective designed to promote empowerment and minimize health risk.

REFLECTIONS AND CONCLUDING THOUGHTS

Using as a benchmark the domains of practice identified by the Royal College of Nursing (2005), now adopted by the NMC with the intention of regulating the role, it is possible to surmise that student ANPs are likely to experience the most dramatic role development in dimensions of practice with which they are less familiar, for example health assessment, diagnostic reasoning and clinical decision-making. Pursuing this argument, it might then be concluded that role development in respect of the education function would be quieter. As noted previously, initial registrants need to be able to demonstrate that they can create and use opportunities to promote the health and well-being of patients, clients and groups (NMC 2004). The voices of student ANPs challenge this expectation. Although it is indeed the case that the individuals who shared their thoughts were familiar with educating both children and families, and a range of adults in different settings, the experience of learning to take up, as a whole, the competencies which define the role can be seen to alter they way in which they are approaching this vital component of professional practice.

The accounts of Wendy, Gloria and Jackie illuminate this further and, in addition, enable understanding to build in respect of the ways in which student ANPs can drive forward government policy in the interests of patients, clients and hard-to-reach groups. Specifically reflecting back on Rollnick et al's (1999) analysis of behavioural change and the risk of creating resistance (Figure 6.2), in different ways, Wendy, Gloria and Jackie can be seen to be forging relationships that have the potential to protect health and minimize risk now and into the future. It is argued that one of the reasons why they are able to do this links to the dynamic interplay between the component parts of the seven domains. Consequently, the education function is not isolated from any of the other domains and the competencies identified therein. This implies that the way in which the ANP takes forward the education function may be different to the way in which a clinical nurse specialist, for example, develops this aspect of their practice. Readers are invited to reflect on this as a possibility, not with the intention of arguing that ANPs are in someway better than their peers. Rather the invitation centres on building an understanding of how and why each of the different elements that comprise the seven domains combine to maximize a role committed to promoting health and minimizing risk in the interests of individuals, groups and society as a whole.

REFERENCES

Adam, J.M. and Ladell, W.S.S. (1953) *Report on field studies on troops of the Commonwealth Division in Korea, winter 1951–1952* (Restricted). London: Scientific Adviser to Army Council.

Ajzen, I. (1991) The theory of planned behaviour. *Journal of Organizational Behavior and the Human Decision Process* 50: 179–211.

American Psychiatric Association (1994) *Diagnostic and statistical manual of mental disorders*, 4th edn. Washington DC: American Psychiatric Association.

Bahrke, M.S. Baur, T.S. Poland, D.F. and Connors D.F (1988) Tobacco use and performance on the US Army Physical Fitness Test. *Military Medicine* 153:229–233.

Barnes, J. (2003) Quality, efficacy and safety of complementary medicines: fashions, facts and the future. Part I. Regulation and quality. *British Journal of Clinical Pharmacology* 55: 226–233.

Barnfather, K.D. Cope, G.F. and Chapple, I.L. (2005) Effect of incorporating a 10-minute point of care test for salivary nicotine metabolites into a general practice-based smoking cessation programme: randomised controlled trial. *British Medical Journal* 331: 999–1002.

Beattie, A (1995) War and peace among the health tribes. In Soothill, K. Mackay, L. and Webb, C. (eds), pp. 11–30. *Interprofessional relations in health care.* London: Edward Arnold.

Becker, M. (1974) *The health belief model and personal health behaviour.* Thorofare, NJ: Charles B. Sack.

Benner, P. (1984) *From novice to expert: excellence and power in clinical nursing practice.* Sydney: Addison-Wesley.

Bickley, L.S. (2003) Techniques of examination. In Bickley, L.S. and Szilagyi, P.G. (eds) *Bates' guide to physical examination and history taking,* 8th edn, pp. 115–208. Philadelphia (PA): Lippincott Williams & Wilkins.

de Bono (1985) *Six thinking hats.* Boston: Little, Brown and Company.

Callam, M.J. Ruckley, C.V. Harper and D.R. Dale, J.J. (1985) Chronic ulceration of the leg: extent of the problem and provision of care. *British Medical Journal* 290: 1855–1856.

Dawson, G. (1994) *Soldier heroes: British adventure, empire and the imagining of masculinities.* London: Routledge.

Dealey, C. (2005) *The care of wounds: a guide for nurses,* 3rd edn. Oxford: Blackwell Publishing.

Department of Health (2001) *The expert patient: a new approach to chronic disease management for the 21st century.* London: DoH.

Department of Health (2002) *Liberating the talents.* London: DoH.

Department of Health (2004a) *Choosing health: making healthy choices easier.* London: DoH.

Department of Health (2004b) *The NHS improvement plan.* London: DoH.

Department of Health (2005) *Long-term conditions model.* DoH. http://www.dh.gov.uk/en/Policyandguidance/Healthandsocialcaretopics/Longtermconditions/index.htm

Department of Health (2006) *Our health, our care, our say.* London: DoH.

Donaldson, L. and Donaldson, R. (2000) *Essential public health.* Berkshire: Petroc Press.

Ebbeskog, B. and Emami, A. (2005) Older patients' experience of dressing changes on venous leg ulcers: more than just a docile patient. *Journal of Clinical Nursing* 14: 1223–1231.

Franks, P.J. and Moffatt, P.J. (1998) Who suffers most from leg ulceration? *Journal of Wound Care* 7: 383–385.

Franks, P.J, Moffatt, P.J. and Connolly, M. (1994) Community leg ulcer clinics: effect on quality of life. *Phlebologie* 9: 83–86.

Goldstein, J.S. (2001) *War and gender: how gender shapes the war system and vice versa.* Cambridge: Cambridge University Press.

Gould, D. (1999) Wound management and pain control. *Nursing Standard* 14: 47–54.

Heatherton, T.F. Kozlowski, L.T. Frecker, R.C. and Fagerstrom, K.O. (1991) The Fagerstrom test for nicotine dependence: a revision of the Fagerstrom tolerance questionnaire. *British Journal of Addictions* 86(11): 19–27.

Home Office (2004) *Paying the Price: a consultation paper on prostitution.* London: Home Office.

Horrocks, J. House, A. and Owens, D. (2002) *Attendances in the accident and emergency department following self-harm: a descriptive study.* Leeds: University of Leeds.

Jones, B.H. Bowee, M.W. Harris, J.M. and Cowan, D.N. (1993) Intrinsic risk factors for exercise-related injuries among male and female army trainees. *American Journal of Sports Medicine* 21: 705–710.

Mills, S. (2001) Regulation in complementary and alternative medicine. *British Medical Journal* 322: 161–164.

Morse, J. (1991) Negotiating commitment and involvement in the nurse-patient relationship. *Journal of Advanced Nursing* 16: 455–468.

NICE (National Institute for Health and Clinical Excellence) (2006) *The public health guidance development process: an overview for stakeholders including public health practitioner, policy makers and the public.* London: NICE.

NMC (2005) *Annex 1 domains of practice and competencies, NMC consultation on a proposed framework for post-registration nursing.* London: Nursing and Midwifery Council.

Oliver, R. and Endersby, C. (1994) *Teaching and assessing nursing: a handbook for preceptors.* London: Baillière Tindall.

Poulton, B. (1991) Factors influencing patient compliance. *Nursing Standard* 5(36): 3–5.

Prochaska, J.O. and DeClemente, C.C. (1982). Transtheoretical therapy: toward a more integrative model of change. *Psychotherapy: Theory, Research, and Practice* 20: 161–173.

Ravaghi, H. Flemming, K. Cullum, N. and Olyaee Manesh, A. (2006) Electromagnetic therapy for treating venous leg ulcers. *Cochrane Database Systematic Reviews* April 19 (2):CD002933.

RCN (2002) *Nurse practitioners: a RCN guide to the nurse practitioner role, competencies and programme accreditation.* London: Royal College of Nursing.

von Restorff, W. and Hebisch, S. (1988) Dark adaptation of the eye during carbon monoxide exposure in smokers and nonsmokers. *Aviation Space Environment Medicine* 59: 928–931.

Robertson, S. and Williams, R. (1998) Working with men: a theoretical base for meeting their needs. *Community Practitioner* 71: 286–288.

Rollnick, S. and Miller, W.R. (1995). What is motivational interviewing? *Behavioral and Cognitive Psychotherapy* 23: 325–334.

Russell, L. (2000) Understanding physiology of wound healing and how dressings help. *British Journal of Nursing* 9:(1): 21.

Rutter, D. and Quine, L. (2002). *Social cognition models and changing health behaviours. Changing health behaviour: intervention and research with social cognition models.* Buckingham: Open University Press.

Shang, A. Huwiler-Muntener, K. Nartey, L. Juni, P. Dorig, S. Sterne, J.A. Pewsner, D. and Egger, M. (2005) Are the clinical effects of homoeopathy placebo effects? Comparative study of placebo-controlled trials of homoeopathy and allopathy. *Lancet* 66: 726–732.

Simpson, N. and Roman, K. (2001) Complementary medicine use in children: extent and reasons. A population-based study. *British Journal of General Practitioners* 51: 914–916.

Stead, L.F. and Lancaster, T. (2005) Group behaviour therapy programmes for smoking cessation. Available from www.mrw.interscience.wiley.com/cochrane/clsysrev/articles/CD002850/frame.html

Stephens, N.G. Parsons, A. Schofield, P.M. Kelly, F. Cheeseman, K. and Mitchinson, M.J. (1996) Randomised controlled trial of vitamin e in patients with coronary disease: Cambridge heart antioxidant study (CHAOS). *Lancet* 347: 781–786.

Tones, K. (1995) Making a change for the better: the health action model. *Healthlines* 27: 17–19.

United Kingdom Central Council (UKCC) (1992) *Scope of professional practice.* London: UKCC.

Weiner, A. (1996). Understanding the social needs of streetwalking prostitutes. *Social Work* 41(1): 97–104.

Wilson, J. and Bunnell, (2007) A review of the merits of the nurse practitioner role. *Nursing Standard* 21(18): 37–40.

7

DOMAIN 5: PROFESSIONAL ROLE

ALISON CRUMBIE

INTRODUCTION

The nurse practitioner role in the UK was first introduced into general practice by Stilwell in the early 1980s (Stilwell 1981, 1985, Stilwell et al. 1987). Since that time the role has developed and changed and there are now numerous examples of nurse practitioners working in diverse and varied roles in both hospital and primary care settings throughout the four countries of the UK. Nurses have moved into the nurse practitioner role to meet the needs of underserved populations (Smith 1992), to enhance the capacity of general practice in areas of poor GP recruitment (Kenny 1997) and to deliver innovative health care services to populations with specific needs (Walsh and Howkins 2002). Examples now exist of nurse practitioners taking on triage roles (Reveley 1999), running minor illness clinics (Marsh and Dawes 1995), accepting same-day clinic appointments (Kinnersley et al. 2000, Venning et al. 2000) operating open access clinics (Salisbury and Tettersell 1988), running bronchiectasis clinics (Sharples et al. 2002), working with farming communities (Walsh and Howkins 2002) and carrying out day case preoperative assessment (Wadsworth et al. 2002). In addition to the diversification into a wide range of clinical areas, nurse practitioners have also been expanding and developing their practice, with many now prescribing independently, ordering radiographs, referring to colleagues in secondary care and taking sole responsibility for whole areas of clinical care with only minimal input from medical colleagues.

The reason the nurse practitioner role has evolved in this way is not only because the government and nurse leaders have encouraged this development but also because nurses themselves have continually worked at developing their professional roles. Nurse practitioner posts have grown and taken shape because clinical nurses have used evidence-based practice to underpin their work with patients; they have researched their own roles and have provided evidence to managers and employers to sustain and develop their work. Nurse practitioners have provided leadership both within the clinical team and within the profession of nursing. The Nursing and Midwifery Council (NMC) competency framework addresses a range of domains of practice which focus on the skills associated with the role; the 'professional role' is the domain which is focused on introducing, developing and establishing advanced nurse practitioner (ANP) practice. The aim of this chapter is to examine the professional role domain with a specific focus on the development of the role, approaches to directing care and methods of providing leadership to others.

DEVELOPS AND IMPLEMENTS THE ADVANCED NURSE PRACTITIONER ROLE

Uses evidence and research to implement the role

In order to implement a new nurse practitioner role, or to make the case for developing the role of an existing nurse practitioner, it is important to be aware of the research that has been conducted on similar roles or in similar areas of practice. There is a growing body of research which examines the nurse practitioner role. Becoming familiar with the existing work can help you to be fully aware of the benefits and pitfalls that lie ahead. Nurse practitioner research originated in the United States in the early 1960s (Hooker and Mayo 2002). In the UK, research into the role of the nurse practitioner commenced with Barbara Stilwell in the early 1980s. Stilwell (1981) provided a description of the pilot project in which she was involved and, later on, an analysis of her role (Stilwell 1985, Stilwell et al. 1987). The analysis included a description of the types of conditions she dealt with, how many required referral for further investigation and the results of patient questionnaires. Patients gave their reasons for consulting with the nurse practitioner including, 'I thought I could talk better to her', 'to save the doctor's time' and 'she's got more time for you'. The conclusions from this study were that the nurse practitioner could deal with one-third of all consultations without referral to a doctor; additional problems were raised in 46% of consultations which mostly involved health education; and most patients made an appropriate choice to consult with the nurse. Stilwell acknowledged that she had 20 minute appointment times and that this was considerably longer than the GP.

Owing to the small number of qualified nurse practitioners in the UK during the 1980s and early 1990s, evaluation of the role was focused on single practitioners (Salisbury and Tettersell 1988, Reveley 1999) or on newly qualified practitioners (South Thames Regional Health Authority 1994, National Health Service Executive 1996, Reveley 1999). Towards the end of the 1990s, nurse practitioner research began to compare the work of the nurses with that of the GP. Concerns were raised that nurses may be acting as cheap alternatives to the GP and therefore could be providing a lesser service to patients and at worst could even be unsafe (Dickson et al. 1996, Crawford 1997). Reveley (1999) carried out an evaluation of the triage role of a single nurse practitioner working in general practice with seven GPs, and Venning et al. (2000) and Kinnersley et al. (2000) reported on randomized controlled trials involving nurse practitioners in general practice. Examples of other studies that used randomized controlled trials to compare the work of the nurse practitioner with doctors in the same setting are Sharples et al. (2002), who examined care in a bronchiectasis clinic, and Cooper et al. (2002), who focused on emergency nurse practitioner services.

In 2002, Horrocks et al. reported on a systematic review of the literature relating to whether nurse practitioners working in primary care can provide equivalent care to doctors. They state that it is important to consider whether nurse practitioners can substitute for doctors by providing safe, effective and economical management of patients. The results of their review demonstrate that patients are more satisfied with care by a nurse practitioner and that the quality of care offered by a nurse practitioner, when compared with a GP, is 'in some ways better' (Horrocks et al. 2002: 821). The authors reported that nurse practitioners tend to have longer consultations and tend to make more investigations, but that there is no difference in the number of prescriptions generated, return consultations, referrals or in patient health status between the two groups.

The research consistently reveals a significant difference between nurse practitioners and doctors in patient satisfaction. The reasons for enhanced patient satisfaction are not clear. Patient satisfaction is a multidimensional construct and components of satisfaction change over time (Fitzpatrick 1993). Patient expectations have been found to affect subsequent patient satisfaction (Merkouris et al. 1999) and it is possible that this plays a role in the increased patient satisfaction with nurse practitioner consultations. Whatever the reason might be for increased satisfaction, the results of the patient satisfaction data in the studies reviewed above would suggest that there is some kind of qualitative difference between nurse practitioners and GPs. There is no information relating to the nature of this difference.

More recently the research has turned to examine the cost-effectiveness of nurse practitioners. Hollinghurst et al. (2006) compared the cost of nurse practitioners in primary care with GPs and found that nurse practitioners were more expensive. This research was based on data that had been collected towards the end of the 1990s before the implementation of independent prescribing and at a time when many nurse practitioners were new to their roles and were having difficulty with patient referrals and liaison with hospital consultants. Many barriers to nurse practitioner practice have now been dealt with and therefore the arguments made by Hollinghurst et al. (2006) need to be reviewed and updated to reflect the current climate. Laurant et al. (2004) carried out a randomized controlled trial and examined what impact the presence of a nurse practitioner had upon the workload of GPs. They concluded that in the short term at least, the GP workload was not reduced and that nurse practitioners should not be considered to be a substitute for GPs; instead, they should be seen as supplementing the work of general practice.

Making yourself familiar with the research that has been carried out on the role of the nurse practitioner in the UK will provide you with a sound basis from which to make your case either to implement or develop the role in your setting. It is important to be aware that several of the studies point to increased patient satisfaction with nurse practitioners and yet, at the same time, you need to treat such a finding with caution because we know so little about the nature of that satisfaction. Equally, it is important to be aware that some researchers have made the claim that nurse practitioners are less economical than GPs, both from a monetary and a time perspective, and yet this research was based upon data collected at the end of the 1990s, when nurse practitioners were unable to prescribe and had difficulty in referring patients.

It is important to ask yourself what you can add to your organization and what impact you can have on patient care. In order to do this, you may need to collect evidence relating to your place of work or your proposed place of work. Identify gaps in care, consider how the nurse practitioner might be best placed to address the gaps and then develop a succinct, articulate argument drawing on all of the available evidence to make your case. Later in this chapter we shall consider how you align such arguments with the strategic vision of an organization and how you might go about marketing such a role.

In summary, before developing and implementing the role of the ANP ask yourself the following questions:

- Why develop the role?
- What can the ANP add to the organization?
- What organizational needs can the ANP address?
- Which gaps in the organization can the ANP address?
- What research has been conducted to support this development?
- In what ways will the introduction of an ANP role benefit patients?

Functions in a variety of role dimensions: health care provider, coordinator, consultant, educator, coach, advocate, administrator, researcher, role model and leader

Nurses who are working at an advanced, expert level will have the flexibility to work in diverse ways to meet the needs of patients, their colleagues and the organizations within which they work. If you stop to analyse a single consultation you might find examples of all of the role dimensions that are listed in this competency, particularly when you are dealing with complex, challenging situations. An example of such a consultation is shown in Scenario 7.1 that demonstrates the breadth of the ANP role in practice.

Scenario 7.1

A 24-year-old woman walked into the consulting room. She was dressed in fashionable clothing, had curly blonde hair and was carrying a large green bag. As usual I greeted her and offered her a seat before I sat down myself to begin the consultation. She blurted out 'I have a sore ear' and then grabbed her bag and started to open it, rummaging through the things inside. I kept quiet and observed her actions. She then put her hands to her face and burst into tears. 'I've not stopped crying for days,' she said, 'My life is in a mess, I have no friends and it's all my fault.' She went on to tell me about her problem with drinking and that she felt she needed to drink heavily to cope with the outside world. She was having black-outs and could not remember what had happened the night before and then felt embarrassed about what she might have said or done. She described her behaviour as being 'some other person' and this really wasn't the way she was. She fluctuated between saying, 'I can't be an alcoholic', and yet realizing that aspects of her behaviour pointed to a problem with drink. The consultation continued with me listening and prompting her to continue to talk and finally she returned to her painful ear.

The outcome of the consultation involved a referral to counselling services, referral for investigations and plans for a follow-up appointment. The consultation required sensitive, skilful communication to help her work through her thoughts and feelings about alcohol. Benner (1984) refers to the ways in which nurses have to work with patients to address culturally uncharted and avoided territory, and alcoholism is an example of this. This is what is meant by the education function (see also Chapter 6).

Such a consultation requires an advanced level of practice to help the patient chart their way through their presenting symptoms, anxiety, depression and substance abuse; it also takes skill to help the patient to express such concerns. When a patient is feeling helpless it is important to be able to be an advocate on their behalf, to provide them with options for support and to facilitate the treatment plan. This requires coordination and administrative ability as it will often involve referral to other agencies.

ANPs will be faced with a wide range of patients with a variety of problems and concerns, and often unwittingly will move through various role dimensions within one consultation. In addition to the specifics of the consultation the nurse practitioner will often provide leadership to others, including students, other health care professionals and other staff in the organization. They will do this by keeping up to date with the latest evidence and keeping themselves informed. Not all ANPs will be actively involved in research but knowing how to access research and how critically to analyse the work will ensure that you remain informed and are able to provide leadership to others.

Interprets and markets the role to the public, legislators, policy makers and other health care professions

The ANP role remains a relatively new concept to the UK public. Some areas of the country have many nurse practitioners working in a variety of clinical settings, other areas have no nurse practitioners. It is, therefore, important to consider every contact with a patient and every contact with another health care professional or manager as an opportunity to promote the role. This type of marketing is known as relationship marketing, which focuses on creating and maintaining long-term relationships with both clients and all other relevant stakeholders. Important issues to consider include how you introduce yourself to each patient, how you approach the subject when the patient asks you 'what is a nurse practitioner?', how you respond when patients or others ask 'when are you going to qualify to be a doctor?' or how you respond when a patient says 'thank you, doctor'. Whatever your approach, it is important always to emphasize to the patient that you are a nurse, not a doctor and in your own words to interpret for each patient exactly what that means.

It may be necessary to consider marketing the nurse practitioner role in a more formal manner. It can be helpful to carry out a SWOT analysis (strengths, weaknesses, opportunities and threats). In marketing terms this is known as the internal audit (strengths and weaknesses) and external audit (opportunities and threats) (see Figure 7.1). You can consider what your strengths and weaknesses might be by considering what you can contribute to your organization, what skills you have to offer and what skills you need to develop. You can then review the organization in which you work and you can consider what external factors will impact significantly on the practice or your place of work in the future. This type of analysis can reveal potential areas for development and can help you to identify how you might be able to contribute to the organization. In turn, this will help you to articulate to others your unique contribution or potential contribution to an area of clinical practice.

It is important to be looking ahead continually and to be aware of developments in policy at a national level. You can then prepare yourself for the future so that you will be adequately prepared to provide clinical care to patients as the health care environment changes in response to strategic shifts at governmental level. In order to

Internal audit	External audit
S **Strengths** What would a nurse practitioner have to offer the organization? What skills would a nurse practitioner have to offer? In what ways could a nurse practitioner benefit patient care? What would be the unique contribution of a nurse practitioner to patient care?	**O** **Opportunities** What are the gaps in your organization? Where is the potential for development? Are there any patient needs that are not being addressed? Is government policy suggesting a change in direction? Is there any funding for the development of new roles?
W **Weaknesses** Could the nurse practitioner have a negative impact upon other members of the health care team? Would the nurse practitioner be too expensive? Do patients understand the role of the nurse practitioner? Do other members of staff within the organization understand the role of the nurse practitioner?	**T** **Threats** Are there any barriers to the development? Is government policy supportive of your proposed development? Is local policy supportive of your proposed development? Are others providing the service you propose? Is your proposal cost effective when compared to others?

FIGURE 7.1 *Example of questions to ask in a SWOT analysis.*

TABLE 7.1 *Sources of information to keep up to date with current trends*

National Health Service (http://www.nhs.org.uk)

National Institute for Health and Clinical Excellence (http:// www.nice.org.uk)

The Department of Health (http://www.dh.gov.uk.org)

The Royal College of Nursing (http://www.rcn.org.uk)

Nursing journals, e.g. *Nursing Standard* (http://www.nursing-standard.co.uk) *Nursing Times* (www.nursingtimes.net)

Medical journals, e.g. *British Medical Journal* (http://www.bmj.com)

Research and development funding (http://rdfunding.org.uk/default.asp)

Queen's Nursing Institute (England and Scotland) (http://www.qni.org.uk)

Colleagues, patients and allied health practitioners

Primary care trusts and hospital trusts (policies, strategy, developments)

Local colleges and universities

Public libraries

Voluntary agencies, not-for-profit organizations and charities

keep yourself in touch with such developments, it is important to keep scanning various websites and to keep reading influential journals. Useful websites and other resources can be found in Table 7.1.

However you choose to market yourself and your role, it is important to remember that every action you carry out in the clinical setting will convey an important message to each member of the public with whom you interact. It is not only a message about yourself but it is also a message about all ANPs.

KEY POINTS

- Familiarize yourself with previous research on the role of the ANP.
- Reflect upon your practice and analyse the complexity of your role.
- Think about the needs of your patient population and shape services to meet those needs.
- Think about the gaps in services and consider how the ANP role might fill those gaps.
- Keep up-to-date with research and policy developments.

DIRECTS CARE

Prioritizes: coordinates and meets multiple needs for culturally diverse patients (see also Chapter 4)

Cultural diversity exists in every area of clinical practice throughout the UK. In some areas the presence of a range of people whose first language is not English makes the issue of cultural diversity obvious. There are examples of great efforts being made by health care teams to address the varied needs of a wide range of cultural groups. An example of this is the Hackney diabetes project, where culturally sensitive educational leaflets, hand-held records, CDs and DVDs were created and training courses were run in Hindi, Turkish, Gujarati, Vietnamese and Urdu (Jesson et al. 2006). In other areas where the patients are mostly white Caucasian, the issue of cultural diversity is less obvious and yet because of the all-pervasive and often unconscious nature of culture (Walsh 2000) if you look carefully enough you will find a wide variety of cultural groups in what appears to be a homogeneous population. An example of this is the nurse practitioner project in farmers' health (Walsh and Howkins 2002). It was recognized that the farming community tended not to access health care services until they were critically ill. They often lived with mental health problems, particularly depression, and would never seek help. The farmers' project aimed to reach out to the farming community by taking services to them rather than expecting the farmers to attend surgeries. A mobile unit was set up with a nurse practitioner and health care assistant. The unit was parked at auction marts and at other places where farmers would congregate and they were encouraged to come into the van to consult with the nurse practitioner if they felt they had any health concerns.

The Hackney project and the farmers' health project are both impressive and obvious examples of nurses reaching out to culturally diverse groups. It is perhaps less obvious that cultural sensitivity is necessary in every single consultation. It is important to speak the 'language' of your patients and to be sensitive to their perspective and their view of the world. An older person might refer to the diet you are suggesting to manage their diabetes as being like 'returning to the rationing of the Second World War' in which case other references to the war and times gone by would be appropriate. A young man might use football analogies to describe his feelings 'I feel like I've kicked a home goal' in which case you can respond with further references to football.

ANPs can reach out to culturally diverse populations in the microcosm of the consultation and at the macro-level of the organization. At the macro-level, services can be shaped in the practice to ensure that no one particular group is alienated and that all groups feel welcomed. One of the best ways of achieving this is to ask patients what they want and to try to understand their perspective.

Uses sound judgement in assessing conflicting priorities and needs

Scenario 7.1 provides an example of a patient attending for a consultation with more than one need. Her reason for booking the appointment was her painful ear but it very quickly became apparent that her major concern was her alcohol problem. This particular consultation required little direction from the nurse practitioner, as the patient very readily shared her concerns and spent most of her time talking about what they both felt was the main reason for her appointment. It is not always so clear and, occasionally, patients will spend a whole consultation talking about their painful knee, their problematic hay fever or their athlete's foot and then, as they are about to end the consultation, they will announce that they have been experiencing some funny pains in their chest recently. This can be particularly likely if the patient is suffering from something they feel embarrassed about, such as erectile dysfunction or dyspareunia and it takes them time to feel safe to share it with another person. The nurse practitioner can use a number of tactics to help chart a way through conflicting priorities and needs. Consultation and communication skills are particularly important here and these are discussed in more detail in Chapter 5. Some useful phrases to help elicit the patient's main concerns and to learn about the patient's agenda can be found in Table 7.2.

If the patient has presented numerous important problems and needs in one consultation, it is sometimes necessary to reflect this list of problems back to the patient and to help them prioritize which issues to tackle first. It may be necessary to explain that you understand that all of the problems are important but you may need to ask the patient to make a follow-up appointment to address the remaining concerns. Such decisions require sound clinical judgement and skilled communication. If you feel that the priority is the patient's uncontrolled blood pressure but he feels the priority is his erectile dysfunction and the effect it is having on his home life, you will need to acknowledge his concerns to demonstrate that you understand his priorities and then you have to work together to address his complex needs.

Builds and maintains a therapeutic team to provide optimum therapy

It is not possible for any one health care professional to deliver all of the care required by a particular patient population. It is, therefore, necessary to develop and to work in teams. There are benefits to teamwork; for example, care given by a group is greater than the sum of its parts, team members are better supported and have increased job satisfaction, rare skills can be made more available to patients, prevention

TABLE 7.2 *Open questions to identify the patient's agenda*

Can you tell me what your main concerns are?
Is there anything else that concerns you?
Is there anything else that is bothering you?
What do you think the problem is?
Is there anything else you would like to add?

and curative work can be better coordinated, team members can learn from each other and the patient receives more efficient care when ill (Pritchard and Pritchard 1994, Blackie 1998). Teamwork can also be a challenge as care offered by different individuals can lead to duplication of effort, lack of direction and a potential threat to the overall view of the patient and the patient's family and carers. The key here is that the nurse practitioner is involved in building and maintaining a *therapeutic* team, one that functions smoothly and seamlessly. An example of such an approach is the TLC (tender loving care) team meeting within a primary health care team.

Scenario 7.2

A group of staff came together to engage in a development called the 'integrated team project'. The idea was that the team would consider what challenges they faced in their work and would carry out a SWOT analysis of their organization. The meetings took place every 2 months over a period of 8 months and over time the idea of the TLC meeting developed. The idea of the TLC meeting is that district nurses, community nurses, social workers, health visitors, practice nurses, nurse practitioners, GPs and Macmillan nurses get together once a week to review all the patients who are in need of TLC. The TLC list is printed off each week by the administrative staff and forms the basis for the meeting. Any patient who is considered to be vulnerable, for whatever reason (new cancer diagnosis, terminal illness, deteriorating dementia and others) is discussed and the team coordinates the care. These meetings allow for networking, the sharing of ideas and perspectives about patients, a forum to review significant events and an opportunity to coordinate care and share the responsibility between practitioners. Meetings can appear to be yet another burden in the working week but if it is obviously useful to everyone and, if the meeting is well managed, runs to time and remains collegial and respectful of each practitioner's input, then people will attend. This improves the efficiency of the team and provides a sound basis for good working relations and ultimately enhances the care of patients and their families.

The TLC meeting provides an example of a therapeutic team operating within the wider primary health care team. Clearly, other teams exist within the wider team, including those that focus on patients with mental health problems and those that focus on organizational issues within the workplace. It is important to recognize the value of such teams and nurse practitioners can play a pivotal role in the support and maintenance of these networks in practice.

Obtains specialist and referral care for patients while remaining the primary care provider

Whether the nurse practitioner works in a hospital or a primary care setting it is going to be important to be able to communicate effectively with colleagues and to be able to refer to specialist practitioners when the patient's condition requires it. Knowing when to refer and when to seek specialist advice requires advanced clinical judgement. Communicating your findings and your reason for the referral requires skill to correspond in a succinct and clear manner. This skill can be learnt and it is well worth practising. Referral letters are an essential part of high-quality clinical care (SIGN 1998).

The purpose of the referral letter is to provide patient information, including demographic details, clinical information and the reason for the referral (SIGN 1998). When writing a letter is important to consider who might be reading it, including administrative staff, the specialist to whom you are referring and the patient and patient's family, who will be quite entitled to read such information at a future date. Some clinicians choose to send copies of referral letters to patients at the point of the referral to enable the patient to be as engaged as possible in the process and to keep them as fully informed as possible. The essential elements of a good referral letter can be found in Table 7.3.

TABLE 7.3 *The essential elements of a referral letter*

Patient demographics
   Date of birth
   Address
   National Health Service number
   Telephone number

Description of the presenting problem
   Reason for referral
   Main presenting symptoms

Related medical information relevant to the problem
Relevant past medical history
Relevant social history
Current medications and relevant past medications
Relevant results of investigations
What the patient's expectations might be (if relevant)

Varying amounts of information will be included in referral letters according to the complexity of the clinical situation. An example of a referral letter is shown below.

Respiratory Consultants
Respiratory Clinic

Dear Colleague

Thank you for seeing this 82-year-old patient with ongoing problems with a productive cough. The problems date back to the end of 2004 when he had the first of several episodes involving a cough that does not respond to asthma medication or antibiotics. This has been an ongoing problem involving periods of exacerbation and periods of improvement. When he has the cough he tends to produce thick, green sputum, which is extremely difficult to expectorate and results in breathlessness.

A number of sputum analyses have demonstrated the presence of a variety of organisms including staphylococcus, *Escherichia coli*, *Haemophilus influenzae* and mixed upper respiratory tract organisms.

On examination in between exacerbations, he is able to speak in full sentences, has relaxed breathing, does not use accessory muscles and his chest size and shape is normal. He has no lymphadenopathy. He has good air entry throughout the chest exam, heart sounds are normal, respiratory rate is 22 per minute and pulse rate is 86 per minute, pulse oximetry is 96%. Chest X-rays have been carried out in 2004 and 2005 and they are normal. His most recent spirometry shows FVC 1.88 L, VC 1.88 L, FEV1 1.38 L, FEV1% 95%, FEV/FVC ratio 82 and PEFR 230.

This patient has never smoked, he has a past history of asthma and a history of cancer of the prostate in 2000. Current medication includes alendhronic acid tablets 70 mg once weekly 30 minutes before food, beclomethasone inhaler 200 µg/actuation two puffs twice daily and salbutamol 200 µg two puffs four times daily as required.

The remainder of his significant active and past medical problems can be found at the bottom of this letter.

In recent months he has tried a mucolytic, which has been helpful in easing the symptoms. Unfortunately, he continues to have distressing exacerbations of the cough, which is just not responding to the normal course of treatments.

Yours sincerely

Nurse practitioner

Medical history: active problems		Significant past		
2005	Hearing loss	2005	Standard chest radiograph	Normal
2004	Osteoporosis	2004	Standard chest radiograph	Normal
2004	Cough	2003	Supraspinatus tendinitis	
2002	Renal impairment	2000	Carcinoma of prostate	
2002	Asthma	1987	Essential hypertension	
1995	Adverse reaction to Micropore			

Acts as an advocate for the patient to ensure health needs are met consistent with patient's wishes

Advocacy is a complex concept that raises a number of moral and ethical dilemmas. It seems to be a reasonably straightforward issue when considered superficially, as it would seem obvious that all nurses should aim to act as an advocate for patients' wishes. The issue becomes less clear when we consider that people who are racists have wishes and might not want to be treated by a doctor or nurse of a certain culture or other patients who are paedophiles may wish to continue to abuse children. Clearly, there are certain circumstances where it is totally inappropriate to act as an advocate for a particular patient. If we set this difficulty aside and we understand that advocacy cannot be seen as a general principle applicable to all patients (Walsh 2000) it is possible to consider times when patient advocacy is an important and necessary function of ANP practice.

According to Baldwin (2003), for advocacy to be required it is first necessary to have a vulnerable patient who is facing conflict and second to have a nurse who is willing to take on the responsibility of advocacy. The nurse must be prepared to understand the patient's wishes and must be proactive as well as reactive in taking on the advocacy role. Often this can result in conflict with other members of the health care team as the nurse speaks on behalf of the patient and tries to make sure that the patient's views are heard. The benefit of advocacy, when it is used appropriately, is that the patient will be empowered, their autonomy will be preserved and their wishes will be acted upon. Scenario 7.3 provides an example of a situation where advocacy was necessary.

Scenario 7.3

A patient with diabetes was attending the regular clinic at the surgery. She was obese and was having great difficulty reducing her weight. The nurse reviewed her in the clinic and found that her HBA1c (glycosylated haemoglobin) was rising and it was time to change her medication. Unfortunately, she experienced severe side-effects with metformin and could only tolerate one 500 mg tablet daily; rosiglitazone had been prescribed previously but she had experienced ankle swelling and breathlessness and this had been stopped for fear of worsening heart failure. She was taking half the maximum dose of gliclazide but she had reported worsening diarrhoea as the dose had increased. It seemed likely that the patient should start insulin and the nurse asked her to think about this.

Immediately after the consultation with the nurse the patient saw the GP about another matter. Because of her weight and rising HBA1c he threatened her with insulin and said she had to change her diet 'or else'. He recommended that she kept a diet diary and asked her to return after a few days. She carried out his wishes and he asked her to change her diet and to return for further blood tests in 6 weeks' time.

When the nurse heard what had happened she spoke with the GP offering an alternative point of view, including the patient's willingness to try insulin. She described the way in which this lady had struggled with obesity for many years and had been unable to make much change to her diet, even though she had received all the information and support from a variety of health care practitioners including other GPs, nurses and the dietician. Eventually the care of this particular patient was handed back to the nurse and over time the patient moved on to insulin. She no longer took oral medication and so the problems with diarrhoea settled completely. Her marriage, which had been under threat because of her diarrhoea and flatulence, settled down and became more harmonious. She remained overweight but her mental health improved.

Scenario 7.3 describes a patient who was vulnerable and disempowered by the GP's actions. She went along with his request as she did not want to upset him although it had no impact on her weight. The nurse needed to be willing to take on the responsibility of advocating for this patient and also needed to be prepared to enter into conflict with the GP. Ultimately, the patient felt empowered to make her own decision, but the whole situation threatened the relationship between the patient and the doctor and the doctor and the nurse. It was important to make sure that the nurse was properly representing the patient's wishes as it was possible that inappropriate assumptions had been made, and in fact some patients might have responded positively to the GP's approach. In this particular case, the patient and the patient's family seemed to benefit from the advocacy role of the nurse practitioner, but this situation does highlight the delicate and complex nature of representing patients' wishes and demonstrates the skill and sensitivity required when acting as the patient's advocate.

Consults with other health care providers and public/independent agencies

There is a degree of autonomy in the nurse practitioner role and nurses who work at this advanced level of practice are expected to take on the responsibility of autonomous decision-making. Although this is an important marker for advanced practice, it is equally important to be aware of the limitations of your practice and to recognize when another health care practitioner can provide the services you cannot. It is therefore important to take every opportunity to become aware of local health care providers and other agencies and to consult with them and refer to them whenever appropriate. Building this network initially takes time and effort, but the patient will benefit as they receive the appropriate advice and support at the appropriate time.

Incorporates current technology appropriately in care delivery

There are numerous ways in which current technology is used in daily practice. The nurse practitioner needs to remain aware of developments both in equipment and in computer software to assist in the delivery of care to patients. For example, ANPs have been at the forefront of bringing spirometry into general practice, which has now become a routine and standard procedure, and nurse practitioners in hospital settings are using endoscopes to carry out investigative procedures. Scenario 7.4 describes how practice was changed in one region after a nurse practitioner used the latest evidence in patients with diabetes.

Scenario 7.4

Having developed a specific interest in people with diabetes, a nurse practitioner spent some time searching for the latest papers relating to the complication of nephropathy. In the process it became apparent that testing for microalbuminuria was important. A positive finding could lead to treatment which would prevent further deterioration of the patient's renal function, and in some cases would reverse the damage that was already present (Panayiotou 1994). On the strength of this, the practice changed its diabetes protocol and started to test all patients for microalbuminuria on an annual basis. As the tests started to arrive in the pathology laboratory, the director noticed there had been an increase in requests for microalbuminuria testing and called the practice to ask what was happening. A discussion with the director of the laboratory ensued and he was sent the relevant papers to provide the evidence to support annual testing for patients with diabetes. He agreed to the testing and gradually the practice became more commonplace across the region and was not met with any further opposition. Microalbuminuria testing is now standard practice in diabetes care and a decade later it has become one of the quality indicators in the new General Medical Services (nGMS) contract in primary care (NHS Confederation and BMA 2006).

In addition to technological advances in testing and investigations, the ANP has a variety of tools on the computer to help support patient care. Expertise in the use of computer systems is critical to facilitate the analysis of practice. Databases can be used to carry out audits, which can lead to changes in clinical practice. Carrying out an audit can help to educate everyone involved in the process; it can enhance teamwork and help people to understand one another's roles in more depth. The audit cycle is outlined in Figure 7.2 and this highlights the need to engage the team in the process and to act upon the findings of the work.

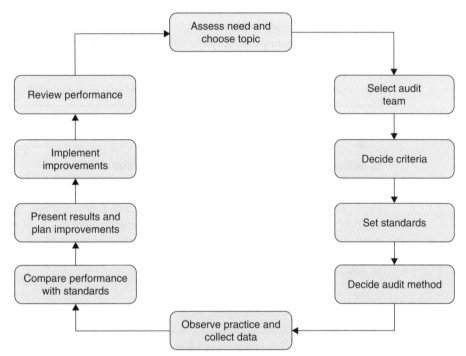

FIGURE 7.2 *Audit cycle.*

Uses information systems to support decision-making and to improve care

The ANP will have a variety of information systems available to assist in the decision-making process. In some instances this can be used in partnership with patients to provide them with the latest evidence and equip them with the necessary information to make an informed choice about their care. The reflective practitioner will regularly review even the most routine conditions encountered in daily practice to ensure that advice given is accurate, current and well informed. Examples of decision-support information systems can be found in Table 7.4.

TABLE 7.4 *Examples of decision–support information systems*

NHS Direct: http://www.nhsdirect.nhs.uk
Patient UK: http://www.patient.co.uk/pils.asp
Prodigy: http://www.prodigy.nhs.uk
Clinical Evidence: http://www.nelh.nhs.uk/clinicalevidence

There are also numerous processes available to the nurse which will be built into the basic clinical computer systems, such as the Framingham risk calculator and automatic electronic checks of drug interactions when prescribing.

KEY POINTS

- Cultural sensitivity can be achieved by working with individual patients and by addressing organizational issues.
- Sensitive professional judgement is required to work with patients who often have complex needs and concerns.
- Develop and maintain good relationships with your clinical team.
- Network with other clinicians who work outside your immediate organization.
- Patient advocacy, used appropriately, is respectful of patients' wishes.
- Keep up to date with technological advances and information technology.

PROVIDES LEADERSHIP

Is actively involved in a professional association

Professional associations can be a source of support, inspiration and education, particularly when nurses are developing and creating new roles. The ANP could find a variety of associations to be beneficial. Active involvement in a local network can be useful in addressing local problems and challenges as it provides a forum for a group of people to form a pressure group to help develop new ways of working and to ensure the group is listened to.

Scenario 7.5

A group of nurse practitioners working within one primary care trust (PCT) decided to develop an informal network to share ideas and experiences and to provide a forum for education and development. The group decided to share significant events at each meeting and to offer support and advice to each other. It became apparent that a shared problem was the difficulty the nurse practitioners had with referral to the radiography departments throughout the trust, with examples of patients being turned away from the radiography department because their request card had not been signed by a GP. Nurse practitioners within the local minor injuries unit had been approved to sign radiography forms and so the nurse practitioners within the general practice setting approached the director of radiology to ask for approval.

A letter was sent from the group to the director, and after several months had lapsed a response was received which stated that the nurse practitioners would have to receive training in radiation safety and would have to provide evidence that they were fully qualified nurse practitioners. In addition, the radiology department wanted to develop a policy on the referral process for non-medical practitioners and requested that each nurse practitioner should develop their own protocol which was countersigned by a GP in their place of practice. The nurse practitioners worked together to develop a protocol for radiograph referrals. Examples of protocols from other areas of the country were found by accessing the Nurse Practitioner Association (NPA) web site (http://www.npa. org.uk). The protocol was adapted by each of the practices and was signed by the GPs. There were long delays while the radiology department reached agreement on a policy for non-medical referrals and this was followed by a further delay while the nurse practitioners waited for the radiation safety training to be provided. Eventually each qualified nurse practitioner in the PCT had submitted the necessary documentation, had attended the training events and had agreed to the radiology department's policy on referral. Finally the nurse practitioners began to sign the radiograph forms and their patients had fewer delays in accessing the care they needed.

Scenario 7.5 provides an example of the way a local group of nurse practitioners used their collective strength to change local practices. They also sought assistance from their colleagues elsewhere in the country who had been through a similar process. The group's links with the national NPA were helpful in achieving this. In order to assist others the local group uploaded a copy of their protocol onto the NPA website so that they in turn could contribute to the development of ANP practice elsewhere in the UK. There are numerous benefits to being involved in a professional association. This is just one small example of how working together can enhance the efficient use of resources within the NHS. Ultimately such collaboration benefits patients who then face fewer delays and are saved from duplicate consultations because the practitioner with whom they are consulting has been provided with the necessary tools to meet their needs. A copy of the protocol can be found in Appendix 2.

Evaluates implications of contemporary health policy on health care providers and consumers

Across the UK the last decade has seen the introduction of many policies which have had major implications for health care consumers. The National Service Frameworks (NSFs) for England and Wales are examples of contemporary health policy that have implications for consumers and providers. For example, the NSF for Coronary Heart Disease (Department of Health 2000) has created a 10-year programme for improving services for heart disease. Standards have been set for the whole of coronary heart disease-related care, from health promotion, emergency care, specialist services and surgery through to rehabilitation. The NSF even provides details of cholesterol targets for people with heart disease, and these set the standard for treatment with cholesterol-lowering medication until the more recent British Hypertension Society Guidelines reduced the targets for lipid lowering even further (Williams et al. 2004). NSFs also exist for health services for children, for renal services, for people with cancer, mental health issues, long-term conditions, diabetes and for older people to name but a few. In Scotland, clinical guidelines are provided by the Scottish Intercollegiate Guidelines Network (SIGN), which aims to reduce variation in practice and clinical outcomes across Scotland (Scottish Intercollegiate Guidelines Network 2006). There are 90 guidelines, ranging from the management of dementia to the management of suspected bacterial urinary tract infection in adults. In Northern Ireland contemporary health policy can be accessed by visiting the

Department of Health, Social Services and Public Safety website (see details below), which provides information on issues such as immunization, waiting lists and sun safety as well as the latest guidance from the chief medical officer and guidelines for the management of a flu pandemic.

In addition to policy relating to specific conditions, the Departments of Health have numerous policy statements relating to broad strategy and direction of travel. For example, the Cumberlege report on community nursing has provided the groundwork for the development of nurse practitioners in the UK by stating that 'the principle should be adopted of introducing the nurse practitioner into primary health care' (Department of Health 1986: 32). In 1991 the National Health Service Executive Management published *Junior doctors: the new deal*, which paved the way for the reduction in junior doctors' hours (National Health Service Executive 1991) and resulted in the development of a need for nurses to advance their roles and to take on some of the work that had previously been the domain of doctors. More recently a government document *Making a difference: strengthening the nursing, midwifery and health visiting contribution to health and health care* (DoH 1999a) recognized the developing role of nurses in the provision of health care.

It can be challenging keeping up to date with all the latest policy developments, and yet many of them have a direct impact upon the work of nurse practitioners and hence upon the care of patients. One method is to regularly access the relevant website for your country. It is also possible to receive regular electronic bulletins from the chief nursing officer by registering your contact details on the Department of Health website (Table 7.5).

Participates in legislative and policy-making activities that influence an advanced level of nursing practice and the health of communities

Policy development occurs at local, regional and national level and there are opportunities for the nurse practitioner to be involved, and indeed to lead the way, at any of these levels. At the local level, policy development is necessary to ensure that local clinical practice remains current and in line with national trends and in accordance with the latest evidence. An example of such a development is the management of hypertension in general practice, which has required regular updates as guidance on the management of hypertension has changed in recent years (Ramsay et al. 1999, Williams et al. 2004, British Hypertension Society 2006). The development of referral guidelines for radiographs outlined above is an example of

TABLE 7.5   *The web sites for the Departments of Health in the four countries of the UK*

England
Department of Health: http://www.dh.gov.uk

Wales
National Assembly for Wales: http://www.wales.gov.uk/subihealth/index.htm

Scotland
The Scottish Executive Health Department: http://www.sehd.scot.nhs.uk/

Northern Ireland
Department of Health, Social Services and Public Safety: http://www.dhsspsni.gov.uk/

the ANP's involvement in policy-making activities at the regional level. At the national level there are opportunities for nurses to comment on developments at the NMC, and in recent years the most obvious example of this has been the consultation on post-registration practice and the proposed competencies for ANP practice (NMC 2005).

Advocates for access to quality, cost-effective health care

Determining the cost-effectiveness of certain health care interventions can be a complex and difficult process. Equally, evaluating the quality of health care can be difficult and may not be as straightforward as it might first appear (see Chapter 8). Nonetheless, it is important for all ANPs to be aware of the cost of particular interventions and to consider whether they are using NHS resources wisely. Certain prescribing habits can have an enormous impact upon the cost of health care and careful analysis of prescribing practice can result in impressive savings for the NHS. Savings can be achieved by making simple switches to generic products with no detrimental effect on the patient. Yet more saving can be achieved by making informed and considered decisions when selecting a drug within a particular class of drugs. An example of this is the selection of an angiotensin-converting enzyme inhibitor (ACEI) for the management of hypertension with no other co-morbidity. The annual cost of ACEI prescriptions per patient can range from £21.79 to £187.41, depending upon the drug selected, and yet there is no proven difference in efficacy between the groups in relation to the reduction in blood pressure (Drugs and Therapeutics Bulletin 1995).

Evaluates the relationship between community/public health issues and social problems as they impact on the health care of patients (poverty, literacy, violence, etc.)

Once again it is necessary for the ANP to take a reflective, analytical stance to consider which public health issues are significant in the patient population with whom they are working. The early nurse practitioners such as Burke-Masters and Stilwell, who provided health care services in areas of poor GP recruitment (Kenny 1997, Barr 2006) are good examples of the ANP not only evaluating the relationship between community health issues and social problems but also acting upon that finding. It is worthwhile considering how easy it is to access your service. Do patients have to pay for taxis because they are unable to park at your surgery? Are patients able to read the educational materials you give them, and if not what impact will that have upon their ability to understand and act upon their treatment plan?

Smoking is a good example of the way in which social issues impact upon the health care of patients. In the UK approximately 28% of men and 24% of women smoke cigarettes (British Heart Foundation 2004). The proportion is highest in the 16–24 age group and declines with age (Department of Health 1999b). Smoking varies within various ethnic groups, for example males from the Bangladeshi and Caribbean communities show particularly high smoking rates: 42% and 34% respectively (British Heart Foundation 2004). Smoking also varies within different social groups; one-third of people in manual households smoke compared with one-fifth in non-manual households, and rates are higher in Scotland than they are in England, Wales and Northern Ireland, and tend to be higher in the north of England and the Midlands than they are in the south (British Heart Foundation 2004). These statistics highlight the impact a person's social group, ethnicity and place of residence will have upon their likelihood of developing health problems associated with smoking. The ANP needs to be aware of these issues and to take note of them when working with patients in their efforts to make lifestyle changes. Clearly a person whose social group routinely engages in smoking is going to have much greater difficulty in stopping smoking than one who is surrounded by motivated, supportive non-smokers.

Actively engages in continuous professional development and maintains a suitable record of this development

The NMC's post-registration education and practice (PREP) guidelines (NMC 2006) aim to ensure that the best possible care is provided for patients by encouraging nurses to reflect on their practice and remain up to date with developments. It is quite clear that thinking about your practice, reflecting on strengths and weaknesses, engaging in lifelong learning, creating a personal development plan and keeping it live are vital to ensure that you keep in touch with current practice and that your patients receive the best possible care. The personal development plan (PDP) is an ideal tool to enable you to highlight the ways in which you meet the NMC's competencies for ANP practice (NMC 2005). It also helps to reveal any areas that could be focused on for development in the coming year.

A good starting point for the personal development plan is to carry out a SWOT analysis on yourself. The SWOT analysis was mentioned earlier in relation to the analysis of the strengths and weaknesses of an organization (see Figure 7.1). When applied to individuals, the SWOT analysis can be used to identify personal strengths and opportunities for development and personal weaknesses and threats to professional progression. You can enlist the help of colleagues to carry out a SWOT analysis, as other people will often have a different perspective to your own. Having carried out a preliminary analysis it is possible then to identify achievable goals and these can be brought together in a development plan. It is important to consider how you intend to achieve the goals and to write down how long you expect it might take you.

Once the PDP has been developed it is then important to share your goals and objectives with your employer, or in the case of nurse partners with a colleague (Crumbie and Kyle 2006). An employer can then consider how your personal plan matches the vision of the organization and will often review your PDP at the time of the annual appraisal. Figure 7.3 provides a summary of the PDP process.

Professional development should be dynamic, live and continuous. It is not simply a process that you have to go through once a year. It is important, therefore, to continually review your objectives and to gradually collect the documentation to demonstrate that you are working towards your goals and the evidence to show which goals you have achieved. Examples of what documentation might support the PDP process can be found in Table 7.6.

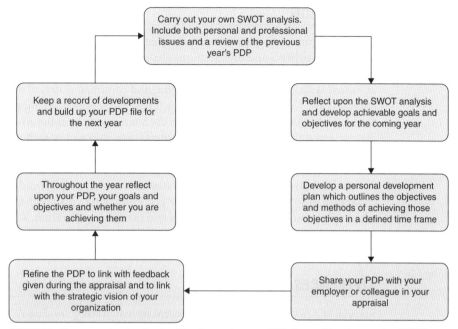

FIGURE 7.3 *The personal and professional development process. PDP, Personal development plan; SWOT, strengths, weaknesses, opportunities and threats.*

TABLE 7.6 *Documentation to support the personal development plan (PDP) process*

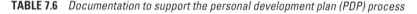

Current PDP
PDP from the previous year
Feedback from colleagues and patients
Significant events
Audits and actions based on the findings
Study days and conferences attended and a record of what you learnt
Courses attended and a record of what you learnt
Involvement in the teaching and support of students
Protocols developed
Involvement in research
Presentations
Publications
Involvement in local charities or other voluntary work

KEY POINTS

- Network with other ANPs both locally and nationally.
- Keep in touch with the direction of local and national policy changes.
- Consider the cost-effectiveness of your practice.
- Consider the public health issues facing your community.
- Keep a record of personal and professional development.
- Personal and professional development should be accurate, relevant and live and this can be achieved through regular reflection and by sharing it with a colleague.

CONCLUSION

The very nature of ANP practice implies that the role should develop and change as the needs of patients and organizations change over time. It is therefore essential to embrace change and to be prepared to be flexible and dynamic. This relies upon the advanced skills of reflection and evaluation and continual efforts to update your clinical skills. You need to remain in touch with latest policy developments at both the local and the national level and with the latest research on the advanced role of the nurse practitioner. The role also involves leadership and as such you are not only keeping in touch and updating your clinical work in line with national trends, but you are also leading the way by using critical reflection, evaluation, the views of patients and carers and a review of the latest evidence to propose and implement changes in practice. Development of the professional role is a never-ending process which, when carried out with sensitivity and careful consideration, will have a lasting benefit to your organization and will ultimately, and most importantly, improve the care of the patients with whom you work.

REFERENCES

Baldwin, M. (2003) Patient advocacy: a concept analysis. *Nursing Standard* 17: 33–39.

Barr, F. (2006) Celebrating 20 years of nurse practitioners. *Independent Nurse* 28 August: 26–27.

Benner, P. (1984) *From novice to expert.* California: Addison Wesley.

Blackie, C. (1998) Community health care nursing in primary health care: a shared future. In *Community health care nursing*, Blackie, C. (ed.), pp. 83–104. Edinburgh: Churchill Livingstone.

British Heart Foundation (2004) Coronary heart disease statistics. http://www.heartstats.org/ (accessed on 17/03/06).

British Hypertension Society (2006) NICE/BHS hypertension guideline review 28 June 2006 http://www.bhsoc.org/NICE_BHS_Guidelines.stm (accessed on 16/08/06).

Cooper, M. A., Lindsay, G. M., Kinn, S. and Swann, J. (2002) Evaluating emergency nurse practitioner services: a randomized controlled trial. *Journal of Advanced Nursing* 40: 721–730.

Crawford, M. (1997) In debate. Delegation: should nurses do the GP's job? *Surgery OTC Review* August: 4.

Crumbie, A. and Kyle, L. (2006) Nurse partnership: the challenge of appraisal. *Primary Health Care* 16: 14–16.

Department of Health (1986) *Neighbourhood nursing: a focus for care. A report of the community nursing review.* London: HMSO.

Department of Health (1999a) *Making a difference: strengthening the nursing midwifery and health visiting contribution to health and health care.* London: HMSO.

Department of Health (1999b) *Health survey for England. Cardiovascular disease 1998.* London: DoH.

Department of Health (2000) *The national service framework for coronary heart disease.* London: DoH.

Dickson, N. Pearson, P. Emmerson, P. Davison, N. and Griffith, M. (1996) Are nurse practitioners merely substitute doctors? *Professional Nurse* 11: 325–328.

Drugs and Therapeutics Bulletin (1995) Who needs nine ACE inhibitors? *Drugs and Therapeutics Bulletin* 33(1): 1–3.

Fitzpatrick, R. (1993) Scope and measurement of patient satisfaction. In *Measurement of patient's satisfaction with their care,* Fitzpatrick, R. and Hopkins, A. (eds), pp. 1–17. London: Royal College of Physicians.

Hollinghurst, S. Horrocks, S. Anderson, E. and Salisbury, C. J. (2006) Comparing the cost of nurse practitioners and GPs in primary care. *British Journal of General Practice* 56: 530–535.

Hooker, R. and Mayo, H. (2002) Doctoral dissertations on nurse practitioners: 1970–2000. *Journal of the American Academy of Nurse Practitioners* 14: 276–284.

Horrocks, S. Anderson, E. and Salisbury, C. (2002) Systematic review of whether nurse practitioners working in primary care can provide equivalent care to doctors. *British Medical Journal* 324: 819–823.

Jesson, A.M. Karar, P. Sanal, E. and Cox, L. (2006) Coping with diabetes project, Hackney diabetes centre. *Practical Diabetes International* 23: 62–65.

Kenny, C. (1997) Fighter pilots. *Nursing Standard* 93: 14–15.

Kinnersley, P. Anderson, E. Parry, K. Clement, J. Archard, L. Turton, P. Stainthorpe, A. Fraser, A. Butler, C.C. and Rogers, C. (2000) Randomized controlled trial of nurse practitioner versus general practitioner care for patients requesting 'same day' consultations in primary care. *British Medical Journal* 320: 1043–1048.

Laurant, M. Hermens, R. Braspenning, J. Sibbald, B. and Grol, R. (2004) Impact of nurse practitioners on workload of general practitioners: randomized controlled trial. *British Medical Journal* 328: 927–933.

Marsh, G.N. and Dawes, M. L. (1995) Establishing a minor illness nurse in a busy general practice *British Medical Journal* 310: 778–780.

Merkouris, A. Ifantopoulos, J. Lanarva, V. and Lemonidou, C. (1999) Patient satisfaction: a key concept for evaluating and improving nursing services. *Journal of Nursing Management* 7: 19–28.

National Health Service Executive (1991) *Junior doctors: the new deal.* London: National Health Service Executive Management.

National Health Service Executive (1996) *Nurse practitioner evaluation project: final report.* Uxbridge: Coopers and Lybrand.

NHS Confederation and BMA (2006) Revisions to the GMS contract 2006/7. Delivering investment in general practice. http://www.nhsemployers.org (accessed on 15/08/06).

NMC (2005) *Consultation on a framework for the standard of post registration nursing.* http://www.nmc-uk.org/aFrameDisplay.aspx?DocumentID=933 (accessed on 24/07/06)

NMC (2006) *The PREP handbook.* http://www.nmc-uk.org/aFrameDisplay.aspx?Document ID=1636 (accessed on 24/07/06)

Panayiotou, B. (1994) Microalbuminuria: pathogenesis, prognosis and management. *The Journal of International Medical Research* 22: 181–201.

Pritchard, P. and Pritchard, J. (1994) *Teamwork for primary and shared care.* Oxford: Oxford Medical Publications.

Ramsay, L.E. Williams, B. Johnston, G.D. MacGregor, G.A. Poston, L. Potter, J.F. Poulter, N.R. and Russell, G. (1999) Guidelines for management of hypertension: report of the third working party of the British Hypertension Society. *Journal of Human Hypertension* 13: 569–592.

Reveley, S. (1999) The role of the triage nurse practitioner in general medical practice: an analysis of the role. *Journal of Advanced Nursing* 28: 584–591.

Salisbury, C. J. and Tettersell, M. J. (1988) Comparison of the work of a nurse practitioner with that of a general practitioner. *Journal of the Royal College of General Practice* 38: 314–316.

Scottish Intercollegiate Guidelines Network (2006) What is SIGN? http://www.sign.ac.uk/about/introduction.html (accessed on 26/10/06).

Sharples, L.D. Edmunds, J. Bilton, D. Hollingworth, W. Caine, N. Keogan, M. and Exley, A. (2002) A randomized controlled crossover trail of nurse practitioner versus doctor led outpatient care in a bronchiectasis clinic. *Thorax* 57: 661–666.

SIGN (1998) Report on a recommended referral document. http://www.sign.ac.uk/guidelines/fulltext/31/section1.html (accessed on 08/08/06).

Smith, S. (1992) The rise of the nurse practitioner. *Community Outlook* November/December: 16–17.

South Thames Regional Health Authority (1994) *Evaluation of nurse practitioner pilot projects: summary report.* London: Touche Roche Management Consultants.

Stilwell, B. (1981) Role expansion for the nurse. *Journal of Community Nursing* 5: 17–18.

Stilwell, B. (1985) Opportunities in general practice. *Nursing Mirror* 161: 30–31.

Stilwell, B. Greenfield, S. Drury, M. and Hull, F. M. (1987) A nurse practitioner in general practice: working style and pattern of consultations. *Journal of the Royal College of General Practice* 37: 154–157.

Venning, P. Durie, A. Roland, M. Roberts, C. and Leese, B. (2000) Randomized controlled trial comparing cost effectiveness of general practitioners and nurse practitioners in primary care. *British Medical Journal* 320: 1048–1053.

Wadsworth, L. Smith, A. and Wateman, H. (2002) The nurse practitioner's role in day case surgery preoperative assessment. *Nursing Standard* 16: 41–44.

Walsh, M. (2000) *Nursing frontiers. Accountability and the boundaries of care.* Butterworth-Heinemann, Oxford.

Walsh, M. and Howkins, D. (2002) Lessons from a farmers' health service. *Nursing Standard* 16: 33–40.

Williams, B. Poulter, N.R. Brown, M.J. Davis, M. McInnes, G.T. Potter, J.P. Sever, P.S. and Thom, S.McG, (2004) The BHS Guidelines Working Party (2004) British Hypertension Society Guidelines for Hypertension Management – BHS IV: Summary: *British Medical Journal* 328: 634–640.

FURTHER READING

Rashotte, J. (2005) Knowing the nurse practitioner: dominant discourses shaping our horizons: *Nursing Philosophy* 6: 51–62.

An excellent article which challenges us to think about the nurse practitioner role and how we define it.

Reveley, S. Walsh, M. and Crumbie, A. (2001) *Nurse practitioners developing the role in hospital settings:* Oxford: Butterworth-Heinemann.

A useful text for nurses who are considering developing the role in hospital settings. There are good case studies in this book highlighting some of the barriers and how these were overcome.

Walsh, M. (2005) *Nurse practitioners; clinical skills and professional issues.* Oxford: Butterworth-Heinemann.

A useful text for beginning nurse practitioners. Legal issues are considered alongside clinical skills.

8

DOMAIN 6: MANAGING AND NEGOTIATING HEALTH CARE DELIVERY SYSTEMS

DAVE BARTON

INTRODUCTION

This chapter reviews the advanced nurse practitioner (ANP) domain of 'managing and negotiating health care delivery systems' (NMC 2006a). As such, it offers a student ANP an introduction to this domain, it details the domain's competencies and then, by reference to clinical scenarios, it reviews the range and diversity of evidence that can be gathered for use in the portfolio. Thus, a central focus of this chapter is that of 'clinical evidence', what is it, how may it arise, and where the student ANP may identify and find it in any clinical situation. However, from the outset it is implicit that, although this chapter will suggest and describe possible sources and examples of clinical evidence, a student ANP must (when recording these evidences in practice and in their portfolio) accord with local and national guidelines that pertain to confidentiality issues.

To begin with, it is necessary to review the nature of this domain, what it is really about, and to consider why it is a domain that is of serious concern for a student ANP. For example, what is meant by the domain title that states that an ANP has to 'manage and negotiate health care delivery systems'? At face value, this may seem a simple assertion, but it will quickly become apparent that it is weighed down with ambiguous meanings. Reviewing the domain title will lead to questions on the differences (and similarities) between the terms 'managing' and 'negotiating'. Are they quite separate terms, or are they closely linked, and if they are linked, is their relation context (theory) based or practice (clinically) based? Is 'managing' the same as 'management', or is one the result of the other, where managing is viewed as a process that arises from management? Is management primarily a process that maintains an organization's function and aim, or can management challenge an organization's function? In contrast, can negotiation be interpreted as a process that arises from management and/or as a process that seeks to maintain the status quo, or to challenge it and initiate change?

Consider also what is understood by the term 'health care delivery systems'. This somewhat 'designer' management term provides a diversity, and a wealth, of meanings and interpretations, ranging from focused 'micro' practical issues (such as drug protocols, care plans, specific therapeutic regimes), through to the more 'macro' global systems (health service initiatives, national service frameworks and targets, management structures, business strategies) that enable large health care organizations (hospitals/community services) to function. Indeed, health care delivery systems are not confined to the traditional health service organizations, but will include social, educational, private and voluntary organizations.

Now consider in more detail the term 'delivery': the inclusion of this term within this domain is significant in its own right, and should draw a student ANP's attention to an expectation of health care as a consumer service, a service that must 'deliver' a social outcome and need. By inference, if an expectation is that a service should deliver (a service, a product), then another possibility is that it could fail to deliver that service! Consequently, this investigation of the domain title has introduced the concept of customer expectation, service and organizational efficiency and quality, and resultant quality assurance needs.

It may appear that this deconstruction is simply playing with words, but it is important to understand how easy it is for this domain to be misunderstood. Thus, we must unpick and develop our understanding of the underlying theoretical and practical concepts if a student ANP is to collect evidence meaningfully on this domain – evidence that will contribute to insights and abilities as a future ANP. What may at first have appeared to be a rather bland domain emerges, in reality, as a complex and diffuse matrix of professional and organizational concepts (Figure 8.1).

Figure 8.1. models this matrix of concepts, revealing the continuous interactions between the varying levels of organizational influence on management of change and stability in health care delivery. Central to this constant organizational interplay is

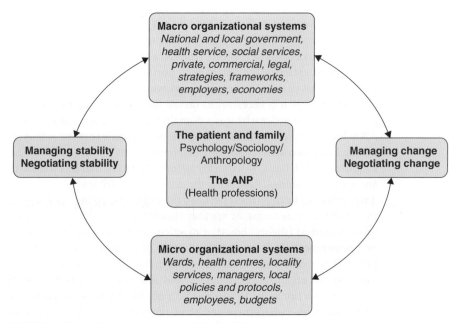

FIGURE 8.1 *The matrix of managing and negotiating health care.*

the patient (and their family). Although they exist in the wider social context, influenced by the complexities of society, of culture of individuality, it is their interaction and dealings with health care organizations, and with health care professionals (specifically the ANP), that is of concern here.

Definitions in health care are rarely comprehensive, and are subject to constant change as the world of clinical work is constantly evolving. However, I offer the following definition, as it may be of use, and give the reader a foundation for the domain's meaning.

> Managing and negotiating health care delivery systems is an advanced nurse practitioner domain concerned primarily with the practitioner's ability to identify the scope and range of organizational structures, health care roles, health care rules and regulation, health care groups, strategies, protocols, material resources and human resources, and selectively utilize them to the advantage of the patient or client group.

Using this definition enables a perspective of this domain as one that focuses on the wide-ranging social and management structures of health care organizations. Despite its broad scope, it is a competency domain that is core for a student ANP in interpreting and understanding the wider practice standard for advanced nursing practice. The aim of this chapter is to tackle those issues, to examine clinical practice in such a way that a student ANP can identify and evidence their own skills within this domain. To that end, the chapter structures itself naturally around the domain's explicit themes and components, most specifically into the two core areas of 'managing' and 'negotiating'. It also directly links this professional domain to the Knowledge and Skills Framework (DoH 2004a), enabling a student ANP to make judgements on their professional activity within that of the national framework for health care professionals.

KEY POINTS

- A general overview of the ANP domain of 'managing and negotiating health care delivery systems'.
- Deconstructing the domain meaning.
- The scope of influence – from focused 'micro' practical issues to 'macro' global systems.
- Acknowledging the continuous interactions between organizational management of change and stability in health care delivery.

THE ANP: MANAGING AND NEGOTIATING HEALTH CARE DELIVERY

The demand for evidence-based clinical practice in health care is also a demand that a student ANP should examine the range of factors that influence their clinical decisions. However, the literature also suggests that there are differences between the culture, research base and decision-making processes of clinicians and health care managers (Walshe and Rundall 2001). Thus, whereas health care managers encourage the clinician's use of an evidence-based approach towards clinical interventions, there exists a difference between the factors that influence the clinician's decision-making, and the factors that influence the health manager's decision-making. A student ANP can use this domain to analyse and acknowledge those differences, and, where possible, explore their integration so that a more holistic process of managing and negotiating health care needs can result.

ANPs are intimately involved in managing care, making decisions daily, not only about individual patient's care needs but also about the environments in which their patients are nursed. Thus, it is perfectly reasonable to view management of health care delivery as concerned with maintaining the specifics of a patient's needs, overcoming organizational, professional and role barriers, and ensuring that a wider health organization functions as it should (Jones 2005). Why then would an ANP also wish to 'negotiate' about a process that is essentially focused on maintenance and stability? The answer is simply that the process of maintaining (managing) a system's stability requires that occupational demands, stresses and strains that affect a system's normal functioning be identified, be best utilized or (if necessary) be prevented (Furlong and Smith 2005). It follows that in any system that involves humans – and most systems do involve humans in one way or another (Handy 1996) – the process of managing organizational aims and occupational and role demands, stresses and strains will require the manager to negotiate with others.

ANPs make complex decisions about their patient's care, and those decisions can actively challenge, or change, the status quo, resulting not only in changes in specific care management but also in more general changes to the patient's health care environment (Trnobranski 1994, Williams and Valdivieso 1994, Rasch and Frauman 1996, Hunt 1999, Pearson and Peels 2002, Barton 2006). The concept of change is a core construct and theme for a student ANP, who should understand that decision-making is 'in effect' the initiation of change, and change is facilitated by negotiation with individuals, groups and organizations. These negotiations relate to the transitional systems that professionals use to enact their health care role, or relate to the organizations and regulations that govern groups of individuals in a health care context (Williamson 1996, Swansburg and Swansburg 2001, West 2001, Newbold 2005). Thus, the link between change, managing and negotiation is clear, and may be described in one of two ways:

1 'Managing' as a process that aims to maintain the current function of a health care role, system or organization. This requires negotiation to defend that health care role, system or organization from unwanted change agents and optimize its current performance.
2 'Managing' as a process that seeks to initiate change to a health care role, system or organization. This requires negotiation to prepare that health care role, system or organization for change, and negotiation that aims to overcome resistance, and optimize new outcomes.

Of course, nothing is ever quite that simple! An ANP may engage in a multitude of managing (management) activities that require a blend of negotiations that seek to provide stability and change all at once. To compound that difficulty, an ANP has to consider the many national and local competency and skill frameworks, all of which place great emphasis on health care management. Simply put, an ANP cannot be content with being a good clinician and a clinical expert, they must also acknowledge their role as a health care manager who affects and effects care systems and patient care, at both micro- and macro-level.

It is for these reasons that this domain has such importance to the ANP role.

KEY POINTS

- The demand for the student ANP to examine the organizational factors that influence their clinical decisions.
- Using the domain to analysis and acknowledge the managing and negotiating of health care needs.
- Understanding the context of 'managing' and 'negotiating'.

THE SCENARIO AND ANALYSIS STRUCTURE

For convenience, the remainder of this chapter considers the two main features of this domain ('managing' and 'negotiation') separately. But first the Nursing and Midwifery Council's (NMC) advice on portfolio evidence is briefly reviewed. Following this, 'managing' and 'negotiation' are individually examined and explained by:

- detailing the competency domain and its links to the KSF;
- presenting a case history;
- examining the case history, considering arising issues and how they relate to the competency framework;
- describing the range of evidences that could be collected for your portfolio of advanced nursing practice.

The portfolio evidence

The Nursing and Midwifery Council has offered the following advice regarding the production of a clinical portfolio of evidence (NMC 2006b).

> A good portfolio is a systematic collection of robust evidence, which demonstrates that the competencies for accreditation have been met. It should contain:
>
> - Evidence which is credible, verifiable, consistent, has sufficient coverage and quality, and arises from more than one source (i.e. it is corroborated). Note that anything that might allow patient/client identification should be removed/obliterated from the evidence.
> - Synthesis of the evidence to show attainment of competencies, together with signposting for the assessor – i.e. you must present the evidence so that the assessor is easily guided through it and shown how it demonstrates that the competencies are met.
> - Evidence of learning through the experience of gathering and interpreting evidence. We do not expect that the evidence will show 'perfect' practice – one of the key attributes of being a professional is lifelong learning, and so the portfolio should contain a reflective commentary on what further learning is required and action points for improving practice.
>
> In other words, it is not enough merely to provide the raw evidence; you will need to analyse, interpret and assess it. You should consider the source of the evidence, what to do with the information you find there, and your own and others' assessment of whether it shows you meet the standards and criteria for accreditation.

Evidence could include written narratives, observational and oral evidence (accounts from managers and colleagues). Try to include a balance of sources of evidence, appropriate to your setting. The main thing is to provide clear evidence of having met the competencies. Evidence could include any of the following, some of which are explained in more detail further on:

- personal development plan
- 360° feedback and personal reflections on this
- patient records (clinical notes)
- direct observation of care, action plans
- patient stories
- excerpts from reflective diary
- critical incident reviews
- notes from action learning sets
- audio tapes
- posters
- videos
- taped discussions.

NMC (2006b)

KEY POINTS

■ Structuring the analysis.
■ Using a portfolio.

'MANAGING' HEALTH CARE DELIVERY SYSTEMS

Consider now the 'managing' aspect of this domain. Review carefully the domain's content on management listed in Appendix 1.

The management aspect

Now consider the case history in Scenario 8.1. Make notes on how you think this may relate to the above domain descriptions.

Scenario 8.1

Albert is 76 years of age, a retired Welsh-speaking skilled, manual engineer, a homeowner with no mortgage or outstanding financial loans, and he has a good pension. Albert has been admitted to hospital acutely short of breath following a slow, 12-month, deterioration in his respiratory health. He was previously an assertive, independent and healthy man who enjoyed his hobbies, his sport and his caravan holidays. He has been married for 40 years to his wife Jane. Jane has recently found her health limited by severe arthritis. They have four adult children: three daughters and one son; they all live within easy distance of their ailing elderly parents' home. In addition, Albert and Jane have numerous grandchildren.

Albert has been an unrepentant heavy smoker all of his life, and has only in the last year ceased his habit. He only agreed to go to hospital after his daughters found him distressed and cyanosed at home. Following admission, investigations revealed a degenerative and untreatable lung disease. The prognosis is generally poor.

Initially admitted to a general medical ward, Albert's condition deteriorates and he is transferred to a high dependency unit for escalation of respiratory support. Aggressive, non-invasive respiratory therapy improves Albert's condition, although he is severely limited in his physical ability during any exertion and dependent on high concentration and continuous oxygen therapy. He is however eating well, drinking and able to enjoy watching television. Nevertheless, under a 'brave' exterior, Albert is very anxious about his condition and his future.

Albert's wife and children are seen by the physicians who inform them of his poor prognosis. They point out that further escalation of respiratory support, or resuscitation, would not be advisable. They also indicate that Albert could be returned to a general ward with the intention to discharge him home with suitable support as soon as possible.

As the allocated patient pathway manager, and as an ANP, you are charged with Albert's future management.

The management scenario analysis

A student ANP will encounter (and need to examine and record) many similar clinical scenarios to this, and will be expected to analyse and critically appraise them. To do this it will be helpful to make a list (a 'domain review'), commenting as relevant on each point of the domain. In this instance, this list will enable identification of essential aspects of the relationship between the clinical scenario and the breadth and depth of a student ANP's 'managing' skills. Using Albert's scenario, this domain review would look something like Table 8.1.

The management portfolio of evidence

This scenario presents a typical 'chronic respiratory disability' in an elderly patient, an all too common clinical pathology and presentation (British Thoracic Society 2001, Health Development Agency 2004) that presents familiar and distinctive care management challenges. It is certain that the local health care and social services will have previously encountered similar clinical presentations.

What is immediately apparent from this scenario (and its subsequent analytical summary/domain review) is that it provides a student ANP with a wealth of opportunities for collecting evidence on direct and indirect clinical management decisions and outcomes. Albert's case history and clinical needs are not unusual in the health care world (British Thoracic Society 2001, Health Development Agency 2004), and prospectively can be met by the implementation and management of existing resources. His needs are an example of how, if all went well, a health care and social service system, and a coordinated clinical management infrastructure should mobilize and support his needs. Of course, it is also possible that Albert's case could, by contrast, exemplify how the health care and social service system could fail his and his family's needs. Whichever the case, the student ANP should explore the

TABLE 8.1 *The managing domain (management systems/organizations/professional regulators)*

Competency	ANP domain review
Demonstrates knowledge about the role of the ANP.	It is evident that Albert's prospective 'care needs' present me with a health care management challenge. This will require considerable coordination, and as an ANP, I should be able to utilize my breadth and depth of skill to enable the specific and general management of Albert's future care.
Provides care for individuals, families, and communities within integrated health care services.	Albert's care needs are diverse and wide-ranging, and will require contribution from numerous health care professionals and other social services. This will require a holistic coordinated management approach – a care package that is integrated and subsequently evaluated.
Considers access, cost, efficacy, and quality when making care decisions. Maintains current knowledge of their employing organization and the financing of the health care system as it affects delivery of care.	As I have identified that Albert's care will require 'joined-up' thinking and 'joined-up' action there follows a need for efficient and quality health care with a multiagency approach. However, as an ANP, I will have to be aware of, and account for, familiar resource issues and limitations, and the consequent demand for realistic objectives. There will be a need for health care planning collaborations, an awareness of available services, key communication contacts, and acknowledgement of the patient's statutory rights.
Participates in organizational decision-making, interprets variations in outcomes, and uses data from information systems to improve practice. Manages organizational functions and resources within the scope of responsibilities as defined in a job description. Uses business and management strategies for the provision of quality care and efficient use of resources. Demonstrates knowledge of business principles that affect long term financial viability of an organization, the efficient use of resources, and quality of care.	It follows that Albert's care plan will have to be realistic, have achievable outcomes, and will require regular reassessment once implemented. As an ANP, I will need to bring into play all my knowledge and understanding of the national and local health care and social services both in the secondary and primary care sectors. I will have to use this knowledge to influence decision-making, both with key individuals, decision makers, budget holders, and committees. My local knowledge is built on a foundation of wider strategic issues, and this will enable me to develop and deliver a care package tailored to Albert's specific needs – a plan that is sustainable and flexible. This will require pro-action, planning, thinking in the long-term and careful evaluation of outcome.
Demonstrates knowledge of, and acts in accordance with, relevant regulations for this level of practice and the NMC Code of Professional Conduct; standards for conduct, performance and ethics.	As an ANP, I will use my knowledge and insight of professional and ethical guidance to expedite positive health care outcomes for Albert and his family. This is particularly significant for Albert in the light of the medical decision to not escalate respiratory support or institute resuscitation.

available evidence, recording the process of managing Albert's care from outset to conclusion, observing, recording, analysing and collating.

Albert's scenario is, within the auspice of this domain, generally focused on the ANP's 'management' of the health care system to enable his prospective care. The demand is that an ANP engages in logical and systematic care planning and implementation, using existing resources and previous experience, rather than engaging in negotiation of new untested resources. However, it cannot be assumed that demands for 'negotiating care' will not arise, and the student ANP should also explore and utilize such evidence as it arises. Consequently, sources of evidence from this scenario abound.

Albert's scenario highlights how a student ANP can reflect on both the patient (family) experience and the personal experiences (Albert's and the ANP's) of encountering the management structures that surround such a case. Examples of evidence could be:

- records (written, audio, video) of formal and informal encounters with Albert and his family;
- narrative accounts (field notes of family stories, interview transcriptions);
- patient letters;
- records of interactions (and outcomes) with medical and non-medical hospital professionals;
- records of interactions (and outcomes) with primary care or non-hospital medical or non-medical professionals;
- records of interactions with non-professionals (support and voluntary);
- case reviews;
- records of physical examination and findings (objective structured clinical examination, OSCEs);
- any other related documentation;
- records relating to formal committees, strategic individual's decisions, multiagency interventions.

These data sources can be analysed and presented in the portfolio in a range of ways:

- written critical reflections on encounters with multiagency organizations, including analysis of their interface with, and contribution to, Albert's care;
- content analysis of narrative accounts, interview transcripts, video or audio tape recordings of meetings or consultations;
- decision-making analysis and outcome evaluation;
- a case study with specific attention to obstacles and resource issues that arise, and with consideration to the family's expectations of the service provision;
- OSCE reports;
- a clinical diary (field notes);
- theme or topic analysis (e.g. written discussion on chronic condition management, family dynamics, pharmacological interventions);
- reference to appropriate theoretical or research evidence or reference to strategic legislation (i.e. Community Care Act 1990, Chronically Sick and Disabled Person's Act 1970).

I suggest below specific issues that may arise from Albert's scenario that could be used as sources of evidence to help structure a student ANP's reflections or analysis of Albert's and his family's needs and experience of health care system management:

- the provision of professional and practical assistance in the home (community nurses, care assistants, specialist nurses);
- the provision of emergency support and contacts (out-of-hours services);

- planning for financial assistance/money management;
- the provision of facilities outside the home (shopping, laundry, prescription delivery);
- the provision of transport and mobility assistance;
- the provision of home adaptations (O_2 therapy/respiratory aids)/disabled facilities (mobility aides)/home maintenance and repairs;
- planning for respite care, holidays;
- the provision of groceries, meals, laundry, domestic housework;
- the provision of radio, television, or computer facilities.

Patients and families, faced with planning for long-term care, or terminal care, in the home, are often bewildered by the array of bureaucracy that is needed to implement such a care package. There is often an assumption that the health and social services will efficiently and spontaneously mobilize, putting in place the support, both human and material, that will allow them to achieve the best care for their loved one (O'Connor et al. 2000). This expectation (which may or may not be met) will provide opportunities for a student ANP to discuss, record and critically reflect on the reality of the family's experience, or on other related evidence. These critical reviews on care management can be variously grounded by a student ANP in the core disciplines that underpin the health care professions, adopting perspectives on psychology, sociology, anthropology, epidemiology, pathology, pharmacology, etc. These perspectives will enable a critical analysis of the core themes of clinical resource, economics and politics and managing (or management of) care in relation to its impact on patient and family outcome. Confusion, anxiety, anger, financial concerns, grieving and hope are just a few of the many human reactions that may be observed. The portfolio content should explore how clinical management (care management) implicates itself in the understanding of human responses (Janzen 2006).

In addition to the human response, the complexity of health and social care organizations, with their multiple interfaces between professional groups, care sectors, and fiscal needs, presents a student ANP with a considerable challenge, and a rich evidence resource. Encounters with management decisions, management groups (committees), clinical specialists, clinical decisions (and their prospective conflict with fiscal strategies), lines of communication between sectors and service providers, all may be recorded, analysed from numerous theoretical perspectives and presented as evidence of a developing awareness of the implication of 'managing' and the ANP role (Figure 8.2). This will provide a counterpoint to the human outcome of the health care management system, and this should be carefully mapped, demonstrating the contrast between what may seem a simple demand for a community care package, and the reality of complex service delivery. Such an analysis should reveal an underlying knowledge of organizational psychology, occupations, professional roles, health organization, health strategies and resource restraints.

KEY POINTS

- Using and analysing a management case history.
- A management portfolio of evidence.
- Identifying key issues and exploring them in more depth.

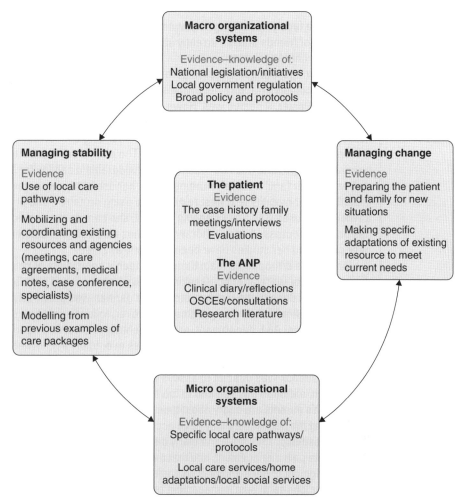

FIGURE 8.2 *Mapping the data matrix of managing Albert's health care. OSCE, objective structural clinical examination.*

'NEGOTIATING' HEALTH CARE DELIVERY SYSTEMS

Having reviewed the 'managing' aspect of this domain, let us now move on to consider the 'negotiating' aspect. The domain's content on negotiating is listed in Appendix 1.

Negotiating

Now consider the following scenario and make notes on how you think this may relate to the domain descriptions in Appendix 1.

Scenario 8.2

Janeen is a 16-year-old Indian woman. She lives at home with her parents who run a successful small business. She has two older brothers and one younger brother. The family is a traditional extended one with, many uncles, aunts and cousins. The family has strong links with family members in India. Janeen has a wide group of friends and is currently studying for her exams in the local secondary school sixth form.

One year ago, Janeen suffered a fracture to her right leg while horse riding. Although a complex fracture, following surgical reduction under anaesthetic and a period in plaster, it healed well. However, it transpired that Janeen had sustained nerve injury that resulted in residual and severe neuropathic pain in her leg. Janeen had described the pain as commencing almost immediately following her surgery to reduce the fracture. The pain is constant, intensely burning in nature, and this has resulted in considerable disability for Janeen and distress for her family. Since returning home, her use of her leg is severely limited and her mobility is at best restricted to using crutches, and at worst she is a wheelchair user. She finds sleeping difficult, she cannot concentrate and she has become depressed and withdrawn. She has also become isolated from her peer group and her studies have been seriously affected.

Initially the orthopaedic team thought Janeen's complaints of pain were exaggerated, or were attention-seeking behaviour because of possible family problems; this despite the family protests that Janeen was previously a happy, active and well-adjusted young woman. However, following several desperate visits to the local A&E department, and an eventual referral to a neurologist, investigations revealed nerve injury, and it was eventually acknowledged that the pain was classically neuropathic in nature. Janeen was informed that the long-term outlook was difficult to assess or predict. She was prescribed Gabapentin, although this seemed to have little effect.

Janeen's parents are angry about their daughter's pain and disability, and suspect that the nerve injury may have occurred when the fracture was repaired under anaesthetic. They are particularly distressed that their daughter has received no adequate pain management, and that they have had to fight to get any acknowledgment of her symptoms. In addition, they have received no hospital referrals for long-term pain management or rehabilitation service, and they have received no community assistance regarding Janeen's educational or home needs. Although sympathetic, local GPs have been able to offer very little.

As the community-based ANP, you are charged with Janeen's future care management.

The negotiating scenario analysis

This scenario presents an uncertain and unpredictable future for a young woman and her family. Janeen's case history, although certainly not unique, is not a common clinical presentation. Her needs demand specialist support, specialist knowledge and rehabilitative care interventions, with prospective flexible and negotiated care management (Dickey and Deatrick 2000). What is certain is that the general health care and social service system will not be geared to respond swiftly to her needs, and creative and specialist care planning will be necessary.

The student ANP will need to seek out and study clinical scenarios such as Janeen's, even when they are relatively uncommon in their own area of clinical practice. Such cases present unusual challenges, and a student ANP will (as before) be expected to analyse and critically appraise them, as this will enable wider appreciation of the context of complex negotiated care management. Again, it will be helpful to list essential aspects of the relationship between the clinical scenario and the breadth and depth of a student ANP's 'negotiation' skills (a 'Domain review'). In Janeen's scenario, this would look something like Table 8.2.

The negotiation portfolio of evidence

It is unclear whether Janeen's pain and resulting disability is transient (her youth being a positive feature in her possible recovery), or whether her symptoms are in fact the early stage of a long-term chronic pain problem. Thus, uncertainty is a key feature of this scenario. Consequently, unlike the previous scenario (Albert's), a key

TABLE 8.2 *The negotiating domain (management systems/organizations/professional regulators)*

Competency	ANP domain review
Collaboratively assesses, plans, implements, and evaluates care with other health care professionals, using approaches that recognize each one's expertise to meet the comprehensive needs of patients.	Janeen's problems are extremely diverse and complex, and I will only be able to address these using a multiagency and multiprofessional approach. A key feature of this care planning will be the patient's acknowledgement (or not) of her health status uncertainty, and the subsequent demand for a flexible care-plan that may be long term.
Undertakes risk assessments and manages risk effectively.	As an ANP, I will formally have to assess Janeen's risk factors, and these will include physical, social and psychological factors. This assessment will guide the means, mechanisms and resources of management that I will need to identify, develop and implement.
Participates as a key member of a multiprofessional team through the development of collaborative and innovative practices.	A key feature and aim of the intimate relationship between myself, as an ANP, with Janeen and her family will be that difficult process of helping them to learn, evolve, adapt and negotiate with a disability that will affect them all.
Participates in planning, development, and implementation of public and community health programmes. Participates in legislative and policy-making activities that influence health services/practice. Advocates for policies that reduce environmental health risks.	As an ANP, I will use my knowledge in enabling organizational and resource innovations that can advantage Janeen. This will require me to explore, develop, and use knowledge of local and national legislation and regulation. Examples of areas I need to use are those of pain management, education resource, education legislation, and related disability legislation and rights.
Advocates for policies that are culturally sensitive.	Any negotiation that I institute to provide Janeen and her family with support and services must be culturally sensitive to her ethnic background, and as an ANP, I will have to use my knowledge and expertise of such issues – both national and local – to promote this to best effect.
Advocates for increasing access to health care for all.	A core feature of any care plan I devise will be its accessibility and effective translation into use to support Janeen and her family.

feature of Janeen's care management is the need for an ANP to engage in wide-ranging and complex decision-making negotiations on potential health interventions and their possible outcomes.

A student ANP will need to reflect on Janeen's personal experiences, on her cultural background, on her family and on the multiple individuals, professionals and organizations that will impact on the negotiations that will seek to enable specific health care outcomes (Ndiwane et al. 2004). However, as a convenience, with this scenario it may help to view the evidences that may arise from two distinct perspectives. First, there is the evidence that will arise directly from the patient and family, and, second, there will be evidence that arises specifically from the possible interventions of the health care and social service organizations.

Consider the patient and family first. The realization of (or arrival of) chronic disabling pain is a traumatic experience for an individual and their family, no matter how well health care management and communication is handled. Indeed, in a case such as Janeen's, the social labelling that arises from the concept of chronic pain or 'disability' could lead her (and her family) to reject or deny this, and instead to focus on immediate and acute features of her symptoms, seeking quick cures and resolutions, where no such outcomes may be possible. This may hamper care planning and require extensive negotiation with Janeen and her family in enabling some form of acceptance of her current condition. However, this may prove difficult, as it will also have to be acknowledged that Janeen's symptoms may resolve in due time, and, as such, her pain and disability may be transient. This uncertainty will surely leave Janeen and her family in an uncertain place, with an uncertain diagnosis, and with uncertain outcomes. This can then also lead to a lack of social recognition of Janeen's current and immediate health problems (Dickey and Deatrick 2000, Kyngas et al. 2000).

This scenario demands that a student ANP reflects on Janeen's experience (as a young teenage woman) of her pain, and that they reflect on the impact of this on Janeen's family, as this is no less significant and will feature in the totality of her compliance with future care and rehabilitation (Kyngas et al. 2000). Chronic pain (particularly when the sufferer is a young family member) affects the whole family: parents, brothers, sisters, aunts, uncles and grandparents. A consequence of this is that care management and subsequent support cannot be confined to the patient alone. For example, brothers and sisters can feel that the additional care needs of their sibling may result in a lack of time for their needs. Parents may struggle to meet the new demands of Janeen's care, these combined with the existing demands of work and day-to-day living can lead to additional unforeseen relationship pressures at home.

Now consider Janeen's care needs with a view to the challenges they present to the health care and social service organizations. These organizations will quickly realize that Janeen's problems are uncertain, possibly long term, and that health outcomes are unclear. They will also recognize that they will not be able to offer immediate solutions to her problems and this lack of predictive outcome may result in hesitancy in identifying and devoting material resources. As a previously fit and healthy young woman, with a relatively recent presentation of an indeterminate pain complaint, it could be predicted that the health care and social service system will not respond to her needs without specific care management negotiation. Such negotiations will require the use of knowledge and skills that ensure the best use of the health care and social service systems that are available. An ANP will (where necessary) need to adapt resource delivery. This scenario is an example of how health care systems should respond to negotiation if they are to meet difficult or unexpected needs. Of course, the evidence collected may or may not demonstrate such outcomes, and, as before, sources of evidence from this scenario will abound.

What is most apparent in terms of portfolio development is that a student ANP can draw from clinical evidence that will focus on wide-ranging negotiation skills in a multiagency and multiprofessional context. Within the scope of this domain, those negotiations will be associated with the organizational structures that affect Janeen's care needs. Examples of evidence are similar, but not necessarily identical, to those listed in the previous (Albert's) scenario. In Janeen's case they could include:

- records (written, audio, video) of formal and informal encounters with Janeen and her family;
- records of narrative accounts (field notes of family stories, interview transcriptions);
- records of family stories;
- patient letters;
- records of interactions (and outcomes) between Janeen and her family with medical and non-medical hospital professionals, for example pain specialists (consultants or others), surgical and rehabilitative specialists (consultants or others) physiotherapists, occupational therapists and specialist nurses;
- records of interactions (and outcomes) between Janeen and her family with primary care or non-hospital medical or non-medical professionals, for example GPs, practice and community nurses and specialist health visitors;
- records of interactions with social and educational service professionals, for example specialist educational needs officer or assessor, disability allowance staff, social security benefits advisors, clinical psychologists, education authority personal, social workers and home tuition services;
- records of interactions with non-professionals (support and voluntary), for example information and advice centres, and specialist support groups;
- summaries of professional case reviews;
- records from health documentation (medical notes);
- records of exposures to, and the outcomes of, strategic individual decisions and multi-agency interventions.

These data sources can be evidenced by

- written critical reflections on encounters with multiagency organizations with analysis of their interface with, and contribution to, Janeen's care;
- content analysis of narrative accounts, interview transcripts, video or audio tape recordings of meetings or consultations;
- decision-making analysis and outcome evaluation;
- field note records of the student ANP'S relationship with Janeen and her family will be crucial as clinical evidence, with particular attention to the family's adaptation and expectations of the service provision;
- a case-study, with specific attention to negotiations required between the range of professional agencies;
- recording of the bureaucratic obstacles and resource (financial) issues that may arise;
- OSCE and consultation reports;
- a clinical diary (field notes);
- theme or topic analysis (e.g. written discussion on neuropathic pain, family and adolescent dynamics, pharmacological interventions);
- reference to appropriate theoretical or research evidence or reference to strategic documentation (i.e. DoH Community Care Act 1990, the DoH Children Act 2004b).

I suggest below specific issues that may arise from Janeen's scenario that could be used as sources of evidence to help structure a student ANP's reflections or analysis of her and her family's needs and experience of health care system management:

- the provision of professional and practical assistance in the home – pain management (medication, mechanical pain-relieving aids, home modifications);
- the provision of, or support provided in acquiring, pain management specialists, physiotherapists, counselling, disability living allowance;
- the practicalities and ease of access to specialists (the components of the multidisciplinary service);
- the provision of, or support provided in acquiring, access to facilities outside the home (youth clubs, support groups, community or ethnic networks);
- educational authority assistance (access to college, home tuition services, special education packages, distance learning and information technology access);
- travel and other mobility assistance (wheelchair, disabled parking permits).

Janeen's scenario exposes the predicaments that arise from chronic and disabling pain in young patients. Her pain and subsequent disability is indeterminate, and there is no intervention or 'cure' that will suddenly remove her problems. Coping with this difficulty can (will) engender emotions of change and loss, a common manifestation in situations where health problems cannot be resolved. An ANP will identify these (classically) as denial, anger, bargaining, depression and acceptance (Kubler-Ross 1981), and can search for manifestations of these in the data. If identified, it will be necessary to examine and analyse their presentation using the theoretical perspectives alluded to earlier, psychological, sociological and anthropological. Observing Janeen and her family can give rise to a critical analysis of the core themes of clinical, resource and political aspects of the features of negotiating advanced care. The portfolio content should explore how clinical negotiation implicates itself in the understanding of observed human responses.

A key theme that also underpins Janeen's care management, and that can usefully structure the collection of portfolio evidence, is the demand for a flexible and responsive multiprofessional and multiagency team (RCN 1999, Eccleston et al. 2003). Health and social care organizations – despite their multiple interfaces, multiple professional groups, care sectors and considerable resources – cannot predict and plan prospectively for all possible health care needs. Acknowledging this opens the way to negotiate care planning, as the resources for such care packages exist, but are not tailored to the nuances of unusual specific patient needs. This process of negotiation provides the prospective advanced clinical nurse with a rich portfolio resource.

Encounters with negotiated decisions, flexible case reviews, clinical decisions that involve multiple professional groups and specialists, financial barriers and the development of new lines of communications may all be recorded, analysed and presented as evidence of a developing awareness of the implication of 'negotiating' and the ANP. As with the management component of this domain, a student ANP must present this evidence so that it contrasts the human outcome of the health care negotiation with the reality of complex service delivery. The evidence should reveal insights into individual and organizational psychology on the mechanisms of multi-professional working, and the mechanisms for manipulating health strategies and resource restraints to advantage patient care (Figure 8.3).

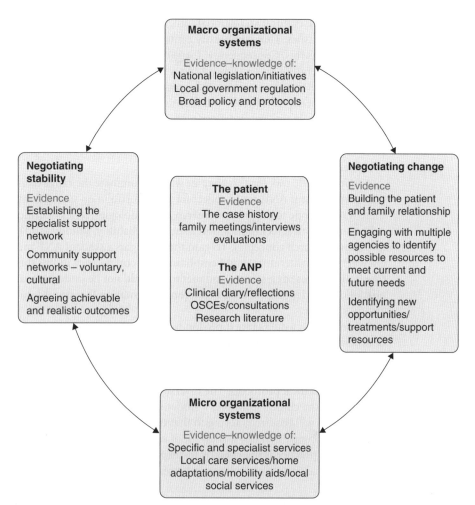

FIGURE 8.3 *Mapping the data matrix of negotiating Janeen's health care. OSCE, objective structural clinical examination.*

KEY POINTS

- Using and analysing a negotiating case history.
- A negotiation portfolio of evidence.
- Identifying key issues and exploring them in more depth.

CONCLUSION

This chapter has sought to explain the nature of the domain of 'Managing and Negotiating Health Care Delivery Systems'. I hope that the reader now sees that to achieve that in its entirety would be a prodigious task of many volumes. Health care delivery systems are not simple or singular concepts, but are, in reality, complex organizations, comprising intricate social orders that are dependent on wide-ranging political, social, cultural and demographic influences as well as extensive regulation and resource issues. That complexity cannot be examined in any depth in a chapter such as this. Consequently, I suggest that a student ANP also reviews the theory and literature on social psychology that relates to organizations and social order, and explores the concepts underpinning the health professions and their work. Far from dry, this theory will illuminate the politics of health care and explain much of our daily activity in delivering care. It is (I hope) now evident that although a domain such as this may at first seem marginal or peripheral to the core clinical work of an ANP, it is in reality an integrated part of their ability to practice effectively.

A more specific task for this chapter was to illuminate the range of evidence and data that a student ANP could collect for their portfolio on such a domain. Again there was no scope to delve into research methodologies, styles of critique, data collection analytical techniques, and issues on reliability, validity (and other important research concepts). To gain these insights a student ANP must search elsewhere in the literature, and I emphasise that competency in this theoretical foundation of research science and method should not be underestimated, as the portfolio of evidence should be a coherent presentation that should stand the test of critical scrutiny.

Consequently, a deliberate omission from this chapter is that of specific examples of evidence or data. It has not included an example of an interview or consultation transcription, a reflective narrative, an OSCE report or reflection, examples from patient notes, or specific descriptions of committee structures, community reviews or examples of local protocols. The diversity of such evidence will (ultimately) be particular to the clinical examples a student ANP selects for inclusion in their portfolio and will require tailoring to that end. The expectation that a student ANP will be developing the skills of analysis, of critical appraisal and of independent and autonomous practice is matched by the expectation that they will select and use evidence in the same way, and not seek prescriptive templates for a portfolio structure.

The chapter has used two clinical case histories, the first a common scenario and the other a less common scenario, as a means to draw the student's attention to the wide array of evidence that can be gained with only a little creative and critical thought, but with a great deal of systematic and thorough planning. A basic analysis of these scenarios has demonstrated that clinical work and clinical care are intimately related to the complex systems of organization that enable that work.

Finally, it has to be acknowledged that these scenarios (or any clinical case), are not exclusive to this domain or any other domain, and one would expect a student ANP in reality to use their own clinical cases to compile data and evidence to illuminate aspects of all the domains described in this book. The chapter has sought to reveal that the ANP can explore these situations and collate data in many forms.

KEY POINTS

- The domain's complexity.
- The range of evidence and the student's practice context.
- A demand for wider methodological and theoretical reading.

REFERENCES

Barton T.D. (2006) Nurse practitioners – or advanced clinical nurses? *British Journal of Nursing* 15(7): 370–376.

British Thoracic Society (BTS) (2001) *A statistics report from the British Thoracic Society.* London: BTS.

Department of Health (1970) *Chronically Sick and Disabled Person's Act.* London: HMSO.

Department of Health (1990) *National Health Service and Community Care Act.* London: HMSO.

Department of Health (2004a) *The NHS Knowledge and Skills Framework (NHS KSF) and the development review process.* London: HMSO.

Department of Health (2004b) *The Children Act (Every Child Matters).* London: HMSO.

Dickey, S. and Deatrick, J. (2000) Autonomy and decision making for health promotion in adolescence. *Journal of Pediatric Nursing* 26(5): 461–467.

Eccleston, C. Malleson, P. and Clinch, J. (2003) Chronic pain in adolescents: evaluation of a programme of interdisciplinary cognitive behaviour therapy. *Archives of Disease in Childhood* 88(10): 881–885.

Furlong, E. and Smith, R. (2005) Advanced nursing practice: policy, education and role development. *Journal of Clinical Nursing* 14(9): 1059–1066.

Handy, C.B. (1996) *The age of unreason.* London: Arrow Books.

Health Development Agency (HDA) (2004) The smoking epidemic in England. London: NICE.

Hunt, J.A. (1999) A specialist nurse: an identified professional role or a personal agenda? *Journal of Advanced Nursing* 30(3): 704–712.

Janzen, J.A. Silvius, J. Jacobs, S. Slaughter, S. Dalziel, W. and Drummond, N. (2006) What is a health expectation? Developing a pragmatic conceptual model from psychological theory. *Health Expectations* 9(1): 37–48.

Jones, M.L. (2005) Role development and effective practice in specialist and advanced practice roles in acute hospital settings: systematic review and meta-synthesis. *Journal of Advanced Nursing* 49(2): 191–209.

Kyngas, H. Skaar-Chandler, C. and Duffy, M. (2000) The development of an instrument to measure compliance of adolescents with a chronic disease. *Journal of Advanced Nursing* 32(6): 1499–1506.

Kubler-Ross, E. (1981) *On death and dying.* New York: Alfred Knopf Publishing.

Ndiwane, A. Miller, K.H. Bonner, A. Imperio, K. Matzo, M. McNeal, G. Amertil, N. and Feldman, Z. (2004) Enhancing cultural competencies of advanced practice nurses: health care challenges in the twenty-first century. *Journal of Cultural Diversity* 11(3): 118–121.

Newbold, D. (2005) Health economics and nursing management. *Journal of Nursing Management* 13: 373–376.

Nursing and Midwifery Council (2006a) *Mapping of the competencies to the Knowledge and Skills Framework.* Available at: http://www.nmc-uk.org/aFrameDisplay. aspx?DocumentID=1668 (accessed on 09/06).

Nursing and Midwifery Council (2006b) *APEL guidance for applicants seeking NMC registration for ANP – Draft 5.* London: NMC.

O'Connor, S.J. Trinh, H.Q. Shewchuk, R.M. (2000) Perceptual gaps in understanding patient expectations for health care service quality. *Health Care Management Review* 25(2): 7–23.

Pearson, A. and Peels, S. (2002) The nurse practitioner. *International Journal of Nursing Practice* 8(4): S5–S10.

Rasch, R.F.R. and Frauman, A.C. (1996) Advanced practice in nursing: conceptual issues. *Journal of Professional Nursing* 12(3): 141–146.

Royal College of Nursing (1999) *The recognition and assessment of acute pain in children.* London: RCN Institute.

Swansburg, R.C. and Swansburg, R.J. (2001) *Management and leadership for nurse managers.* Sudbury, MA: Jones and Bartlett.

Trnobranski, P.H. (1994) Nurse practitioner – redefining the role of the community nurse. *Journal of Advanced Nursing* 19(1): 134–139.

Walshe, K. and Rundall, T.G. (2001) Evidence-based management: from theory to practice in health care. *The Milbank Quarterly* 79(3): 429–457.

West, E. (2001) Management matters: the link between hospital organisation and quality of patient care. *Quality in Health Care* 10: 40–48.

Williams, C.A. and Valdivieso, G.C. (1994) Advanced practice models: a comparison of clinical nurse specialist and nurse practitioner activities. *Clinical Nurse Specialist* 8(6): 311–318.

Williamson, O.E. (1996) *The mechanisms of governance.* Oxford: Oxford University Press.

FURTHER READING

Advanced practice: scope of practice, role development

Ament, L. (2005) Clinical education in managed care for advanced practice nurses: a case example. *Nurse Education in Practice* 5(6): 36–44.

This report reviews managed care as a major component in the current practice environment of APNs. Professional nursing organizations are using the managed care concepts. The paper describes how a nurse practitioner project used managed care theory and practice.

Bryant-Lukosius, D. DiCenso, A. Browne, G. and Pinelli, J. (2004) Advanced practice nursing roles: development, implementation and evaluation. *Journal of Advanced Nursing* 48: 519–529.

This paper reviews issues influencing the introduction of advanced practice nursing roles. There is emphasis on the environmental factors that undermine the roles, and limited use of evidence-based approaches to guide their development, implementation and evaluation.

Daly, W. and Carnwell, R. (2003) Nursing roles and levels of practice: a framework for differentiating between elementary, specialist and advanced nursing practice. *Journal of Clinical Nursing* 12: 158–167.

This is a very useful review of the nature of advanced roles for nurses. It gives particular attention to the confusion regarding role titles, the nature and boundaries of practice, the levels of practice, the levels of clinical autonomy, and preparation for these roles.

Offredy, M. (1998) The application of decision-making concepts by nurse practitioners in general practice. *Journal of Advanced Nursing.* 28(5): 988–1000.

This paper reviews the evidence that suggests that the development of new nursing roles and responsibilities associated with higher level practice in the UK need to be accompanied by the appropriate legal framework and policy infrastructure if the development is to succeed. This is particularly so in relation to changes in the interface between nursing and medicine.

Pearson, A. and Peels, S. (2002) Advanced practice in nursing: international perspective. *International Journal of Nursing Practice* 2002(8): S1–S4.

This paper compared management decisions and patient outcomes between patients managed through the nursing triage system and those who received conventional GP care. It provides a wealth of useful debate and referencing. The research found that patients who were treated by a nurse had more positive outcomes, indicating that nurse management is as effective as that provided by GPs.

Woods, L.P. (1999) The contingent nature of advanced nursing practice. *Journal of Advanced Nursing* 30(1): 121–128.

This paper examines the issues faced by advanced nurse practitioners in the UK as they attempt to implement a new role in practice. It reveals that, whilst the passage from experienced nurse to ANP can be considered highly individual and complex, practitioners appear to move through three discrete stages during the transitional process. A conceptual model is presented which illustrates the contingent nature of advanced nursing practice.

Health policy and organizations

Davies, C. (2004) Political leadership and the politics of nursing. *Journal of Nursing Management* 12: 235–241.

This paper provides a critical examination of the concept of political leadership as it has recently developed in the field of nursing. This enables a number of questions to be posed concerning where nursing fits in relation to current health policy on workforce change. The paper offers an interesting and critical insight on how far the historical neglect of nursing in policy arenas has been overcome.

Davies, H.T.O. Nutley, S.M. and Mannion, R. (2000) Organizational culture and quality of health care. *Quality in Health Care* 9: 111–119.

This paper offers a useful theoretical discourse on health policy in relation to the assessing and improvement of the quality of health care. The paper explores cultural change in health care perceptions and the impact of this on health services and structural reorganization.

Donaldson, C. Currie, G. and Mitton, C. (2002) Cost effectiveness analysis in health care: contraindications. *British Medical Journal* 325: 891–894.

This paper guides potential users of economic evidence through issues and definitions that relate to common economic concepts and terms. It offers a general definition of what health economics is and of what the discipline of economics seeks to achieve, and outlines the basic criteria and concepts underlying economic evaluation before going on to define some of the methods used in regard of cost and benefit.

Douglas, H.R. and Normand, C. (2005) Economic evaluation: what does a nurse manager need to know? *Journal of Nursing Management* 13(5): 419–427.

This paper considers how health economists can assist nurse managers, using the concepts and tools of economic evaluation. Four principal methods; cost-minimization, cost-effectiveness, cost-utility and cost-benefit analysis, are reviewed. The paper provides a systematic framework to analyse health care decisions. In the current context of competition for scarce resources, it suggests that nurse managers need to embrace these techniques.

Mitton, C. and Patten, S. (2004) Evidence-based priority-setting: what do the decision-makers think? *Journal of Health Services Research and Policy* 9(3): 146–152.

This paper offers an interesting examination on the perspectives of decision-makers when using evidence to support priority-setting. The paper notes that decision-makers used a mix of soft and hard forms of evidence in priority-setting, but also that barriers to the use of evidence in priority-setting included crisis-orientated management, time constraints and a lack of skills.

Venning, P. Durie, A. Roland, M. Roberts, C. and Leese, B. (2000) Randomized controlled trial comparing cost effectiveness of general practitioners and nurse practitioners in primary care. *British Medical Journal* 320: 1048–1053.

This paper offers a useful comparison of the cost effectiveness of GPs and nurse practitioners as first point of contact in primary care. The results revealed that clinical care and health service costs of nurse practitioners and general practitioners were similar.

9

DOMAIN 7: MONITORING AND ENSURING THE QUALITY OF HEALTH CARE PRACTICE

NICOLA WHITEING

INTRODUCTION

The National Health Service (NHS) has seen a rapid change in how health care is delivered, resulting in role changes and alternative professional competencies for nurses. There has been a realization that the major health improvements needed in the NHS cannot be made without advanced nursing skills and roles (Walsh and Crumbie 2003). There is a need, however, to ensure quality in the development and implementation of these roles and continuous evaluation of their success. Quality of care, and how it should be measured and maintained, is a subject that has been actively written about in the nursing literature since the 1980s (Hyrkäs and Paunonen-Ilmonen 2001). The UK Government has also put quality high on the political agenda through the introduction of clinical governance (DoH 1998) and the NHS Plan (DoH 2000).

This chapter will explore how the advanced nurse practitioner (ANP) can meet the domains and competencies of monitoring and ensuring the quality of their own advanced practice role and also the advanced practice culture within the wider organization. Each competency also fits into the knowledge and skills framework, as shown in Appendix 1.

PROFESSIONAL, ETHICAL AND LEGAL CONSIDERATIONS

Incorporates professional/legal standards into advanced clinical practice

It is inevitable that as the ANP, or aspiring ANP, expands their role, an increased number of activities previously performed must be delegated to other members of the health care team. There are legal issues surrounding the delegation of such activities and if the ANP delegates inappropriately or provides inadequate supervision they are at risk of litigation. The ANP must, therefore, ensure that they are confident that the person carrying out the activities is competent to do so and must provide adequate supervision to ensure patient safety (Dimond 2003). Such competence of practitioners must be in line with organizational protocols and the competency must be assessed and documented. These competency-based documents, etc., should be gathered and used as evidence for the advancing role in practice.

Clear, comprehensive record-keeping is part of the professional responsibilities of all registered nurses, not least the ANP undertaking advanced practice. The ANP must ensure that records comply with standards set out by the Nursing and Midwifery Council (2007) and the employing organization, and that audit is undertaken of documentation to ensure high standards (Dimond 2003). As discussed later in this chapter, records should be kept relating to the advanced practice role itself, role definition, and clinical supervision and these should act as a resource to the ANP in building their portfolio.

Acts ethically to meet the needs of the patient

The more complex and demanding advanced nursing practice becomes, the more nurses must reflect on the professional, ethical and legal implications of their work (Humphris and Masterson 1998). Greater legal and professional accountability has been highlighted with advanced practice (Poysner 1996) and as a greater level of responsibility is assumed with ever increasingly complex patient health needs, the ANP must assume a greater level of responsibility (Jones and Davies 1999). It is, therefore, vital that ANPs clearly define their professional scope of practice while identifying possibilities and limitations of the role (Furlong and Smith 2005) and clearly define and document levels of accountability (Jones and Davies 1999). Should the ANP feel unqualified or inexperienced to perform an activity they should seek help from a more experienced practitioner as necessary. Membership of a trade union, special interest groups and professional bodies is important in supporting the ANP, both in their professional development and also in ensuring that their practice does not expose patients to any unnecessary risk (Tingle 2002).

Assumes accountability for practice and strives to attain the highest standards of practice

ANPs are personally and professionally accountable for their practice and as such must ensure that they have the competence to undertake and perform advanced practice activities to the same reasonable standard as the person that would normally have undertaken and been entrusted with those activities (e.g. a doctor). Difficulties will arise when ANPs are poorly prepared for their roles, with insufficient knowledge and skill to perform the functions of the advanced nursing role (Jones and Davies 1999). Indeed, in law, being inexperienced is no defence and the ANP, at whatever level in their development, will be judged by the same standards as more experienced colleagues unless they have sought the advice of someone more experienced than they are (Furlong and Glover 1998, Jones and Davies 1999, Tingle 2002). In working alongside other members of the multidisciplinary team (MDT), procedures and protocols can be adapted to reflect the ANPs legal accountability and aid protection against claims of clinical negligence (Tingle 2002).

KEY POINTS

- As practice becomes more advanced the ANP must reflect on the professional, ethical and legal implications of her work.
- The professional scope of practice and clear lines of accountability must be defined.
- Delegation of work to others by the ANP must be appropriate, with provision of adequate supervision and competency assessments.
- Comprehensive record keeping is paramount.

EVALUATING RESPONSES TO HEALTH CARE AND REVISING PRACTICE

Actively seeks and participates in peer review of own practice

In developing the role of the ANP and advanced nursing practice within organizations, a key element is rigorous evaluation to examine how well the role is working and why, and to investigate problem areas in order that action can be taken to address them (Walsh and Reveley 2001, Bryant-Lukosius and DiCenso 2004). In addition, the ANP, as leader and teacher, must continuously drive quality initiatives to revise care delivery strategies and improve the quality of care. Indeed, the NHS Plan states that the NHS will be driven by a cycle of continuous quality improvement (DoH 2000) and with the introduction of clinical governance prior to the NHS Plan the government's determination is reflected to ensure that health care is of a high quality. It is not only the organization that holds responsibility for meeting the clinical governance agenda and ensuring high standards and quality but also each individual practitioner. Thus, the ANP has a responsibility to gain evidence as to the effectiveness of services provided.

There are a number of ways in which the ANP can begin to examine and ensure high quality care delivery. Clinical governance is the main vehicle for the continuous improvement to quality of patient care and high standards (Scally and Donaldson 1998) and provides a framework in which the ANP can address quality issues within the organization. Clinical governance encompasses a range of quality improvement activities of which organizations must provide evidence as to their performance (Cranston 2002):

- clinical effectiveness;
- risk management;
- information technology (IT) strategy;
- practice development (lifelong learning);
- clinical audit;
- health and safety;
- research and development.

The ANP plays a vital role in contributing to clinical governance reports and also in compiling the department/specialty clinical governance portfolio outlining existing achievements in addition to short-, medium- and long-term planned goals. The portfolio can be used as evidence for the ANP's contribution to the monitoring and ensuring of quality health care within this domain.

Evaluates the patient's response to the health care provided and the effectiveness of care

In examining high-quality care delivery, the patients' response to the health care provided and its effectiveness must be evaluated. Patient records provide the ANP with valuable data to evaluate their response to the health care that has been/is being provided and the effectiveness of such health care. It is important that the ANP identifies variances from plans of care and works with others to analyse and resolve them where possible. There are a variety of ways in which patient care and best practice can be documented, including policies, protocols, pathways, guidelines and standards (Parsley and Corrigan 1999). These often mean different things to different professional groups and can cause confusion and lead to duplication of documentation. One method of documentation introduced as a way of improving both patient outcomes and multidisciplinary communication is the integrated care pathway (ICP) (Currie and Harvey 1998, Kinsman 2004). The ICP provides a good example of how documentation can be used to improve outcomes and Scenario 9.1 demonstrates how the use of an ICP addresses these domains and can develop practice.

Scenario 9.1

A care pathway has been used for patients undergoing total knee replacements for 6 months. On monitoring the length of stay (LOS) for these patients it was seen that those patients having their surgery on a Friday were averaging an extra 2 days LOS. Within the unit, physiotherapy services were available Monday to Friday for elective orthopaedic patients and it was felt that there was a link between those patients having surgery on a Friday and not having physiotherapy over the weekend and an increased LOS.

As such, a physiotherapy service was implemented on a Saturday and Sunday morning for all of those patients who had undergone surgery on a Friday. In addition, although some nursing staff were mobilizing patients bed to chair, other more junior staff did not feel happy to do this. The ANP and physiotherapy staff organized some teaching on rehabilitation within the first 2 days post-operatively for all nursing staff. In addition, the nursing section of the care pathway was adapted to include some of the physiotherapy aspects so that nursing staff got used to providing this rehabilitation as part of their working day.

As a result of the changes implemented, a LOS of 5 days was achieved for all patients, including those who had operations on a Friday.

Interprets and uses the outcomes of care to revise care delivery strategies and improve the quality of care

Care pathways are increasingly being used within the UK as a tool for managing patient outcomes and care processes (Currie and Harvey 1998). The care pathway is a multidisciplinary tool that outlines the course of events for the treatment of patients undergoing similar procedures, for example hip replacement, hysterectomy and angiogram (Currie and Harvey 1998, Parsley and Corrigan 1999). Events are placed on a timeline that ranges from hours, days and weeks or in stages dependent on where the pathway is being used. For instance, for the patient in ITU (intensive treatment unit) the care pathway's events may be in hours, whereas care pathways for those patients with a mental illness may be sequenced weekly, or in stages or phases. In all cases, the number of sequenced events is equal to or less than the designated length of stay.

The care pathway enables one documentation tool to be used among all members of the multidisciplinary team, facilitating better communication. Members of the team can see how the patient is progressing within different areas and can use the tool to communicate with each other. In addition, an important aspect of the care pathway is that patients can be directly involved in their own care. The pathway is used in conjunction with the patient, giving them ownership over their care (Reveley and Carruthers 2001) and empowering them to look at their own progress and goals that they will be expected to achieve prior to discharge/transfer.

Care pathways have, however, been criticized as being too prescriptive and not allowing for individual patient care, thus the ANP must work with patients to ensure that their own individual needs are written into the care pathway. Staff should also be taught not to use the pathway as a protocol but to continue to look at the patient and use their own clinical judgement when planning care alongside the pathways.

The pathway should be a working document and continuously developed among members of the MDT to ensure that as research evidence becomes available it is translated into the pathway as applicable. As well as keeping up-to-date with research evidence being published, the ANP needs to audit patient outcomes using the pathways, monitoring any variances. Variances are deviations that the patient makes away from the pathway and are usually caused by one or more of the following: the patient does not achieve the event, for example they develop a physiological problem; the practitioner omits or delays a treatment; and, finally, problems caused by the system such as lack of resources, policies, procedures (etc.). These variations should be monitored for the frequency of their occurrence and their causes.

In measuring best practice and evaluating patients' responses to the health care provided, the ANP should also participate in other, perhaps more general, audits. In line with government documents (DoH 1993a, 1994) the importance of audit has been recognized and implemented. Many professional groups have undertaken their own unidisciplinary audit work; however, the importance of multidisciplinary audits has been recognized (DoH 1993a). It is acknowledged that if genuine benefits to patients are to occur, all members of the MDT need to be involved in improving care and it is for this reason that a multidisciplinary audit must be undertaken.

Actively seeks and participates in peer review of own practice

The ANP's role in audit needs to consist not only of participating in clinical audits but also in audits evaluating and monitoring the quality of their own role and practice within the organization. An outcomes audit of those patients managed by the ANP will demonstrate effectiveness of the role and resources (Griffiths 2003) through keeping simple records of activity, referrals, trends and outcomes. Another way of monitoring the quality of the role is by using peer audit through which a group of people of equal qualification and grade assess the performance of their peers (Kemp and Richardson 1999). It is particularly useful when examining professional performance for promotion and the developing ANP may wish to use peer audit material in their portfolio as evidence of their commitment to continuously developing their own practice.

Whichever audit is being undertaken several models are available to assist the ANP and they should experiment with different models to find one which they are confident in using. Gillies (1997) proposed that clinical audit follows a cycle of activity signposting a number of key stages within the audit process. Other models have illustrated similar stages in different ways, such as using spirals to visualize the proposed methods. The ANP may find the following stages helpful when undertaking audit (Parsley and Corrigan 1999).

- *Selection* – Decide on what quality issues need to be examined and prioritize them. Define your objectives and choose an appropriate methodology.
- *Planning* – Develop your data collection strategy: who is going to be doing what and what are the deadlines. Identify any resource implications that there may be.
- *Implementation* – Start to implement your audit plan, keep records of all meetings, activities and critical events. Analyse all data collected and if any changes are required these need to be made. Report your findings to those involved and ensure that they are distributed throughout the organization.
- *Evaluation* – Assess your audit project against your original objectives set in stage one. Have they been met? What has been learnt at each stage of the process? Identify what improvements have been made and what may have impeded their success. Take on board what was done well and what could have been improved for future audit projects.

The process should then be repeated and with each audit cycle, quality is improved, demonstrating a cycle of continuous improvement.

Achieving successful audit is not without its difficulties (Johnston et al. 2000) and as such the ANP should foster an environment for audit demonstrating its value in developing quality in clinical care and also in professional advanced practice roles. Multidisciplinary audit should be encouraged and staff training programmes should be reviewed to incorporate training in audit processes. Relevant staff should be involved in the audit process to assist in the successful adoption of change behaviours and communication across the organization must take place to ensure that best practice is not confined to one area but shared among others. The ANP should attend and participate in monthly audit meetings in which projects are discussed, developed and results presented. These meetings should be multidisciplinary in attendance and may be confined to a specialty or may be larger across the organization.

Another resource available to the ANP is the continuous quality improvement (CQI) model that provides an alternative to the more rigid research methods for evaluating quality, focusing not just on organizational problems and reducing errors but also on seeking new and innovative ways of working (Parsley and Corrigan 1999). The process embodies principles of teamwork, empowerment, process monitoring and improvement, customer service and strategic planning (Dickerson 2000), which enable effective solving of problems that in turn provide improvements for practice (Kemp and Richardson 1999). Organizations may have several projects being undertaken at any one time by various CQI groups.

Once variations in health outcomes or revisions to care delivery strategies have been identified, an intrinsic function of advanced nursing practice is that of change agent (Heath and Jagger 2003, Bryant-Lukosius et al. 2004). A change in practice may need to be implemented as a result of an external force, such as a national guideline, policy or framework. The ANP must be aware of advances in practice beyond that of their own organization and understand how these advances will influence them and others in the organization. In addition, the ANP constantly needs to reappraise practice and seek more effective and efficient ways of doing things and influence others to do the same. This in turn, will bring about opportunities to change ways of practising.

In implementing any type of change, such as a new guideline, protocol or care pathway, it is well documented that its success is linked with the involvement of all staff in the change process from the beginning (Andrews 1993, Cutcliffe and Bassett 1997). The ANP must collaborate and consult with health care providers and decision-makers from the beginning regarding a change in practice. It should be accepted that individuals see things in different ways and therefore people will respond differently to change: some readily and with enthusiasm and others resisting any suggestions of participating in or accepting a change in practice. A number of models have been presented which will help the ANP understand the different ways in which people within the organization may react to a planned change and what the ANP can do to help bring them on board to accept a change in behaviour. Further reading on these models can be sought through change management or leadership texts and the ANP is advised to learn more about these models prior to attempting any changes to increase the likeliness of success.

Heath and Jagger's (2003) five-point framework described below is a simple and useful starting point for those new to change management.

- What? Have a clear vision of what is to be changed and what is to be achieved; be very focused.
- Who? Consider those that should be involved in the change but also those that will ultimately be affected by the change. Consider who needs to lead the change; the ANP may not be the most appropriate person.
- Why? Is the proposed change necessary? Do the advantages of changed behaviour outweigh the costs? Consider and document the driving and restraining forces (Lewin 1951) or undertake a SWOT (strengths, weaknesses, opportunities and threats) analysis (Morrison 2003) for any proposed change.
- How? A successful change is planned, considering the aims and objectives of the projects, methods to be used, resources required, key tasks to be completed and by whom, timescales and review dates.
- When? Be realistic in what can be changed in the allocated timescales, prioritize activities and lay them out on a Gant chart for all team members and other staff to see.

Plans compiled for a change in practice should be used as evidence in meeting competencies within this domain regarding the revision of care delivery strategies.

KEY POINTS

- Evidence must be collected through audit, to evaluate the effectiveness of the ANP.
- Best practice should be measured and the patients' responses to the health care provided evaluated. This can be done through reviewing patient documents, policies and guidelines.
- The ANP should act as change agent leading by example and creating an environment open to change.

WORKING WITHIN THE HEALTH CARE TEAM

Collaborates and/or consults with members of the health care team about variations in health outcomes

Advanced nursing practice provides an opportunity to redefine parameters for practice between nurses and other members of the health care team (Dunn 1998). Therefore, a key component of advanced practice is working in collaboration with the multidisciplinary team in ensuring continuity and coordination of patient care (Stanton et al. 2005). Patients present with complex health care needs and it is crucial that the ANP is able to communicate effectively and consult with other team members, striving to improve collaboration among the health care team (Donagrandi and Eddy 2000).

As previously discussed, ANPs are accountable for their practice and it is likely that they will provide a large percentage of activities for the patient. However, it is essential that they draw upon other MDT members and their services, as well as using critical thinking, current research and diagnostic reasoning in order to administer good quality care while ensuring efficient usage of resources (Cox 2004). This will enable the ANP to manage episodes of care and help to eliminate the fragmented care (Wayman 1999, Donagrandi and Eddy 2000) that is often seen as the patient moves between departments and professionals. In order that the ANP works well as a member of the MDT, the ANP must educate and inform other professionals about the role, what the ANP's scope of practice is and about any advances in advanced practice.

Following assessment of the patient and identification of actual or potential health problems, the ANP should devise a plan of care in conjunction with other members of the MDT. Short-term and long-term goals should be delineated and the plan reviewed and revised as the patient progresses. Where variations from the planned care or goals occur, the ANP must work with others to analyse and resolve them where possible. If the management and care delivery for the patient exceeds the ANP's scope of practice, they must seek help and support from more experienced or senior colleagues. It is for this reason that relationships with other health care professionals are crucially important for successful liaison and coordination of patient care.

The use of the ICP discussed previously provides an excellent platform for enhanced collaboration and communication between the MDT. It is particularly helpful for seeing where in care provision patients are presenting variations from expected health outcomes. Where patterns in these variations can be seen, MDT members should meet and examine where in the service problems lie, and work towards addressing these issues.

Evaluates patient follow-up and outcomes, including consultation and referral

In addition to multidisciplinary collaboration in the ANP's own organization, there need to be links between acute, primary and tertiary care to ensure smooth transition between areas during referral or discharge. There is also a need for both the novice and experienced ANP to network with the wider health and social care network within their own organization and outside it, so as to appreciate wider issues. The ANP needs to learn to manage more than just the patient's presenting complaint but also to appreciate the need for prevention or treatment of health issues (Evans et al. 2005). By having an awareness of the roles of other health care team members and between acute, primary and tertiary settings, the ANP will learn to refer appropriately and evaluate variations from health with positive outcomes.

Examples of collaborative working, such as minutes from meetings, joint projects or effective referral systems, should be used as evidence for the advanced practice role.

Many advanced practice roles within the UK are adopting the role of case manager similar to that of the United States. Indeed the role of the community matron outlined by the Department of Health (2004) describes a role in which the ANP provides case management for people with severe (three or more long-term health care conditions) and complex health care needs. This case management approach aims to provide systematic proactive care to prevent unplanned hospital admission and premature admission to long-term care facilities and to expedite hospital discharge (Evans et al. 2005). The ANP through Domain 3 facilitates the patient's journey through the health care system, arranging for consultation with specialists or specialized services and ensuring that transfers to more appropriate level of care areas are made when needed.

Despite the patient's location within the health care system the ANP has responsibility for scheduling and following up on tests, procedures and treatments, negotiating primary care and/or acute care resources and monitoring patient outcomes. Chapter 5 has discussed the ANP's role within the assessment, diagnosis, treatment, referral and discharge of the patient under care, and Scenario 9.2 shows an example of how the ANP works as a case manager, referring at the appropriate time and following up on all tests ordered despite the patients location within the system.

Following the end of a patient care episode, as a way of monitoring the quality of services, the ANP should track the progress of patients once they have left his or her care. This will be easier for some ANPs than others, dependent on where they are working. For the ANP in the GP surgery, follow-up and progress tracking will be easier; however, for the ANP working in an A&E department or walk-in centre this will be much more difficult. Where possible, however, particularly if a patient is experiencing a new service, the ANP should follow up with a phone call, to ensure that they are progressing well and to monitor such factors as complication rates, readmission to services and satisfaction with services. To gain a true picture the ANP may need to consult with other members of the health care team, such as the primary care team, depending on what patients report. Records of follow-up conversations with patients, comments noted and any actions taken should be kept by the ANP.

Scenario 9.2

Mr Baker is due to undergo a hip replacement in 4 weeks' time. He has come to the pre-assessment clinic to attend the education class, have his fitness assessed for surgery and ask any questions regarding his forthcoming surgery/aftercare. Neil is an ANP and has been assigned to act as case manager for Mr Baker. Neil takes a thorough health history from Mr Baker and then carries out a physical examination of his systems. During the cardiac assessment, it is noticed that Mr Baker has a cardiac murmur and with no previous history it is decided that he ought to undergo an echocardiogram prior to being deemed fit for surgery. The anaesthetist on call for the clinic is contacted because Neil is not yet confident which murmurs should be further investigated. The anaesthetist comes to see the patient while he is still in clinic.

Once the anaesthetist has agreed that Mr Baker does need an echocardiogram, Neil ensures that Mr Baker is told exactly what has been found, reassures him that there is nothing to worry about but that the echocardiogram is needed prior to surgery. He is sent home and told that a date for the appointment will be sent to him in due course.

Following Mr Baker's consultation Neil completes a written referral for his patient to have his echocardiogram carried out. He also writes to the GP to ensure that he is aware of what has been found and completes all of his own documentation. The scheduling team are also told that this gentleman's surgery may be postponed for a short period of time while waiting for the appointment; they can therefore look for potential patients to fill the slot at a later date.

Three days after Mr Baker's consultation, all of his blood tests and microbiology swabs are reviewed and documented. As soon as Neil hears that the appointment has been allocated, he contacts Mr Baker to ensure that he has received notification and to answer any questions that he may have. He is also informed that all other tests carried out were satisfactory. Neil ensures that all documentation is complete and arranges for the notes to be sent to relevant departments.

Following the echocardiogram, Mr Baker is given the go ahead for surgery. The anaesthetist is shown the report and both Neil and the anaesthetist document that the Mr Baker is fit for surgery. Neil rings the patient to tell him that all is well and to answer any questions that he may still have. The scheduling team are told that the patient is fit for operation on the planned date and the GP is updated by letter.

On the day of surgery Neil visits Mr Baker in pre-surgery prior to his operation. Once he is satisfied that Mr Baker is prepared for surgery he hands over care to the ANP covering theatres and post-operative care, ensuring that all relevant communication from both pre-assessment and collaboration with other departments and primary care are clearly documented.

KEY POINTS

- To ensure continuity and coordination of patient care, the ANP must work in collaboration with the MDT.
- If the patient's management and care delivery exceeds the ANP's scope of practice, help and support should be sought from more experienced or senior colleagues.
- The ANP should network with the wider health and social care network outside of his or her own organization.

EVIDENCE-BASED PRACTICE

Promotes and uses an evidence-based approach to patient management that critically evaluates and applies research findings pertinent to patient care management and outcomes

The concept of using research in practice is not a new one; however, there is now much more of an emphasis on a systematic approach to the analysis of research, using the information to influence practice and then analysing and evaluating the outcomes on patient care (Munro 2004). Evidence-based practice (EBP) is a key component of clinical governance with the notion of EBP being driven through various government documents, aiming for a health service in which clinical, managerial and policy decisions are no longer based on tradition or ritual but on sound and pertinent information. National Service Frameworks (NSFs) and the National Institute for Health and Clinical Excellence (NICE) have a role in providing evidence on best practice. In England and Wales, NSFs have currently been established for coronary heart disease, mental health, older people, diabetes, renal and children's services and, in addition, England also has NSFs for cancer services and long-term conditions. The ANP should have an awareness of the content of those that are applicable within the area of the organization in which he/she works.

Various definitions of EBP exist. NICE (2002: 70) defined EBP as 'the conscientious, explicit, and judicious use of current best evidence … in making and carrying out decisions about the care of individual patients'. Evidence-based practice is a broad term and is an extension of evidence-based medicine, to include all disciplines of the health care team (DeBourgh 2001).

In leading on the development and implementation of EBP, the ANP is in an ideal position. Through the role of a practice leader and through the direct provision of patient care, the ANP has a direct influence on patient outcomes (DeBourgh 2001). The ANP should actively participate in efforts to design, implement and evaluate changes in health care systems and gather evidence to this effect for their portfolio. Evidence-based practice should also be promoted within the organization as an effective and efficient approach to improving the quality of patient care (DeBourgh 2001).

A number of authors have discussed the contribution that patients/clients can make to health care systems (Closs and Cheater 1999, DeBourgh 2001, Griffiths 2003). The community matron, mentioned earlier, is ideally placed to look at how patients self-manage their long-term conditions and take these observations into account when making decisions about future care for them and others. A key element is in the adaptation of patient care packages and pathways to allow for consideration of individual patient needs and preferences when making health care decisions. This approach counteracts arguments that EBP and the implementation of ICPs leads to 'prescriptive' approaches to patient conditions, not allowing for sufficient flexibility towards the individual patient's care. The ANP can establish or join existing public–patient involvement groups both within their own specialty and also the wider organization. These groups are useful in obtaining the views of users, particularly when setting up new services. As part of the author's previous role in the setting-up of an independent treatment centre, user views were obtained over a period of a year regarding visiting hours, meals, transport, infection control procedures and design and layout of the centre. Such user group involvement by the ANP can be gathered and used as evidence.

Monitors current evidence-based literature in order to improve quality care

Evidence-based practice enhances the health care environment and facilitates competent clinical practice, innovation and a commitment to progressing nursing as a profession (DeBourgh 2001). Practice will be more appropriate, timely and acceptable to the patient, the team and the organization and with EBP so high on the health care agenda at present it is an ideal time for the ANP to develop skills in this area (Griffiths 2003).

There are many practices based on tradition or practitioner preferences that should be changed to EBP. There are, however, only a limited number of practices that can be changed within a particular time-frame and therefore the ANP alongside colleagues must decide which areas should be addressed first. It is important that the ANP has an awareness of the organization's EBP/research and audit strategy both in taking forward EBP and to avoid duplication between other members of the multidisciplinary team. Knowledge gained through organizational strategies and working alongside others will enable the ANP to access appropriate resources that are available, such as other people and finances, and ensure that EBP is part of a strategy that is introduced successfully over time.

There are a number of ways in which the ANP can begin to get involved in the implementation of EBP and also assist other staff too. A few suggestions are listed below.

- *Clinical practice committees* – Used as a forum to develop, implement and review clinical practice guidelines, policies, procedures and care pathways. The ANP acts as chair or participant in the forum, identifying practice/professional issues or concerns, coordinating the team in writing new guidelines and the monitoring of outcomes. Outcomes include guidelines produced and implemented based on published national standards/guidance, clear improved patient outcomes, including patient satisfaction and effective resource utilization of the ANP.
- *Multidisciplinary meetings/staff meetings* – Used to develop care pathways, discuss unit targets and review new equipment. Provides a good opportunity for the ANP to promote his or her role as an active leader/participant within the organization among all members of the multidisciplinary team. Within their own staff meetings, the ANP has the opportunity to discuss with other nursing staff opportunities that they may feel important to investigate and to feed back information on other organizational developments and guidelines to be implemented. The ANP can again promote their own advanced practice role.
- *Clinical governance forums* – Opportunity for the ANP to meet with managers as well as fellow clinicians/practitioners in discussing activities within the clinical governance

agenda; in particular, focusing on research and audit, patient satisfaction, and training and development. Like the multidisciplinary meetings, the clinical governance forum gives the new ANP knowledge about what strategies are in place to assist with developing and implementing EBP within the organization and to share resources/workload.

- *Research and audit committees/meetings* – In line with the organization's commitment to clinical governance and EBP, a research strategy is developed and implemented. New research and audit ideas are put forward and developed as appropriate. Also concerned with the implementation of research findings, publications, conference presentations and the sharing of best practice. In addition to carrying out their own research, the ANP helps other members of staff to develop an important issue into a piece of research with sound methodology; the ANP is able to ensure that the findings of any research will be transferred into practice as appropriate.
- *Project management* – ANPs can act either as a lead of or as a participant in projects that may be carried out within the organization or in conjunction with another organization. This enables EBP to be developed, best practice to be shared among other departments and/or organizations and the role of ANP to be promoted and developed.
- *Collaboration with universities* – The ANP may find it useful to link with a local university, both to support advanced practice programmes in which research skills will be prominent and to work in collaboration on research projects. It can be time-consuming initiating a piece of research, particularly if the ANP has minimal experience. Linking with a research team within a university can help to get the project started and increase the likelihood of the research being used once completed (Griffiths 2003).
- *Clinical supervision* – The advantages of clinical supervision are discussed later in this chapter. Clinical supervision sessions will highlight issues that are worthy of further investigation. If it is expected that clinical supervision sessions may bring up topics to warrant further investigation, this must be established within the ground rules prior to its use.
- *Teaching* – A large part of the role of the ANP is to act as teacher for both staff and patients. Although formal courses within universities are important, so too is the demonstration of applied clinical practice by the ANP. The ANP therefore has a role in ensuring that evidence-based knowledge learnt by nurses through courses is translated into practice. What is learnt must be supported in clinical practice by examining the most effective and efficient clinical practices. Many staff may read journal articles as part of a course and although they are encouraged to reflect on their own practice it often stays at that level. The ANP has an important role in assisting staff to formulate questions and access evidence to answer them (DeBourgh 2001).
- *Expert role modelling* – The ANP, as an expert role model, provides structure and support for staff to develop in confidence to integrate new practices and use new information and evidence to perform more effectively (DeBourgh 2001). Staff observing the ANP communicating and working effectively with other members of the MDT, managing complex situations, demonstrating accountability and advancing clinical practice, will also develop these attributes and abilities (Wiseman 1994).

It is often difficult, once the evidence is gathered, to know where to start in including it in clinical practice. This was an area that Flemming (1998) addressed through the suggestion of a five-stage process:

- areas of concern from practice are converted into focused, structured questions;
- the focused questions are used as a basis for literature-searching in order to identify relevant external evidence from research;

- the research evidence is critically appraised for validity and generalizability;
- the best available evidence is used alongside clinical expertise and the patient's perspective to plan care;
- performance is evaluated through a process of self-reflection, audit or peer assessment.

KEY POINTS

- The ANP must promote EBP within their organization.
- Views of service users should be sought where possible in evaluating and developing services.
- The ANP should take an active role in promoting and implementing EBP through participation in a variety of forums/committees.

CONTINUING PROFESSIONAL DEVELOPMENT

Accepts personal responsibility for professional development and the maintenance of professional competence and credential

Continuing professional development (CPD) underpins quality in the NHS, enhancing patient care (Bartle 2000, Wood 2004). Earlier in this chapter the increasing demands on individuals to exercise personal and professional accountability were highlighted. Together with the necessity to demonstrate high quality, effective and efficient interventions, the importance for the ANP of undertaking CPD cannot be underestimated (Clouder and Sellars 2004). Following the ANP's initial advanced training and preparation, clinical competence must be maintained and he or she must keep professionally up to date (Bousfield 1997, Harris and Redshaw 1998, Ball 1999). On return to the workplace, the ANP will need time to reflect and consolidate newly acquired knowledge, refine new practical skills and revert from learner to carer (Harris and Redshaw 1998).

The NMC supports lifelong learning and CPD, noting that it is more complex than merely keeping up to date. An enquiring approach to practice and issues that impact on practice is required (NMC 2002). Although lifelong learning is essential to assure the quality service the government is striving towards, the ANP needs to take control of her own CPD (Wood 2004), establishing both personal priorities for professional growth and career satisfaction and also those of the employing organization. It is easy for ANPs to become 'too busy' to establish their own specific growth and thus becoming restrained and frustrated in their role (Hockenberry-Eaton and Kennedy 1996).

The personal development plan (PDP) is often used as part of an organization's appraisal process; however, it can also be easily developed by practitioners for use within their own portfolio. In developing the PDP, the ANP should consider their strengths and weaknesses within the role that they are in or are striving to grow into. Strengths should be continued and developed and weaknesses can be addressed through setting some short-, medium- and long-term goals. These should be realistic and not too ambitious too soon (Buckingham and Palmer 2003), identifying the resources and support required to meet them and highlighting the ways in which the ANP and the organization will know that they have been achieved. A mentor chosen by the ANP is useful in helping to develop and work through the PDP, giving advice and direction as necessary.

CPD can take many forms and consists of far more than attending higher education courses. For the purposes of this chapter CPD is discussed in two areas: professional development with the organization in mind, for example research, public speaking; and professional development for the individual, for example attending higher education programmes.

Professional development for the organization

There are now many opportunities for ANPs to obtain positions that allow time to pursue writing, research, public speaking, teaching and consulting. Indeed, the NMC domains and competencies discussed throughout this book reflect these roles. In addition to the patient and staff teaching role that is undertaken within the organization, the ANP may want to make links with their local higher education institution (HEI) and undertake teaching within specialist courses that are running. Preparing a lesson can facilitate learning and ensures that the ANP is always aware of current evidence within the subject matter.

Another effective way both to enhance professional knowledge and also support the profession is through writing for publication (Buckingham and Palmer 2003). The ANP should select journals which he or she feels comfortable to write for and about a subject that interests them and in which they can demonstrate knowledge. In addition to writing about their subject specialty, the nursing literature needs more evidence on the advanced practice role, and the ANP should share their experiences or their research into their role. Editors are available to help and support the production of papers, and as such the ANP should use them as a resource in addition to colleagues who have experience in writing for publication.

Approaching journal editors to sit on the editorial or advisory board is a useful way of developing skills in the peer reviewing of papers and developing skills in research techniques and writing. Another useful introduction to publications is to contact a journal's book review editor and offer to review and comment on books recently published (Buckingham and Palmer 2003).

ANPs must continue to increase their clinical and professional knowledge and expertise by keeping updated with new knowledge in their specialty area. There are now a large number of local and national conferences available for staff to attend as part of their own professional development. Although attendance at these equips the ANP with up-to-date knowledge and fresh ideas to take back to their organization, the ANP also has a role as a speaker at such events. A good way to begin to be involved in conference presentation and speaking is to submit a poster presentation for consideration. Poster presentations enable the ANP to share their work with others but do not involve public speaking with large numbers of people, which often puts potential presenters off. As confidence grows, the ANP will develop from speaking to small groups or running workshops to giving presentations to a larger number of delegates. Again, subject matter varies but every opportunity should be used to promote the advanced practice role and share best practice.

From experience, ANPs who use their expertise in ways such as those outlined above in addition to their normal clinical work not only contribute to CPD for the organization but also may find their role more satisfying and as a result are encouraged in their professional growth (Hockenberry-Eaton and Kennedy 1996).

Professional development for the individual

ANPs not only need to have core skills and competencies in the diagnosis, treatment and care of patients, but, as this book has discussed, need to be able to form genuine partnerships with patients and work effectively in multidisciplinary teams. The recognition of causes of unsafe practice and an ability to act on them, to be able to assess the quality of care and identify ways of improving it, and to act as educator are just some of the other skills the ANP must possess (Donaldson 2001). In order that the ANP maintains his or her professional credibility in these areas, they need to be seen to be participating in these roles and also to take personal responsibility for maintaining competence and seeking the necessary supervision of practice as required (Dimond 2003).

This can be done through attending study days and short courses on topics such as clinical skills, research, time management, publishing and management skills (Bamford and Gibson 2000). Courses undertaken at other organizations or at a university will equip students with the knowledge and clinical skills to take back to their workplace. The new knowledge and skills that are obtained on courses must be developed and consolidated with the support of an appropriate mentor. It is not good enough that courses are undertaken and written in the ANP's portfolio; they must be used to enhance quality patient care and organizational processes.

The ANP should also consider other ways of developing knowledge and practice. Arrangements could be made to shadow another member of clinical staff or to obtain a rotation or secondment opportunity (Buckingham and Palmer 2003), which may be particularly useful for the practitioner considering moving into an advanced practice role. The use of reflection as a tool to examine and grow in practice, reading journals and accessing information on the web and joining national or regional organizations (Hockenberry-Eaton and Kennedy 1996) are other ways of participating in CPD. Active participation in special interest groups, seminars and other professional forums provides a platform for discussion and may be particularly beneficial if the ANP is primarily working alone. Concern has been raised that nurses are at risk of becoming professionally isolated in extended roles (Jones et al. 2001), and the use of such groups give ANPs the opportunity to meet, chat and learn from others in an informal way (Buckingham and Palmer 2003). All of the activities described above can be used as evidence within the ANP's portfolio.

All nurses are now required to keep a portfolio of practice in line with NMC requirements to meet with Post Registration Education and Practice (PREP) (NMC 2004). However, although the portfolio is a requirement, it also has advantages in collecting and presenting evidence of CPD, with Jasper (1998) supporting their use in advancing practice. Many definitions of the portfolio exist, notably that it represents learning, progress and achievement over time (Wenzel et al. 1998, Karlowicz 2000); acts as a personal and professional development tool aimed at encouraging reflection and self-direction in identifying learning needs (Calman 1998); and is concerned with the evidence of good practice (Redman 1994, Coffey 2005) (see also Chapter 10).

With portfolios being used as an assessment method, accreditation of prior learning and as a measure of competence by professional and academic institutions, it is advisable that the developing ANP works towards maintaining a portfolio to demonstrate their own personal and professional development and also to identify self-development needs. It is through the collection of this evidence that the ANP's personal and professional growth (Price 1994) and their growing accountability and autonomy (Joyce 2005) will be demonstrated. As such, the portfolio should be continuous and dynamic in nature (Alsop 2003, McMullan et al. 2003), constantly changing as the ANP undertakes new experiences and learning through the monitoring of practice and participating in continuous quality improvement methods. This should not be a collection of items in a folder but should demonstrate that the ANP has reflected and critically examined situations and that this in turn demonstrates learning (McMullan et al. 2003).

In developing the portfolio with advanced practice in mind, the domains and competencies discussed within this book should be addressed. The following list may be helpful in thinking about what might be included within the portfolio:

- evidence of knowledge, skills and understanding, demonstrating good practice under each of the domains and competencies;
- collection of evidence-based practice development initiatives that the ANP has implemented/participated in;
- reflections of past and present activities and experiences that subsequently demonstrates learning;
- features of the ANP's professional career demonstrating personal growth and development within roles

Further reading regarding collecting evidence for the portfolio can be found in Chapter 10.

KEY POINTS

- Clinical competence must be maintained following initial advanced training and preparation.
- Establish personal and professional objectives through a PDP.
- Keep a portfolio of evidence for work at an advanced level of practice.

THE ANP'S ROLE IN MAINTAINING HIS OR HER OWN PROFESSIONAL COMPETENCE

Engages in clinical supervision and self-evaluation and uses this to improve care and practice

In improving quality in health care and addressing CPD for the ANP clinical supervision has become popular. Throughout the early 1990s the UK government identified clinical supervision as a national initiative within the strategy '*A vision for the future*' (DoH 1993b), defining it as 'a formal process of professional support and learning which enables individual practitioners to develop knowledge and competence, assume responsibility for their own practice and enhance consumer protection and safety of care in complex situations'. One of the drivers behind clinical supervision as a target within the strategy was the apparent need for practitioners to receive support within their day-to-day practice, and a view that clinical supervision could assist in sustaining safe standards of clinical practice. A decade on, alongside the views above, clinical supervision has had greater emphasis put on its role within CPD (Wood 2004) and is supported by professional bodies such as the Nursing and Midwifery Council (NMC 2006) as a way of both evaluating and improving patient/client care and also in contributing to meeting the PREP (CPD) standard (NMC 2004). Clinical supervision provides practitioners with an opportunity to share working practice in detail, develop the ability to continuously monitor the quality of their work and receive feedback and guidance from a more experienced practitioner of their choice (Proctor 1991).

For the ANP, developing a new role, or indeed the practitioner striving towards becoming an ANP, clinical supervision is of great importance in helping to develop and apply new knowledge, to manage the emotional aspects of the role and finally to develop standards of clinical practice (Kaur 2003, Wood 2004). It is hoped that through being supervised and also through acting as a supervisor for more junior staff, the ANP will demonstrate a reduction in the number of complaints (Goorapah 1997) and promote standard setting and audit (Gorzanski 1997, Hyrkäs and Paunonen-Ilmonen 2001, Teasdale et al. 2001, Kaur 2003, Wood 2004).

Work by Proctor (1991) asserted three main functions of clinical supervision: formative, restorative and normative. Formative supervision is concerned with the practitioner developing their skills and knowledge and updating these. The ANP reflects and draws upon his or her own strengths, weaknesses and abilities in gaining new skills and knowledge. Restorative supervision provides the ANP with personal support to help deal with professional problems that may arise within work. The clinical supervision sessions enable the ANP to explore personal feelings and discuss alternative ways to tackle clinical and/or professional situations in a safe environment. The final function, the normative function, is concerned with managerial aspects of practice, promoting high-quality care, reducing risk and meeting organizational objectives. Proctor's work (1991) has been influential in nursing, suggesting that through clinical supervision the quality of nursing care can be raised, increasing the competence of nurses and providing them with support (Teasdale et al. 2001).

Various approaches to clinical supervision can be used, all of which can be seen to be of benefit to the ANP. One-to-one supervision, group supervision and network supervision can all be used, either on their own or in combination (Hyrkäs and Paunonen-Ilmonen 2001, Kaur 2003, Winstanley and White 2003, Edwards et al. 2005). Indeed, at various times in the ANP's development and career, it may be more suitable to have one type of supervision over another. In establishing a new role and focusing on developing clinical skills, the ANP may benefit from one-to-one supervision from a medical colleague of the same specialism. For professional and leadership issues the ANP may find that one-to-one supervision with another more experienced ANP from another specialty provides the support and guidance that is needed.

Group supervision can be formulated with a group of like-minded nurses from a particular specialty, such as a cardiology directorate, or from a group of ANPs working in different specialities across an organization. Clinical supervision is becoming more common among a variety of professional groups (Hawkins and Shohet 2000), and the ANP, particularly in primary care settings, may find it beneficial to take a multidisciplinary approach to supervision. The ANP should, however, be aware that clinical supervision can be seen to be different things to different professions and as such the supervisor should ensure that all supervisees are familiar with the aims, objectives and process of clinical supervision. Group supervision is seen to offer the additional benefits of advice and support from other members of the group that one-to-one supervision does not offer (Edwards et al. 2005).

At times a solitary ANP role within a specialty or organization can be isolating and as such the ANP may benefit from clinical supervision in the form of a network of other ANPs in a specialty across a region. This can be particularly useful for developing roles and sharing ideas; however, travel arrangements and diary commitments must be considered in establishing if it is going to be a long-term practical solution.

In looking at the work of Proctor (1991) these three approaches to clinical supervision can be seen as relevant in addressing the formative, restorative and normative functions of clinical supervision. All three functions are important and a balance of the three needs to occur, although one particular function may dominate at a particular time as can be seen in Scenario 9.3. Whichever form of clinical supervision is undertaken, it is hoped that the ANP will be able to manage the stresses of his or her new role and those that are associated with developing the role.

Actively seeks and participates in peer review of own practice

In selecting an appropriate supervisor, the ANP must ensure that the supervisor has the appropriate level of skills to facilitate their needs and that the ANP will feel confident and comfortable taking part in open discussions within the sessions. Kaur (2003) wrote that when choosing a supervisor the ANP should consider the potential supervisor's ability to share their expertise, skills, knowledge and experience, the ability to question critically and challenge the ANP, the ability to communicate and facilitate and the ability to bring new perspectives to situations in helping the ANP move on in their practice. It is well documented that if the supervisee chooses their own supervisor, supervision is far more successful (Sloan 1998, Winstanley and White 2003, Edwards et al. 2005).

Edwards et al. (2005) carried out a study evaluating the effectiveness of clinical supervision with their results reflecting previous studies. The length and frequency of sessions are important in determining a successful outcome. Sessions should not last less than 45 minutes and occur at least once every 4 weeks (Butterworth et al. 1997); sessions lasting over an hour achieve the most success (Edwards et al. 2005).

Accepts personal responsibility for professional development and the maintenance of professional competence and credential

Clinical supervision is not only critical to the developing ANP but also to ensuring continuing quality of the service and optimal standards of care (Clouder and Sellars 2004). Within the role of leader and supervisor the ANP must also provide members of perhaps more junior staff with supervision and place clinical supervision high on the organization's agenda for moving a quality service forward. The ANP must start and finish sessions on time, create a facilitative, comfortable environment, minimizing interruptions. They must maintain the focus of the session providing skilled support to enable the supervisee to explore issues and reach their own decisions (Kaur 2003). Ground rules regarding length of sessions, confidentiality and documentation must be established prior to any clinical supervision beginning.

Evaluation of the effectiveness of clinical supervision must take place (Kaur 2003, Edwards et al. 2005). Although this may be difficult to achieve, the ANP needs to draw on evaluative measures, such as complaints records, incident reports, observation of clinical/professional practices and discussions with staff and colleagues. Clinical supervision is a significant support mechanism for all staff involved in care delivery (Kaur 2003). Acting both as a supervisor and as a supervisee, the ANP will be able to highlight professional and clinical issues, take steps to evaluating practice and make improvements, ultimately improving the quality of patient care.

Scenario 9.3

Sandra has just started in her first advanced practice role in a busy trauma and orthopaedic unit, and although she has undertaken a nurse practitioner course has not been using her skills autonomously. ANP roles are new to the organization and only one other ANP has been employed, working in cancer services.

The consultants and business managers want Sandra to set up some point of referral clinics for patients with osteoarthritis and low back pain, to which GPs will refer patients direct. It is expected that Sandra will examine the patients, order relevant tests/investigations, refer on to physiotherapists or surgeons as necessary and establish a treatment plan as appropriate. These clinics will be the first nurse-led clinics within the organization.

In addition to the clinics, Sandra is responsible for providing clinical care to patients across the unit, educating and training all members of nursing staff and she has a role as a leader and researcher.

To begin with, Sandra is going to need support in developing the skills and knowledge she has learnt during her nurse practitioner course so that she can apply them to her practice. In addressing this formative function of clinical supervision, Sandra finds one-to-one supervision with a medical colleague beneficial, giving her a chance to discuss cases that she is responsible for and any difficulties she may be experiencing with, for example, her assessment techniques. The ANP role is new to her organization so in terms of setting up the role and developing it there is going to be little experience to draw on from within her own organization. Therefore, networking with a group of ANPs who are already in established posts will not only address the restorative function offered by clinical supervision but may also contribute towards some of her formative needs too.

As her role develops and she begins to feel more comfortable, Sandra may feel that she no longer needs such frequent one-to-one sessions with her consultant and that she now needs to focus on the organizational objectives, risk management issues and managerial aspects, thus a general manager or director of nursing may be in a better position to meet the normative function through a supervisory role in the clinical supervision sessions. This could be carried out either on a one-to-one basis or with a group of senior nurses across the organization.

> ## KEY POINTS
>
> - Clinical supervision is of benefit to the ANP in developing and applying new knowledge.
> - Network with other ANPs outside of the organization to develop the role and share ideas.
> - The ANP should act as supervisor to other staff and place clinical supervision high on the organization's agenda.

THE ANP'S PRACTICE AND QUALITY IMPROVEMENT

Monitors quality of own practice and participates in continuous improvement

This chapter has suggested ways in which the ANP can evaluate and improve quality in health care; however, the ANP also has a role in evaluating his or her own practice and role within an organization. ANP roles are innovative and exciting developments that provide nurses with an opportunity to work at an advanced level of practice (Furlong and Smith 2005). Although these changes are welcome, ANPs must ensure and demonstrate that outcomes are being improved and that patient needs are being met. In a climate in which health care must be cost-effective, ANPs need to be able to justify their role through evaluation and outcomes research (Ball and Cox 2003, Furlong and Smith 2005).

In evaluating and developing the role, data must be obtained to establish how well the role is working, and why, and to investigate any problem areas that there may be in order that action can be taken to rectify them (Walsh and Reveley 2001). There are a number of ways in which the ANP and other staff members can evaluate the role in advanced practice services, a few of which will be discussed below.

Research

It is important and beneficial that ANPs become familiar with a variety of research methodologies and work in a research capacity not only to monitor and continuously improve the quality of the advanced nursing service but also to contribute to the implementation of EBP as previously documented. Managers will often compare the new service provided by the ANP to previously existing medical services. These two services are very different by the very nature of the ANP role and evaluation of the service cannot be judged on the same markers. The ANP, for example, will spend longer in a consultation than medical colleagues due to the holistic approach that the ANP will apply. Although this may have cost implications, the extra time spent on health education, addressing emotional and social needs of the patient and counselling cannot have a price put on it in contributing to the patient's peace of mind (Walsh and Reveley 2001).

When establishing an advanced practice service within the organization, clear goals and objectives must be ascertained prior to its commencement (Walsh and Reveley 2001, Furlong and Smith 2005, Lloyd Jones 2005). These are important data against which further research can be benchmarked, and ensure that the correct research data are gathered (Walsh and Reveley 2001). A variety of research approaches beyond the scope of this chapter can be used by the ANP in collecting qualitative and quantitative data. Of interest, however, and worthy of mention here particularly for the novice researcher is that of action research.

Action research has become increasingly popular among nurse researchers and offers a means to narrow the gap between evidence and practice (Hart 1995, 1996, Clark 2000, Reed 2005). Unlike more traditional approaches to research, action research moves away from carrying out research 'on' people to undertaking it 'with' and 'for' people (Hart 1996, Clark 2000). Nursing literature has documented the apparent reluctance of nurses to translate research findings into their practice; often because they are unable to see the relevance to their practice and feel that the research has been carried out by people who are far removed from the real world of nursing practice (Clark 2000). Action research encourages people to participate in the research process and for them to highlight and subsequently investigate issues that are relevant to their own situation and make changes (McNiff et al. 1996, Denscombe 1998, Clark 2000, Reed 2005). As the word 'action' implies, the research is driven by the motivation of the researcher(s) with the clear intentions of implementing changes.

Action research methodologies are underpinned by four characteristics: collaboration between researchers and practitioners, the solution of practical problems, change in practice and the development of theory (Clark 2000). Many advantages and disadvantages have been cited within the literature. It addresses practical problems in a positive way, feeding results back into practice. Owing to action research being carried out at a very micro-level, however, it does mean that results cannot be generalized to other areas and research may be restricted by what is permissible and ethical within the ANP's workplace setting (Denscombe 1998, Reed 2005). Participating in action research enables the ANP to constantly reappraise his or her own performance and practices, and as such ensure that both they and the organization are constantly evolving and striving for excellence.

Whatever type of research the ANP decides to implement or participate in, it is important that evidence is produced to establish the effectiveness of the ANP role. It is only through concrete evidence that opposition to the developments will be overcome and trust managers will continue to invest in such services (Walsh and Reveley 2001, Lloyd Jones 2005).

Patient satisfaction

Many patient satisfaction surveys are carried out either via a questionnaire or through a telephone conversation. Although patient satisfaction surveys are useful in obtaining data relating to quality of services, they can be problematic in that the data can be subjective. Surveys of patient experience consistently give an overoptimistic view of the quality of care received and often do not highlight areas of poor care delivery (Staniszewska and Henderson 2005). Indeed, Mahon (1996) noted that although patients may be willing to rate quality they do not always have clear reasons for their evaluations. Patient satisfaction is also dependent on the patient's own level of expectation regarding the care that they receive, which, in turn, is dependent on educational, social and cultural factors (Walsh and Reveley 2001). In trying to overcome some of these factors, the ANP may find it useful to arrange for telephone follow-up to be instigated. This will allow the data gatherer to speak in much greater depth with the patient to obtain a better understanding of their experience and rephrase or explain questions to the patient to aid their understanding. Whether a questionnaire or telephone follow-up is used, it is advisable that the data are not returned to the ANP or that the ANP does not carry out the telephone follow-up, so as to decrease any bias (Cormack 2000).

Although some of the problems with patient satisfaction surveys have been highlighted, the ANP should note their importance as an evaluation method. Other audit outcomes will not be able to measure patient satisfaction, and it is an important area of information to be gathered in terms of the quality of service that is being provided. In addition to patient satisfaction, the ANP may find the following list helpful in providing ideas for evidence to collect in evaluating the service and role:

- how the ANP service compares with existing medically led services, e.g. cancellation rates, complication rates, length of stay, referral rates, numbers of investigations/tests ordered;
- nurse practitioner activity and impact elsewhere in the organization/UK;
- achievement of predetermined objectives/goals;
- ANP's personal and professional development;
- development of protocols/guidelines/pathways;
- research activity;
- professional networking, e.g. conferences, national forums, etc.

Audit trails

Audit has been discussed at length earlier in this chapter, but it is helpful to note here that the ANP will find it helpful to produce audit trails of activity within his or her service. The ANP needs to keep simple records of activity, referrals, trends and outcomes and produce activity and outcome reports to service managers as applicable.

Feedback

In monitoring their own practice, feedback from others within the ANP's own organization and also external to it can be useful. This may take the form of informal discussions and feedback through meetings or networking forums, or it may be more formal feedback, making use of such methods as the 360° feedback. This method has been used among managers for some time and is now becoming more popular in other areas. Individual and team performances can be assessed against defined competencies or it can be used as an individual appraisal tool. Either way, anonymous feedback is obtained from a variety of sources, peers, managers, staff and 'customers', and fed back to the individual (Peiperl 1999, Brett and Atwater 2001). The feedback is compared with the individual's own ratings as to their performance and they are given the opportunity to focus on their strengths, plan for improvement and practice key behaviours. Many people find this method beneficial as they are receiving feedback from more than one person who may have little knowledge of their role; others can feel very 'exposed' and may expect more positive feedback than they have received. Brett and Atwater (2001), however, argue that this is positive in terms of motivating the individual to change in their behaviour.

In addition to evaluating the role of the ANP, ANPs must develop the role and continue to demonstrate its effectiveness in clinical care. ANPs need to provide strong leadership by communicating messages about advanced practice: its purpose, scope and education. Other departments and organizations will need guidance about introducing advanced practice roles and the support required for their successful implementation and outcomes (Bryant-Lukosius et al. 2004). Many ANP roles are introduced without appropriate planning and thought about how the roles will work within the organization. Preparation for advanced practice functions is vital, both so that the ANP can fulfil any legal duty and also so that patients are sufficiently protected and receive the best possible care (Harris and Redshaw 1998, Jones and Davies 1999).

Once ANPs are in post, they must be continuously supported and not left to find where they fit within the organization; with the appropriate support, many more benefits for both the ANP and the organization may become apparent (Walsh and Reveley 2001). Without appropriate planning and systematic efforts to develop and evaluate ANP roles, many barriers will inhibit developing the full potential of the ANP role (Bryant-Lukosius et al. 2004). Bryant-Lukosius and DiCenso (2004) recommended that to improve the introduction of ANP roles there was a need to clearly define the role, support the development of the role as a nursing one, promote the use of the ANP's knowledge, skills and expertise, create supportive environments and provide rigorous and ongoing evaluation of the role and predetermined outcomes-based goals.

KEY POINTS

- The ANP must demonstrate that outcomes are being improved and patient needs are being met in a cost-effective way.
- The ANP should become familiar with research methodology.
- Clear goals and objectives must be ascertained prior to the commencement of an advanced practice service.
- To monitor their own practice, ANPs should welcome feedback from a variety of personnel.

CONCLUSION

This chapter has discussed ways in which the competencies within the domain of monitoring can be met and the quality of advanced health care practice can be ensured. The NHS plan (DoH 2000) states that the NHS will be driven by a cycle of continuous quality improvement and, therefore, the ANP must not only provide safe, high-quality care but also constantly see and create opportunities for improvement (Donaldson 2001). Clinical governance provides an ideal framework in which ANPs can ensure and monitor the quality of services, focusing on clinical effectiveness, risk management and their own professional development and lifelong learning.

Suggestions have been put forward for ways to gather data regarding quality and ways to implement changes in practice. Patient records, outcomes and satisfaction data should be used to constantly evaluate practice and strive for quality. The importance of ANPs' own professional development has been highlighted, outlining ways in which they can participate in CPD activity, promoting a positive effect both for the ANP and also for the organization. As advanced practice roles expand, research and other evaluative methods must be undertaken to evaluate their effectiveness and best practice shared not only within the organization but also nationally. It is only by carrying out such activities that advanced nursing practice will continue to develop and ultimately increase the quality of health care.

REFERENCES

Alsop, A. (2003) Reflecting on practice and portfolio development. In *Core skills for nurse practitioners*, Palmer, D. and Kaur, S. (eds), pp. 174–184. London: Whurr Publishers.

Andrews, M. (1993) Importance of nursing leadership in implementing change. *British Journal of Nursing* 2: 437–439.

Ball, C. (1999) Revealing higher levels of nursing practice. *Intensive and Critical Care Nursing* 15(2): 65–76.

Ball, C. and Cox, C. (2003) Part 1: Restoring patients to health – outcomes and indicators of advanced nursing practice in adult critical care. *International Journal of Nursing Practice*, 9(6): 356–367.

Bamford, O. and Gibson, F. (2000) The clinical nurse specialist: perceptions of practising CNSs of their role and development needs. *Journal of Clinical Nursing* 9(2): 282–292.

Bartle, J. (2000) Clinical supervision: its place within the quality agenda. *Nursing Management* 7(5): 30–33.

Bousfield, C. (1997) A phenomenological investigation into the role of the clinical nurse specialist. *Journal of Advanced Nursing* 25(2): 245–256.

Brett, J. and Atwater, L. (2001) 360° feedback: accuracy, reactions and perceptions of usefulness. *Journal of Applied Psychology* 86: 930–942.

Bryant-Lukosius, D. and DiCenso, A. (2004) A framework for the introduction and evaluation of advanced practice nursing roles. *Journal of Advanced Nursing* 48: 530–540.

Bryant-Lukosius, D. DiCenso, A. Browne, G. and Pinelli, J. (2004) Advanced practice nursing roles: development, implementation and evaluation, *Journal of Advanced Nursing* 48: 519–529.

Buckingham, L. and Palmer, D. (2003) Lifelong learning. In *Core skills for nurse practitioners*, Palmer, D. and Kaur, S. (eds), pp. 202–214. London: Whurr.

Butterworth, T. Carson, J. White, E. Jeacock, J. Clements, A. and Bishop, V. (1997) *It is good to talk: An evaluation study in England and Scotland*. Manchester: School of Nursing, Midwifery and Health Visiting, University of Manchester.

Calman, K. (1998) *A review of continuing professional development in general practice. Report by the Chief Medical Officer*. London: Department of Health.

Clark, J. (2000) Action research. In *The research process in nursing*, 4th edn, Cormack, D. (ed.), pp. 183–197. Oxford: Blackwell.

Closs, S. and Cheater, F. (1999) Evidence for nursing practice: a clarification of the issues. *Journal of Advanced Nursing* 30(1): 10–17.

Clouder, L. and Sellars, J. (2004) Reflective practice and clinical supervision: an interprofessional perspective. *Journal of Advanced Nursing* 46(3): 262–269.

Coffey, A. (2005) The clinical learning portfolio: a practice development experience in gerontological nursing. *Journal of Clinical Nursing* 14(8b): 75–83.

Cormack, D. (2000) *The research process in nursing*, 4th edn. Oxford: Blackwell.

Cox, C. (2004) *Physical assessment for nurses*. Oxford: Blackwell.

Cranston, M. (2002) Clinical effectiveness and evidence-based practice. *Nursing Standard* 16(24): 39–43.

Currie, L. and Harvey, G. (1998) Care pathways development and implementation. *Nursing Standard* 12(30): 35–38.

Cutcliffe, J. and Bassett, C. (1997) Introducing change in nursing: the case of research. *Journal of Nursing Management* 5: 241–247.

DeBourgh, G. (2001) Champions for evidence-based practice: a critical role for advanced practice nurses. *Acute and Critical Care Nursing* 12: 491–508.

Denscombe, M. (1998) *The good research guide*. Buckingham: Open University Press.

Department of Health (1993a) *Clinical audit: meeting and improving standards in healthcare*. London: HMSO.

Department of Health (1993b) *A vision for the future. Report of the Chief Nursing Officer*. London: HMSO.

Department of Health (1994) *The evolution of clinical audit*. Leeds: Department of Health.

Department of Health (1998) *A first class service: quality in the new NHS*. London: HMSO.

Department of Health (2000) *The NHS plan: a plan for investment, a plan for reform*. London: HMSO.

Department of Health (2004) *NHS Improvement Plan 2004: Putting people at the heart of public services*. London: HMSO.

Dickerson, P. (2000) A CQI approach to evaluating continuing education: processes and outcomes. *Journal for Nurses in Staff Development* 16(1): 34–40.

Dimond, B. (2003) *Legal and ethical issues in advanced practice*. In *Advanced nursing practice*, 2nd edn, McGee, P. and Castledine, G. (eds), pp. 184–199. Oxford: Blackwell Publishing.

Donagrandi, M. and Eddy, M. (2000) Ethics of case management: implications for advanced practice nursing. *Clinical Nurse Specialist* 14(5): 241–249.

Donaldson, L. (2001) Safe high quality health care: investing in tomorrow's leaders. *Quality in Health Care* 10: 8–12.

Dunn, L. (1998) Creating a framework for clinical nursing practice to advance in-the West Midlands region. *Journal of Clinical Nursing* 7: 239–243.

Edwards, D. Cooper, L. Burnard, P. Hannigan, B. Adams, J. Fothergill, A. and Coyle, D. (2005) Factors influencing the effectiveness of clinical supervision. *Journal of Psychiatric and Mental Health Nursing* 12: 405–414.

Evans, C. Drennan, V. and Roberts, J. (2005) Practice nurses and older people: a case management approach to care. *Journal of Advanced Nursing* 51(4): 343–352.

Flemming, K. (1998) Asking answerable questions. *Evidence Based Nursing* 1(2): 36–37.

Furlong, E. and Smith, R. (2005) Advanced nursing practice: policy, education and role development. *Journal of Clinical Nursing* 14: 1059–1066.

Furlong, S. and Glover, D. (1998) Legal accountability in changing practice. *Nursing Times* 94(39): 61–62.

Gillies, A. (1997) *Improving the quality of patient care*. Chichester: John Wiley.

Goorapah, D. (1997) Clinical supervision. *Journal of Clinical Nursing* 6(3): 173–178.

Gorzanski, C. (1997) Raising the standards through supervision. *Modern Midwife* 7(2): 11–14.

Griffiths, M. (2003) *Evidenced-based care, research and audit*. In *Core skills for nurse practitioners*, Palmer, D. and Kaur, S. (eds), pp. 57–60. London: Whurr Publishers.

Harris, A. and Redshaw, M. (1998) Professional issues facing nurse practitioners and nursing. *British Journal of Nursing* 7: 1381–1385.

Hart, E. (1995) Developing action research in nursing. *Nurse Researcher* 2(3): 4–14.

Hart, E. (1996) Action research as a professionalizing strategy: issues and dilemmas. *Journal of Advanced Nursing* 23: 454–461.

Hawkins, P. and Shohet, R. (2000) *Supervision in the helping professions*. Buckingham: Open University Press.

Heath, T. and Jagger, K. (2003) Change management. In *Core skills for nurse practitioners*, Palmer, D. and Kaur, S. (eds), pp. 24–42. London: Whurr.

Hockenberry-Eaton, M. and Kennedy, L. (1996) Promoting accountability in advanced nursing practice. *Journal of Paediatric Health Care* 10(2): 92–94.

Humphris, D. and Masterson, A. (1998) Practising at a higher level. *Professional Nurse* 14(1): 10–13.

Hyrkäs, K. and Paunonen-Ilmonen, M. (2001) The effects of clinical supervision on the quality of care: examining the results of team supervision. *Journal of Advanced Nursing* 33: 492–502.

Jasper, M. (1998) Using portfolios to advance practice. In *Advanced nursing practice*, Rolfe, G. and Fulbrook, P. (eds), pp. 246–256. Oxford: Butterworth Heinemann.

Johnston, G. Crombie, I. Alder, E. Davies, H. and Millard, A. (2000) Reviewing audit: barriers and facilitating factors for effective clinical audit. *Quality in Health Care* 9(1): 23–36.

Jones, R. Freegard, S. Reeves, M. Hanney, K. and Dobbs, F. (2001) The role of the practice nurse in the management of asthma. *Journal of Primary Care* 10(4): 109–111.

Jones, S. and Davies, K. (1999) The extended role of the nurse: the United Kingdom perspective. *International Journal of Nursing Practice* 5(4): 184–188.

Joyce, P. (2005) A framework for portfolio development in postgraduate nursing practice. *Journal of Clinical Nursing* 14: 456–463.

Karlowicz, K. (2000) The value of student portfolios to evaluate undergraduate nursing programs. *Nurse Educator* 25(2): 82–87.

Kaur, S. (2003) Clinical supervision. In *Core skills for nurse practitioners*, Palmer, D. and Kaur, S. (eds), pp. 160–173. London: Whurr Publishers.

Kemp, N. and Richardson, E. (1999) *Quality assurance in nursing practice*, 2nd edn. Oxford: Butterworth Heinemann.

Kinsman, L. (2004) Clinical pathway compliance and quality improvement. *Nursing Standard* 18(18): 33–35.

Lewin, K. (1951) *Field theory in social science*. New York: Harper and Row.

Lloyd Jones, M. (2005) Role development and effective practice in specialist and advanced practice roles in acute hospital settings: systematic review and meta-synthesis. *Journal of Advanced Nursing* 49(2): 191–209.

McMullan, M. Endacott, R. Gray, M. Jasper, M. Miller, C. Scholes, J. and Webb, C. (2003) Portfolios and assessment of competence: a review of the literature. *Journal of Advanced Nursing* 41(3): 283–294.

McNiff, J. Lomax, P. and Whitehead, J. (1996) *You and your action research project*. London: Routledge.

Mahon, P. (1996) An analysis of the concept 'patient satisfaction' as it relates to contemporary nursing care. *Journal of Advanced Nursing* 24: 1241–1248.

Morrison, D. (2003) *E-learning strategies: how to get implementation and delivery right first time*. Chichester: Wiley.

Munro, N. (2004) Evidence-based assessment: no more pride or prejudice. *Acute and Critical Care Nursing* 15: 501–505.

National Institute for Clinical Excellence (2002) *Principles for best practice in clinical audit*, p. 70. Oxon: Radcliffe Medical Press.

Nursing and Midwifery Council (2002) *Supporting nurses and midwives through lifelong learning*. London: NMC.

Nursing and Midwifery Council (2004) *The PREP handbook*. London: NMC.

Nursing and Midwifery Council (2006) *Clinical supervision*. London: NMC.

Nursing and Midwifery Council (2007) *Record keeping*. London: NMC.

Parsley, K. and Corrigan, P. (1999) *Quality improvement in healthcare: putting evidence into practice*, 2nd edn. Cheltenham: Stanley Thornes.

Peiperl, M. (1999) Conditions for the success of peer evaluation. *The International Journal of Human Resource Management* 10: 429–458.

Poysner, J. (1996) Physicians assistant: legal implications of the extended role. *British Journal of Nursing* 5: 592.

Price, A. (1994) Midwifery portfolios: making reflective records. *Modern Midwife* 4(11): 35–38.

Proctor, B. (1991) *On being a trainer.* In *Training and supervision for counselling in action,* Dryden, W. and Thorne, B. (eds), pp. 49–73. London: Sage.

Redman, W. (1994) *Portfolios for development: a guide for trainers and managers.* London: Kogan Page.

Reed, J. (2005) Using action research in nursing practice with older people: democratizing knowledge. *Journal of Clinical Nursing* 14: 594–600.

Reveley, S. and Carruthers, L. (2001) Setting up a nurse practitioner-led pre-operative assessment clinic in an orthopaedic unit. In *Nurse practitioners developing the role in hospital settings,* Reveley, S. Walsh, M. and Crumbie, A. (eds), pp. 65–77. Oxford: Butterworth Heinemann.

Scally, G. and Donaldson, L. (1998) Clinical governance and the drive for quality improvement in the new NHS in England. *British Medical Journal* 317: 61–65.

Sloan, G. (1998) Clinical supervision: characteristics of a good supervisor. *Nursing Standard* 12(24): 42–46.

Staniszewska, A. and Henderson, L. (2005) Patients' evaluations of the quality of care: influencing factors and the importance of engagement. *Journal of Advanced Nursing* 49: 530–537.

Stanton, M. Swanson, M. Sherrod, R. and Packa, D. (2005) Case management evolution from basic to advanced practice role. *Lippincott's Case Management* 10(6): 274–284.

Teasdale, K. Brocklehurst, N. and Thom, N. (2001) Clinical supervision and support for nurses: an evaluation study. *Journal of Advanced Nursing* 33(2): 216–224.

Tingle, J. (2002) The legal implications of extending nurses' roles. *Practice Nursing* 13(4): 148, 150, 152.

Walsh, M. and Crumbie, A. (2003) Nurse practitioner education: what level? *Nursing Standard* 18(4): 33–36.

Walsh, M. and Reveley, S. (2001) Evaluating the nurse practitioner role in hospital. In *Nurse practitioners developing the role in hospital settings,* Reveley, S. Walsh, M. and Crumbie, A. (eds), pp. 130–143. Oxford: Butterworth Heinemann.

Wayman, C. (1999) Hospital-based nursing case management: role clarification. *Nursing Case Management* 4(5): 236–241.

Wenzel, L. Briggs, K. and Puryear, B. (1998) Portfolio: authentic assessment in the age of the curriculum revolution. *Journal of Nursing Education* 37(5): 208–212.

Winstanley, J. and White, E. (2003) Clinical supervision: models, measures and best practice. *Nurse Researcher* 10(4): 7–38.

Wiseman, R. (1994) Role model behaviours in the clinical setting. *Journal of Nurse Education* 33: 405–409.

Wood, J. (2004) Clinical supervision. *British Journal of Perioperative Nursing* 14(4): 151–156.

10 COLLECTING THE EVIDENCE

SUE HINCHLIFF

INTRODUCTION

This chapter will explore the following topics in its examination of how practitioners can set about collecting their evidence for accreditation of their advanced nursing practice.

• What is accreditation?
• Differences between academic and professional accreditation.
• Supporting the path to professional accreditation.
• Benefits of accreditation.
• What is meant by evidence?
• What constitutes evidence?
• Capturing the evidence.
• Keeping a portfolio.
• Peer review of the evidence.

So far in this book we have looked at the journey towards advanced nursing practice in all its domains.

Now we need to think about how this evidence of what it is like to practise at an advanced level can be captured. There will come points in a practitioner's learning career where he or she needs to provide evidence of having gained competencies, knowledge and skills, and offer that evidence to others who may measure it against standards of, say, clinical expertise. Equally, you may be helping other practitioners to do this as part of their lifelong learning journey. This process of measuring evidence against standards or competencies is part of professional accreditation.

WHAT IS ACCREDITATION?

Accreditation simply means measuring a person, product or place against a set of standards; if it meets those standards, whatever it is can be accredited or recognized in some way for having 'measured up'. Sometimes this may mean that the person, product or place will be recorded somewhere as having been accredited. An example of this would be when one passes the driving test and gains a license and it is recorded in the Driving Standards Agency's records. Equally, accreditation can be used for promotional purposes; for example, a workplace can be recognized as having met the Investor in People or government Chartermark standards, and can advertise itself in this way. However accreditation is recognized or used, it makes the recipient different in some way from others.

In essence, accreditation, whether this is for a person, a product or a place, involves four stages:

- *Standard/competency setting* – this stage involves experts getting together to undertake a values clarification about their area of practice. Their values and beliefs are then grouped into themes, i.e. domains, and standards are set by consensus with the group; the standards are then piloted and amendments are made as necessary.
- *Dissemination of the standards/competencies* with guidance to facilitate the collection of evidence – once the standards are published the accreditation agency should produce guidance for practitioners who wish to be accredited against the standards. This will enable them to collect the evidence in a portfolio to support their claim for accreditation.
- *Comparison of the evidence against the standards/competencies by peers* to ensure compliance – the review of the evidence includes external peer involvement. Peers review the portfolio for compliance with the standards and an external moderator ensures objectivity and the quality of the review process.
- *Review and evaluation* of all stages of the foregoing process in order to effect quality enhancement. The process of accreditation is reviewed through all four stages to ensure that it is doing what it sets out to do, i.e. to measure evidence submitted by practitioners against the agreed standards in a fair and objective way.

Note that a *standard* is a desired and achievable level of performance against which actual performance can be measured, whereas *competencies* refer to the specific knowledge, skills, judgement and personal attributes required for a practitioner to practise safely and ethically in a designated role and setting. One of the characteristics of a self-regulating profession is the development of standards/competencies based on the values of the profession. Note that standards are frequently accompanied by performance criteria, and sometimes by a note to indicate what sort of evidence might show compliance with that standard.

So accreditation implies measurement against a set of standards (or sometimes competencies), but where do these come from? One of the commonest standards is 12 linear inches, a foot, since it was based on the average size of a man's foot. This is called a *gold standard* – it is absolute and never varies.

Sometimes we use *minimum standards* – here we are not necessarily concerned with best practice but with minimum standards for safety. The initial practical driving test is an example of this. You are allowed to have a certain number of errors so long as safety is not compromised in any way. This sort of accreditation is often mandatory in nature.

As a corollary to this, the Advanced Driving Test is based on *standards of best practice*. Although in health care we strive to meet standards of best practice, sometimes our practice needs to be shaped or developed towards this end. Many accreditation bodies use systems that do not 'fail' those who do not fully comply with the standards straight off; they provide feedback which helps to shape the evidence submitted by the applicant so that he or she is guided towards submitting the best sort of evidence to demonstrate compliance with the relevant standards. This approach usually leads to voluntary participation. Note that sometimes, with organizational standards, the challenge may be so great that they not attainable.

Differences between academic and professional accreditation

None of the examples cited so far has come from either academic or professional accreditation.

Academic accreditation

This is usually called validation and it focuses on the student and his/her learning experience and learning outcomes. The student is seen as the end-user and any focus on practice is tangential and through assessment, which is, at some point, summative. The end-point is an award or CATS (credit accumulation and transfer scheme) points for the student, and this award tells of intellectual achievement rather than practice development. There are identified levels of achievement and a strong focus on fitness for award.

Professional accreditation

This allows us to measure what a practitioner does in practice against practice standards using practice methodologies – i.e. it tells us about fitness for practice; it may also tell us about organizational leadership and development.

It demonstrates how propositional knowledge concerning theory, evidence and research, often gained though academic accreditation, can be blended uniquely with personal knowledge and professional experience to impact on practice. The net effect of this is what Titchen and Ersser (2001: 35) describe as 'professional craft knowledge', which they see as 'often tacit and unarticulated and sometimes intuitive'. In this way practice both uses and generates evidence. It makes nursing visible and offers a way for nurses to articulate what is unique about what they do. It focuses on practice development and can be a tool for quality improvement in practice. Ultimately, the patient is the end-user.

Professional accreditation is frequently underpinned by a framework that identifies competencies within domains of practice. It may be set within a career and competency framework with levels similar to those used within academia. For instance, the competent practitioner with some experience might have a diploma or first degree; the expert nurse might have a master's degree and the consultant nurse might be working towards a doctorate.

Evidence of how the practitioner purports to meet the standards is usually collected in a portfolio, which is subjected to the same external peer scrutiny as would occur in the academic world. Note that this portfolio could be submitted as part of an APEL (accreditation of prior experiential learning) claim to a university in order to gain CATS points.

We need both academic and professional accreditation, for they complement each other, and it is the mix that leads to professional craft knowledge and patient benefit. Everybody then gains; the practitioner gains an award and also professional credibility and recognition, the patient gains improved care and the employer gains a more competent nursing workforce.

Supporting the path to professional accreditation

The journey towards professional accreditation is made a lot easier if the person seeking accreditation has someone who can act as a 'critical friend' who can offer both support and challenge along the way. Even an expert nurse needs a companion along the journey. There will be ups and downs, and it is important to have someone who can take an objective view of what is happening.

The accreditation process, by its very nature, causes you to question your practice and this can lead initially to a loss of confidence. This is entirely normal but it is easier to handle the feelings if you can explore them with a respected and skilled colleague who can support you. Support may also include encouraging you to consider different options or helping you to reflect on an issue. You may choose your clinical supervisor or you may have a facilitator or mentor to guide you on your way.

You not only need support but you also need to have your thoughts, reflections, decisions and actions challenged in order to distil the maximum learning from them. This may involve causing you to look at something in a different way. This, too, can be painful and challenge must be offered in a constructive and supportive way – without challenge you will not produce evidence of sufficient rigour and quality.

As you collect your portfolio of evidence your facilitator should be used to test each piece of evidence for its rigour, quality, sufficiency, trustworthiness and the extent to which it demonstrates without doubt that you have achieved the standards or competencies in question.

THE BENEFITS OF PROFESSIONAL ACCREDITATION

The value of accreditation depends on where you are standing. The benefits are obviously different, depending on whether you are a practitioner, an employer or a patient or client.

The patient or client always has to be central to whatever we do in professional accreditation. After all, assuring best practice in educational initiatives for nurses, in nursing practice and in competency development, ultimately improves outcomes for patients and clients. If you were a patient you would feel reassured to know that your primary nurse had been recognized as an expert practitioner; you could be confident that the nurse had achieved certain standards of practice or had reached particular practice benchmarks.

Employers are concerned about value for money, and when offering continuing professional development opportunities to their staff they want to know that the event, short course or resource has been examined against predetermined quality standards and found to be both educationally sound and of appropriate design and content to achieve its purpose. It should also be offered by experts who are recognized as qualified to teach the topic. Accreditation is, therefore, a proxy for assuring all these elements.

Employers are also concerned to offer a service that is fit for purpose and fit for practice. Competency development is key to quality improvement, and accreditation facilitates a constant review of current practice. Practice development provides a basis for collaborative working and offers a structured framework for developing innovations in practice that ultimately increase staff satisfaction – all of which contribute to improved recruitment and retention of the professional workforce.

What are the benefits, then, to practitioners? Well, for one thing, there's a feel-good factor about being accredited – it feels like the achievement that it is. It is something to be celebrated; it could be used in a bid for promotion; it establishes credibility in the area which is accredited.

When a practitioner is accredited as an individual, he or she has to put together a portfolio of evidence of different kinds, demonstrating that the relevant standards have been met. This gives the opportunity to experiment with and experience a range of assessment methodologies, such as 360° review, user narratives, direct observation of care, taped or videoed exchanges, and so on. As mentioned previously, this portfolio of evidence can be used to make an APEL claim to a university for academic credit.

So, if accreditation has a wide range of benefits, what is the downside? Well, accreditation presents a snapshot of a person, educational product or practice area at a point in time. In order for that accolade to continue to hold true, there must be regular review and performance monitoring, and these should be capable of demonstrating growth and further development.

Nobody would deny that it is quite onerous and time-consuming to develop effective standards (Scrivens 1995). Even then, as practitioners develop and as time moves on, the standards can be pushed further towards excellence. Equally, on the part of the person seeking accreditation it can be a lengthy process to put all the required evidence together, but as Scrivens says, 'the greatest value of accreditation lies in the preparation' (p. 56). Accreditation is never a quick fix. Those who are to assess evidence must be rigorously prepared, monitored and continue to be offered development opportunities. For all these reasons, accreditation costs money – but the benefits outweigh those costs.

Here, in summary, then is a list of some of the benefits:

- promotes 'feel-good factor' in the recipient;
- establishes credibility for the person accredited;
- helps to maintain standards;
- offers a 'kite mark' to assure quality;
- facilitates continuous review of current practice by the accreditee;
- puts a value on professional nursing and makes it visible;
- maintains consistency through the setting of standards;
- enhances the recipient's reputation;
- offers a structured framework for innovations in practice;
- is a key to practice developments;
- provides a basis for collaborative working;
- helps to improve patient care;
- aids recruitment and retention through improved job satisfaction;
- offers experience of a range of evaluation methodologies;
- uses peer review – and the expertise of other practitioners;
- promotes a culture of reflection, challenge and support;
- facilitates learning from practice and in practice.

What is meant by evidence?

Evidence is needed to convince peer reviewers that standards have been met, so the evidence must relate directly to the standards. Sometimes standards are very precise; often, though, the standard may be more generic, and in this case they are usually accompanied by criteria for demonstrating compliance. The accreditee is accountable for demonstrating clearly and beyond doubt that the standard has been met.

Evidence should be rigorous, of sufficient quantity and quality, trustworthy and corroborated:

- *Rigour* – evidence must be precisely matched to the standard or competency and the required level. It should not be sloppily expressed; it should reflect person-centred, evidence-based care and reflective analytical practice. It should be consistent.
- *Quantity and quality* – there is sometimes a tendency to submit all the evidence that might exist against a standard 'to be on the safe side'. This is not necessary; all that is needed is a sufficient range of evidence to show unambiguously that the standard has been met. Your mentor/facilitator should be able to help you decide on how much evidence is enough. Quality refers to the depth and soundness and relevance of the evidence – it should not be superficial or lacking in analysis and evaluation.
- *Trustworthiness* – the evidence has to belong to the person who says that they produced it. For this reason most schemes require verification of the evidence by a third party. It should not be invented or fabricated but should represent the truth, even if that does not show best practice. There should be no plagiarism of others' work nor should the portfolio be unduly derivative and lean too much on published sources, even when cited.
- *Corroboration* – demonstrating achievement of a standard should not rest on one piece of evidence. Evidence should be triangulated and come from a number of sources to show without doubt that the standard has been met. For example, 360° review, patient stories and direct observation may be used to satisfy peer reviewers that a standard has been achieved.

Finally, the peer reviewer should be guided through the portfolio by a narrative; instructions to the reader should be clear: you know your portfolio, but the reader needs signposts to guide his or her journey. There should be analysis and interpretation of what the evidence shows, together with your own assessment of the extent to which you meet the standards.

What constitutes evidence?

Evidence is required to show that the person seeking accreditation can meet all of the standards/competencies in question. From the above it follows that a range of different types of evidence must be submitted. Examples that you might consider follow below. Note that many of these methods involve *reflective practice*.

The definition of reflective practice as articulated by Johns (1996: 1135) underpins accreditation:

> a window for practitioners to look inside and know who they are as they strive towards understanding and realising the meaning of desirable work in their everyday practices. The practitioner must expose, confront and understand the contradictions within their practice between what is practised and what is desirable. It is the conflict of contradiction and the commitment to achieve desirable work that enables the practitioner to become empowered to take action to appropriately resolve these contradictions.

To articulate this philosophy, components of accreditation should include, for example, the recording of significant experiences, the use of a model of structured reflection and the maintenance of a learning/reflective diary. Reflection should be used as a means of exploring approaches to clinical supervision and facilitation, clinical effectiveness and clinical governance; together with reflection on the effectiveness of the participant's skills.

Critical incident reflections

Critical incidents can be used to explore key aspects of your work. Keep a note of them as they arise and take some time to reflect on them. Write down your reflections in a way that captures the experience and how you dealt with it and with the other actors in the scenario.

- Perhaps you discussed things with a colleague?
- What happened when you debriefed after the incident?
- How did you feel?
- What skills/knowledge did you use?
- What was it that led you to make the decisions you did?
- Where did your insights come from?
- What triggered your actions, thoughts, feelings?
- What did you handle well?
- What could have been improved?
- What did you learn from the incident?

Try showing your reflections to someone who can offer you some constructive criticisms: they might be able to pick out aspects of your work you had not considered. You might want to use your clinical supervisor or facilitator if you have one.

Direct observation of practice

Ask your clinical supervisor, facilitator or a colleague to observe you in your practice. You might like to ask them to take some notes or reflections to help capture your actions and any outcomes. They might want to ask you questions to tease out why you acted as you did; what was in your head at the time; what other options you had and why you did not choose them. If you use this method over a period of time your observer may be able to alert you to how your practice has developed. This process acts as a form of deconstruction of practice; note, though, that reconstruction must occur for care to continue to be holistic.

Then think about how this might become evidence to demonstrate your particular expertise. It can be used to supplement critical reflection of practice and may help you to expose areas of your practice that you do not normally articulate or recognize.

Remember that your evidence does not have to demonstrate perfect practice, the value lies in critiquing it honestly so that you can do it better next time round and recording your reflections.

Notes of clinical supervision, facilitation

You might want to include some evidence of the joint dialogue you have with your colleagues, team, clinical supervisor or facilitator. Do ask their permission before you include personal notes. Their notes might be used to answer the following questions:

- What has the journey been like in exploring/evaluating/improving clinical practice?
- How have you managed to find the evidence base for your practice?
- How has your understanding of practice developed?
- Has this experience filtered through into other work you do?
- Are there any other people/processes you utilize that help you critique your work?

If you ask your supervisor or facilitator to write up some notes this will add to the trustworthiness and corroboration of your evidence.

360° feedback

Ward (1997) defines 360° feedback (or review) as 'the systematic collection and feedback of performance data on an individual or group, derived from a number of stakeholders in their performance' (p. 4).

360° feedback is a bit like taking photos of a sculpture from every angle rather than simply from the front. This would obviously give you a much better understanding of the piece of work – and so it is with practice. You might wish to think about gathering some feedback about your work from managers, nursing colleagues, clients and others in the multiprofessional team who interface with you. You should also include the views of support staff. You could seek feedback using interviews, discussions, testimonials or a questionnaire, the results of which could be analysed and presented in your portfolio. Remember, your stakeholders should try to identify your strengths and areas where you need to develop further. You, similarly, need to assess yourself and your practice on the same parameters.

Try to use people who are familiar with your work who can help you identify aspects of your practice which you have not been able to articulate or identify yourself.

Remember all the time that whatever evidence you collect has to be mapped against a particular standard or competency – there is no point in including evidence for the sake of it.

User perspectives: patient narratives, patient stories

You might try to get specific user feedback. For instance, you might like to include examples of patients' thank-you letters or you might talk with a patient about how he or she felt about the care offered. You may have other organizational systems in place that capture user feedback; think about how you can include these in your portfolio. Remember that if you are using evidence from patients, make sure that you have the patients' consent and that confidentiality is not breached. It should not be possible to identify patients from any evidence.

Often patient stories provide a vivid – and sometimes harrowing – account of what the period of care was like, and their relationships and fears during this time. From them it is possible to identify the impact that the practitioner has on their care and the culture which characterizes their care environment.

Outcomes

Think about, and demonstrate in the portfolio, how your actions have had an impact on patient care. What might help you to identify this? You might want to access audit trails that detail the route that led to any outcome, or an exchange of emails may show the processes you went through.

Some questions you can think about are:

- What and how people are affected by your interactions and interventions?
- How does practice change in your clinical area?
- How do you impact on others in the team?
- What do peers say about you and your sphere of influence?

This will all help to enable you to capture and verify your contributions to the workplace.

Action learning

This can be described as

> a continuous process of learning and reflection, supported by colleagues,
> with the intention of getting things done.
>
> McGill and Beaty (1998)

You may be part of an action learning set and wish to include some evidence in your portfolio from this process.

Action learning is an approach to individual and group development, traditionally used to develop managerial and organizational effectiveness. Over several months, people work in a small group, usually between 6 and 10 people (an action learning set), to tackle issues or problems that are important to them, and learn from their attempts to change things.

Action learning comprises four elements:

- the person – members join and contribute voluntarily;
- the problem – everyone brings and must 'own' an issue on which he or she wants to act. It does not always have to be a problem, it could equally be a celebration that the member wishes to explore;
- the group or set – colleagues who can help us to 'bottom out' the issue in question;
- the action and the learning – after having analysed the issues, thought through the options and decided what to do, with the help of the set, individuals act to resolve their problems.

Action learning sets meet over a period of time and at regular intervals to help each other think through the issues, create options, agree on action and learn from the effects of that action through providing high challenge and high support. Learning about how groups work is an added benefit. The colleagues in the set may be from the same organization or from different organizations. Each time the group meets they should agree a facilitator if there is not a permanent facilitator who is external to the group.

The facilitator's role is to help the set to develop, to facilitate support and challenge and to help members reflect on their own learning. The main purpose is to help members towards a deeper understanding of themselves and their practice, and increased effectiveness in their work.

In summary, to function effectively, action learning sets need:

- *To meet regularly* – people in the set should decide how many meetings to have, where to hold them, for how long, when to stop, how to evaluate, and so on.
- *Consistent membership* – it is often impossible for every member to be at every meeting of the set, but more than one absence of any one member can reduce the effectiveness of the set. Aim for a minimum of four members and a maximum of ten, with between six and eight being the optimum, with the agreed commitment to attend a certain number of meetings.
- *Ground rules* – people in the set should agree ground rules to govern behaviour. For example, the set might agree that all members have an equal right to the time and attention of the set.
- *A balance of challenge and support* – people in the set should be aware that support is often needed before challenge can be accepted.
- *To review the process* – people in the set need to stop work on problems at intervals and reflect on how well the group as a whole is working.

- *A facilitator* – to help the set to develop, to facilitate the supporting and challenging processes and to help members reflect on their own learning. The main purpose is to help members towards a deeper understanding of themselves and the contexts in which they work, and to increase effectiveness in their work. The facilitator may initiate the running of the set and then hand it over to the set as soon as it is established.

This self-management is a first step in people taking responsibility for their own actions and learning. It is recommended that no more than 3 months should elapse between meetings.

Other methods of collecting evidence

As well as the above, you might also want to include the following, as long as they can be mapped against a particular standard and they are your own work:

- publications;
- patient information leaflets;
- essays or assignments, especially where these are practice based or can show how knowledge is being applied to practice;
- reflections;
- poems, drawings, cartoons that illustrate a particular point;
- action plans;
- reports;
- records;
- letters or emails;
- audit trails;
- learning contracts (see Appendices 4 and 5).

Writing your narrative

It is not enough simply to present your evidence in a portfolio. You need to build up a clear and convincing discussion of what your evidence demonstrates, for you are trying to persuade your peer reviewer that the evidence is fit for accreditation.

Just as a barrister will have to use different pieces of evidence to make a case to persuade a jury of guilt or innocence of a client, you will have to do the same to demonstrate that you have met the standards and competencies in question. You must select your evidence thoughtfully and then link this to particular outcomes, standards or competencies and then seek to persuade your peer reviewer.

For each standard you need to submit your evidence of achievement and write a narrative to argue the case. Remember that a single piece of evidence can be used to demonstrate several competencies.

You might want to include an identification of your strengths and where you need to develop further. Do not forget to articulate aspects of practice which may be taken for granted – things you would not normally think twice about. Be rigorous in putting everything you do under the microscope. Finally, do not be too humble; do not undervalue your own expertise.

Now get out your own portfolio and look at the methods you have used within it to capture evidence of your ability to develop your practice. Have you used all or any of the ways described above? They are not prescriptive, but offered as a variety of methods which might work for some practitioners. You might like to select a way of exploring practice that you have not used before and try it on your own practice.

CAPTURING THE EVIDENCE

So far we have discussed a number of different sorts of evidence that might be submitted in support of the claim for accreditation against a set of standards. All of this evidence is collected and assembled in a portfolio which can be peer reviewed.

Professional portfolios

One of the most commonly used definitions of a portfolio is provided by Brown (1995):

> … a private collection of evidence which demonstrates the continuing acquisition of skills, knowledge, attitudes, understanding and achievement. It is both retrospective and prospective as well as indicating the current state of development and activity of the individual.

The maintenance of a personal professional portfolio serves a number of useful purposes, including:

- valuing yourself and your skills and knowledge both personally and as a professional;
- keeping a record of professional updating for NMC post-registration education and practice requirements;
- providing evidence for performance appraisal;
- the identification of needs during staff development review;
- aiding career management and development;
- providing additional insights into your experience for your current or prospective employer;
- demonstrating independent learning;
- encouraging reflective practice;
- providing a permanent record of achievement over time.

Brown sees a *profile* as:

> … constructed from evidence selected from the personal portfolio for a particular purpose and for the attention of a particular audience.

A portfolio of evidence for accreditation is more than a profile but less than a general personal portfolio of lifelong learning. It is a purposeful and systematic collection of evidence that sets out to demonstrate how its author 'measures up' against the standards or competencies set for the accreditation scheme in question. It is not private and so issues of confidentiality, accountability and the moral and ethical decisions about selection and preparation of material are important.

The standards (usually accompanied by performance criteria) or competencies are determined by experts in the area of clinical practice under consideration.

The portfolio of evidence is assessed for sufficiency and rigour by peers. The process of compilation is frequently facilitated and is seen as a developmental opportunity in itself.

Remember that the rigour with which you compile your portfolio for accreditation may enable you to use it to for academic recognition as well as, for example, providing evidence for an accreditation of prior learning (APL) or an accreditation of prior experiential learning (APEL) submission for academic credit.

The portfolio describes the journey towards the acquisition of the standards, detailing the reflections, insights, knowledge and skills gained along the way. It therefore describes a journey – often over a period of 1 to 2 years, which forms a focused part of the overall lifetime career and learning journey.

Each portfolio will be highly personalized so that what is relevant information to some practitioners will not be significant or pertinent to the clinical situation, experience or learning of others.

What to include in your portfolio

The following are general suggestions; the accreditation scheme that you are following may differ in its guidance and you should follow that.

1 Your CV, which should include:
   - relevant professional details, e.g. NMC registration PIN;
   - membership of professional organizations, e.g. RCN;
   - professional/academic qualifications;
   - employment history;
   - unpaid/voluntary and leisure activities.
2 Descriptions(s): these should include significant operational areas/skills and synopsis of current roles and responsibilities in clinical practice.
3 A supporting letter from your facilitator/manager (or other appropriate senior practitioner). The letter is a statement of verification that the standards/competencies described in your portfolio have been demonstrated in practice and that the evidence is your own work.
4 The next sections should be divided into information about, and evidence to support, each standard or competency that you wish to include in your application for accreditation. It may be useful to use the following format:
   - title of the standard or competency;
   - introduction – a short paragraph introducing the standard or competency – this should cover how you acquired your skill/learning. Refer, where appropriate, to your CV, job description, etc. rather than repeating information. You may want to expand parts of your CV or job description(s) in order to give more detailed contextual information;
   - relevant training – list any relevant training/continuing professional development undertaken;
   - description of skill/learning – this should be a breakdown of the knowledge, skills and abilities you are submitting as evidence in the portfolio. What is required here is not a bald statement of what you have done, but identification of the intellectual activity involved. Ask yourself what decisions you had to take when delivering a particular aspect of care, what factors you had to take into account and, most importantly, if you were doing this again what would you repeat or do differently and why?

You may wish to express your skills/learning/knowledge by the following terms framework:

Knowledge	I am able to list/state/outline, e.g. the key principles or the evidence underpinning, say, wound care.
Understanding	I can discuss/explain/clarify/identify, e.g. the policy of/procedures for, say, maintaining tissue viability.
Application	I can illustrate/demonstrate/apply, e.g. the process of moving and handling a person with paraplegia.
Analysis	I know how to distinguish/contrast/compare/calculate, e.g. the effectiveness of a patient breast awareness programme.

| Synthesis | I am able to organize/set up, e.g. a multiprofessional care conference. |
| Evaluation | I know how to evaluate/appraise/assess/review, e.g. the care planned in relation to the nutrition of a patient having chemotherapy. |

The evidence

A good portfolio is more than a simple collection of paper; it should be a systematic collection and integration of robust evidence, which demonstrates that the standards for accreditation have been met (Pearce 2003, Hull et al. 2005). It should contain:

- Evidence that is consistent, has sufficient coverage and quality, and arises from different sources.
- Synthesis of the evidence to show attainment of standards, together with reader direction, i.e. you must present the evidence so that the reader is guided through it and shown how it demonstrates that the standards are met. To help with this, you may wish to analyse facilitation contracts, records and evaluations.
- evidence of learning through the experience of gathering and interpreting evidence.

Nobody expects that the evidence will show 'perfect' practice; one of the key attributes of being a professional is lifelong learning, and so the portfolio should contain reflective commentary on further learning required and action points for improving practice. In other words, it is not enough merely to provide the raw evidence; you will need to analyse, interpret and assess it. You should consider the source of the evidence, what to do with the information you find there, and your own and others' assessment of whether it shows you meet the standards and criteria for accreditation.

On the other hand, it is vital to remember that it is quality that counts, not quantity. A portfolio may rest on only a small number of sessions, events or projects that have been explored in depth, from a variety of viewpoints, and properly analysed and presented. Peer reviewers recognize that you are probably preparing your portfolio in the context of a busy and often stressful workplace.

Each standard or competency should be substantiated by evidence, which demonstrates the knowledge/skills for which you are seeking accreditation. It may be useful to write a one-page summary indicating how the evidence supports the claim that you have met the criteria. The same pieces of evidence can be used more than once; cross-refer to your CV, job description or other standards/competencies as appropriate.

PEER REVIEW OF THE EVIDENCE

The peer review process facilitates verification of the candidate's claims that he or she has achieved the standards, performance criteria and/or competencies in question. It also provides an opportunity for the candidate to receive detailed developmental feedback on their practice; celebrating the strengths and highlighting areas which would benefit from development.

Peer review may occur at a distance from the person seeking accreditation or face-to-face through a critical review panel. Whatever method is chosen, the portfolio is usually reviewed by a pair of reviewers, at least one of whom is external to where the candidate practices and who does not know the candidate; frequently, both reviewers have no previous knowledge of or connection with the accreditee.

It is common for one of the pair to be an expert in the candidate's area of clinical practice.

A third person is usually involved as a moderator. This person will moderate a percentage of all the portfolios and also any that give rise to concern. Their role is to monitor the outcome of the first review and to quality assure the process. They also evaluate the objectivity of the feedback offered.

The reviewers are chosen for their educational and practice expertise, and for their prior experience of the review process. They are familiar with the standards in question and usually are supplied with review criteria so that all reviewers are tackling the job in a consistent manner.

CONCLUSION

This chapter should have gone some way towards giving you a greater sense of confidence about either preparing your own portfolio or facilitating others in compiling theirs. Remember, there are always people who can help you with both support and challenge in your collection of appropriate evidence. It may be helpful to look at how others have compiled their portfolios – but there is no one right way of doing it – every portfolio is unique. However, the one question you have to ask is: does it show that I can meet the standards/competencies in question? If the answer is yes, then you should merit accreditation.

REFERENCES

I would like to acknowledge the use of a variety of unpublished work, internal papers, systems and processes, reports, etc., that have been developed by both the Practice Development Team and the staff of the Accreditation Unit at the Royal College of Nursing (RCN). The intellectual property belongs to the RCN. The work evolved over time with adaptation by myself and numerous authors whom it is not possible now to identify, but for whose efforts I am grateful.

Brown, R. (1995) *Portfolio development and profiling for nurses.* Lancaster: Quay Publishing.
Hull, C. Redfern, L. and Shuttleworth, A. (2005) *Profiles and portfolios: a guide for health and social care*, 2nd edn. Basingstoke: Palgrave Macmillan.
Johns, C. (1996) Visualising and realising caring in practice through guided reflection. *Journal of Advanced Nursing* 24: 1135–1143.
McGill, I. and Beaty, L. (1998) *Action learning.* London: Kogan Page.
Pearce, R. (2003) *Profiles and portfolios of evidence: foundations in nursing and health care.* Cheltenham, Nelson Thornes.
Scrivens, E. (1995) *Accreditation: protecting the professional or the consumer?* Buckingham: Open University Press.
Titchen, A. and Ersser, S. (2001) The nature of professional craft knowledge. In *Practice knowledge and expertise in the health professions*, Higgs, J. and Titchen, A. (eds), pp. 35–42. Oxford: Butterworth Heinemann.
Ward, P. (1997) *360 degree feedback.* London: Institute of Personnel and Development.

APPENDIX 1: MAPPING OF THE NMC-PROPOSED COMPETENCIES AGAINST THE KNOWLEDGE AND SKILLS FRAMEWORK

Reproduced with permission of the Royal College of Nursing and the Nursing and Midwifery Council

NMC competence	KSF dimension
THE NURSE–PATIENT RELATIONSHIP	
Creates a climate of mutual trust and establishes partnerships with patients, carers and families	C1 L4
Validates and checks findings with patients	C1 L4
Creates a relationship with patients that acknowledges their strengths and knowledge and assists them in addressing their needs	C1 L4 HWB4 L4
Communicates a sense of 'being there' for the patient, carers and families and provides comfort and emotional support	C1 L4
Evaluates the impact of life transitions on the health/illness status of patients, and the impact of health/illness on patients' lives (individuals, families, carers, and communities)	C1 L4
Applies principles of empowerment in promoting behaviour change	C1 L4
Develops and maintains the patient's control over decision-making, assesses the patient's commitment to the jointly determined plan of care, and fosters personal responsibility for health	C1 L4 HWB4 L4
Maintains confidentiality, while recording data, plans and results in a manner that preserves the dignity and privacy of the patient	C1 L4 C3 L4 HWB2 L4
Monitors and reflects on own emotional response to interaction with patients, carers and families and uses this knowledge to further therapeutic interaction	C1 L4 C2 L4
Considers the patient's needs when bringing closure to the nurse–patient relationship and provides for a safe transition to another care provider or independence	C1 L4 HWB4 L4

(Continued)

(*Continued*)

NMC competence	KSF dimension
RESPECTING CULTURE AND DIVERSITY	
Demonstrates respect for the inherent dignity of every human being, whatever their age, gender, religion, socioeconomic class, sexual orientation and ethnic or cultural group	C6 L4 HWB4 L4
Accepts the rights of individuals to choose their care provider, participate in care and refuse care	C6 L4 HWB4 L4
Acknowledges their own personal biases and actively seeks to address them while ensuring the delivery of quality care	C2 L4 C6 L3
Actively promotes diversity and equality	C6 L4
Incorporates cultural preferences, health beliefs and behaviours into management plans as appropriate	C6 L4
Provides patient-appropriate educational materials that address the language and cultural beliefs of the patient	IK3 L3
Accesses patient appropriate resources to deliver care	C5 L2 C6 L4
Supports patients from marginalized groups to access quality care	C6 L4
Spiritual competencies	
Respects the inherent worth and dignity of each person and the right to express spiritual beliefs	C6 L4 HWB5 L4
Assists patients and families to meet their spiritual needs in the context of health and illness experiences, including referral for pastoral services	C6 L4 HWB4 L4 HWB5 L4
Assesses the influence of patients' spirituality on their health care behaviours and practices	C6 L4 HWB4 L4 HWB5 L4
Incorporates patients' spiritual beliefs in the care plan	C6 L4 HWB4 L4 HWB5 L4
Provides appropriate information and opportunity for patients, carers and families to discuss their wishes for end-of-life decision-making and care	C6 L3 IK3 L4 HWB L4
Respects wishes of patients and families regarding expression of spiritual beliefs	C6 L4 HWB4 L4 HWB5 L4
MANAGEMENT OF PATIENT HEALTH/ILLNESS STATUS	
Health promotion/health protection and disease prevention	
Assesses individual's health education/promotion-related needs	HWB1 L4 HWB2 L4 HWB4 L4

NMC competence	KSF dimension
Plans, develops and implements programmes to promote health and well-being and address individual needs	HWB1 L3
	HWB2 L4
	HWB3 L3
	HWB4 L4
	HWB5 L4
	HWB6 L4
Provides health education through anticipatory guidance and counselling to promote health, reduce risk factors, and prevent disease and disability	HWB1 L3
	HWB3 L3
	HWB4 L4
	HWB5 L4
Develops and uses a follow-up system within the practice workplace to ensure that patients receive appropriate services	HWB3 L4
	HWB5 L4
	HWB7 L4
	IK1 L2
Recognizes environmental health problems affecting patients and provides health protection interventions that promote healthy environments for individuals, families and communities	C3 L4
	HWB3 L3

Management of patient illness

Analyses and interprets history, presenting symptoms, physical findings and diagnostic information to develop the appropriate differential diagnoses	HWB6 L4
	HWB7 L4
Diagnoses and manages acute and long-term conditions while attending to the patient's response to the illness experience	C3 L4
	HWB3 L4
	HWB5 L4
	HWB6 L4
	HWB7 L4
Prioritizes health problems and intervenes appropriately, including initiation of effective emergency care	C3 L4
	HWB3 L4
	HWB5 L4
	HWB7 L4
Employs appropriate diagnostic and therapeutic interventions and regimens with attention to safety, cost, invasiveness, simplicity, acceptability, adherence and efficacy	C5 L3
	IK3 L4
	HWB5 L4
	HWB7 L4
	HWB8 L3
	HWB10 L3
Formulates an action plan based on scientific rationale, evidence-based standards of care and practice guidelines	HWB5 L4
	HWB6 L4
	HWB7 L4
Provides guidance, counselling, advice and support regarding management of the health/illness condition	CI L4
	HWB1 L4
	HWB3 L4
	HWB5 L4

(Continued)

(*Continued*)

NMC competence	KSF dimension
Initiates appropriate and timely consultation and/or referral when the problem exceeds the nurse's scope of practice and/or expertise	C1 L4 IK1 L3 HWB6 L4
Assesses and intervenes to assist the patient in complex, urgent or emergency situations	
A. Rapidly assesses the patient's unstable and complex health care problems through synthesis and prioritization of historical and immediately derived data	HWB2 L4 HWB6 L4 HWB8 L4
B. Diagnoses unstable and complex health care problems using collaboration and consultation with the multiprofessional health care team as indicated by setting, specialty and individual knowledge and experience	C1 L4 IK1 L3 HWB8 L4
C. Plans and implements diagnostic strategies and therapeutic interventions to help patients with unstable and complex health care problems regain stability and restore health, in collaboration with the patient and multiprofessional health care team	C1 L4 C3 L4 IK1 L3 HWB3 L4 HWB5 L4 HWB7 L4 HWB8 L4
D. Rapidly and continuously evaluates the patient's changing condition and response to therapeutic interventions and modifies the plan of care for optimal patient outcome	C3 L4 HWB3 L4 HWB5 L4 HWB7 L4 HWB8 L4 HWB10 L3
For health promotion/health protection and disease prevention, and management of patient illness	
Demonstrates critical thinking and diagnostic reasoning skills in clinical decision-making	HWB5 L4 HWB6 L4 HWB7 L4
Obtains a comprehensive and/or problem-focused health history from the patient or carer	C1 L4 HWB2 L4 HWB6 L4
Performs a comprehensive and/or problem-focused physical examination	HWB2 L4 HWB6 L4
Analyses the data collected to determine health status	C1 L4 HWB2 L4 HWB6 L4
Formulates a problem list and prioritized management plan	HWB2 L4 HWB6 L4

NMC competence	KSF dimension
Assesses, diagnoses, monitors, coordinates and manages the health/illness status of patients over time and supports the patient through the process of dying	HWB2 L4 HWB5 L4 HWB6 L4 HWB7 L4 HWB8 L3
Demonstrates knowledge of the pathophysiology of acute and chronic conditions or conditions commonly seen in practice	HWB6 L4
Communicates the patient's health status using appropriate terminology, format and technology	C1 L4 IK1 L3 HWB2 L4 HWB3 L4
Applies principles of epidemiology and demography in clinical practice by recognizing populations at risk, patterns of disease, and effectiveness of prevention and intervention	IK1 L3 HWB2 L4 HWB3 L3 HWB6 L4 HWB7 L4
Acquires and uses community/public health assessment information in evaluating patient needs, initiating referrals, coordinating care and programme planning	HWB2 L4 HWB6 L4
Applies theories and evidence to guide practice	C5 L4 IK2 L3 IK3 L4 HWB7 L4
Provides information and advice to patients and carers concerning drug regimens, side-effects and interaction in an appropriate form	C1 L4 HWB1 L4 HWB5 L4
If legally authorized, prescribes medications based on efficacy, safety and cost from the formulary	HWB3 L4 HWB5 L4 HWB7 L4 HWB10 L4
Evaluates the use of complementary/alternative therapies used by patients for safety and potential interaction	HWB5 L4 HWB10 L4
Integrates appropriate non-drug-based treatment methods into a plan of management	HWB1 L4 HWB5 L4 HWB7 L4
Orders, may perform, and interprets common screening and diagnostic tests	HWB2 L4 HWB6 L4 HWB8 L3
Evaluates results of interventions using accepted outcome criteria, revises the plan accordingly, and consults/refers when needed	C1 L4 IK1 L3

(*Continued*)

(*Continued*)

NMC competence	KSF dimension
	HWB3 L4
	HWB5 L4
	HWB7 L4
	HWB8 L3
Collaborates with other health professionals and agencies as appropriate	C1 L4
	C4 L3
	IK1 L3
Schedules follow-up visits appropriately to monitor patients and evaluate health/illness care	HWB3 L4
	HWB5 L4
	HWB7 L4

THE EDUCATION FUNCTION

Timing

Assesses the on-going and changing needs of patients, carers and families for education based on the following:

A. Needs for anticipatory guidance associated with growth and the developmental stage	C2 L4
	HWB4 L4
	G1 L3
B. Care management that requires specific information or skills	C2 L4
	G1 L3
C. The patient's understanding of their health condition	C2 L4
	G1 L3
Assesses the patient's motivation for learning and maintenance of health-related activities using principles of change and stages of behaviour change	C2 L4
	G1 L3
Creates an environment in which effective learning can take place	C2 L4
	G1 L3

Eliciting

Elicits information about the patient's interpretation of health conditions as a part of the routine health assessment	HWB2 L3
	G1 L3
Elicits information about the patient's perceived barriers, supports, and modifiers to learning when preparing for patient's education	G1 L3
Elicits from the patient the characteristics of learning style from which to plan and implement the teaching	G1 L3
Elicits information about cultural influences that may affect the patient's learning experience	G1 L3

NMC competence	KSF dimension
Assisting	
Assists patients by displaying a sensitivity to the effort and emotions associated with learning about how to care for one's health condition	C2 L4 G1 L3
Assists patients in learning specific information or skills by designing a learning plan that is comprised of sequential, cumulative steps, and that acknowledges relapse and the need for practice, reinforcement, support and re-teaching when necessary	C2 L4 G1 L3 HWB1 L3 HWB4 L4
Assists patients to use community resources when needed	C2 L4 HWB4 L4
Providing	
Communicates health advice and instruction appropriately, using an evidence-based rationale	C1 L4 HWB1 L3 G1 L3
Negotiating	
Negotiates a jointly determined plan of care, based on continual assessment of the patient's readiness and motivation, re-setting goals and optimal outcomes	C2 L4 HWB4 L3 G1 L3
Monitors the patient's behaviours and specific outcomes as a guide to evaluating the effectiveness and need to change or maintain educational strategies	C2 L4 HWB5 L4
Coaching	
Coaches the patient by reminding, supporting and encouraging, using empathy	C2 L4 G1 L3
PROFESSIONAL ROLE	
Develops and implements the advanced nurse practitioner role	
Uses evidence and research to implement the role	IK3 L4
Functions in a variety of role dimensions: advanced health care provider, co-ordinator, consultant, educator, coach, advocate, administrator, researcher, role model and leader	C2 L4 HWB2 L4 G7 L3
Interprets and markets the role to the public, legislators, policy-maker and other health care professions	C4 L3 G8 L2
Directs care	
Prioritizes, coordinates and meets multiple needs for culturally diverse patients	HWB5 L4 HWB7 L4

(*Continued*)

(*Continued*)

NMC competence	KSF dimension
Uses sound judgement in assessing conflicting priorities and needs	HWB2 L4 HWB6 L4 HWB7 L4
Builds and maintains a therapeutic team to provide optimum therapy	C1 L4 C4 L4 C5 L4 G7 L2
Obtains specialist and referral care for patients while remaining the primary care provider	C1 L4 C4 L3 HWB7 L4
Acts as an advocate for the patient to ensure health needs are met consistent with patient's wishes	C6 L3 HWB3 L2
Consults with other health care providers and public/independent agencies	C1 L4 C4 L3
Incorporates current technology appropriately in care delivery	HWB6 L3 HWB7 L3
Uses information systems to support decision-making and to improve care	C5 L4 IK3 L4

Provides leadership

Is actively involved in a professional association	C2 L3
Evaluates implications of contemporary health policy on health care providers and consumers	C4 L3 HWB1 L4 G2 L2 G7 L2
Participates in legislative and policy-making activities that influence an advanced level of nursing practice and the health of communities	C4 L3 HWB1 L4 G2 L2
Advocates for access to quality, cost-effective health care	C4 L3 C6L3
Evaluates the relationship between community/public health issues and social problems as they impact on the health care of patients (poverty, literacy, violence, etc.)	C4 L3 HWB1 L3
Actively engages in continuing professional development and maintains a suitable record of this development	C2 L3

MANAGING AND NEGOTIATING HEALTH CARE DELIVERY SYSTEMS

Managing

Demonstrates knowledge about the role	C3 L3

NMC competence	KSF dimension
Provides care for individuals, families, and communities within integrated health care services	C5 L3 HWB7 L4
Considers access, cost, efficacy, and quality when making care decisions	C5 L3
Maintains current knowledge of their employing organization and the financing of the health care system as it affects delivery of care	C5 L3 G4 L2
Participates in organizational decision-making, interprets variations in outcomes, and uses data from information systems to improve practice	C5 L3 IK2 L2
Manages organizational functions and resources within the scope of responsibilities as defined in a job description	C5 L3 IK2 L2 G5 L3
Uses business and management strategies for the provision of quality care and efficient use of resources	C5 L3 G5 L3
Demonstrates knowledge of business principles that affect long-term financial viability of an organization, the efficient use of resources, and quality of care	C5 L3 G4 L2
Demonstrates knowledge of, and acts in accordance with, relevant regulations for this level of practice and the *NMC code* (NMC, 2008).	C3 L3 C5 L3

Negotiating

Collaboratively assesses, plans, implements, and evaluates care with other health care professionals, using approaches that recognize each one's expertise to meet the comprehensive needs of patients	C1 L4 HWB5 L4
Undertakes risk assessments and manages risk effectively	C3 L4
Participates as a key member of a multiprofessional team through the development of collaborative and innovative practices	G2 L3
Participates in planning, development, and implementation of public and community health programmes	HWB1 L3
Participates in legislative and policy-making activities that influence health services/practice	HWB1 L3
Advocates for policies that reduce environmental health risks	C3 L4 HWB1 L4
Advocates for policies that are culturally sensitive	C3 L3 C6 L3
Advocates for increasing access to health care for all	C3 L3 C6 L3

(*Continued*)

(*Continued*)

NMC competence	KSF dimension
MONITORING AND ENSURING THE QUALITY OF ADVANCED HEALTH CARE PRACTICE	
Ensuring quality	
Incorporates professional/legal standards into advanced clinical practice	C5 L4
Acts ethically to meet the needs of the patient in all situations, however complex	C5 L4 HWB5 L4
Assumes accountability for practice and strives to attain the highest standards of practice	C4 L3 C5 L3
Engages in clinical supervision and self-evaluation and uses this to improve care and practice	C2 L4 C5 L2
Collaborates and/or consults with members of the health care team about variations in health outcomes	C5 L3 HWB5 L4
Promotes and uses an evidence-based approach to patient management that critically evaluates and applies research findings pertinent to patient care management and outcomes	C5 L3 HWB7 L4 G2 L4
Evaluates the patients' response to the health care provided and the effectiveness of the care	HWB5 L4
Interprets and uses the outcomes of care to revise care delivery strategies and improve the quality of care	C4 L3 C5 L3 HWB7 L4
Accepts personal responsibility for professional development and the maintenance of professional competence and credentials	C2 L4 C5 L2
Monitoring quality	
Monitors quality of own practice and participates in continuous quality improvement	C5 L4
Actively seeks and participates in peer review of own practice	C2 L4
Evaluates patient follow-up and outcomes, including consultation and referral	C5 L3 HWB7 L4
Monitors current evidence-based literature in order to improve quality care	C5 L3 G2 L4

REFERENCE

NMC (2008) *The code. Standards of conduct, performance and ethics for nurses and midwives.* London: Nursing and Midwifery Council.

APPENDIX 2: NURSE PRACTITIONER RADIOGRAPH REFERRAL GUIDELINES

1 Eligibility criteria of nurse practitioners

Referrer to be a formally recognized nurse practitioner (NP) who has completed a first degree/post-graduate diploma/MSc or a recognized programme in nurse practitioner studies

Referring NP will undergo annual appraisals with another trained NP colleague

Referrer has attended the 'Basics of Ionizing Radiation' course and is registered with the X-ray department

2 Criteria for requests

All X-ray referrals will meet the standards outlined by the RCR Working Party[1]

Referrer will ensure correct biographical information is entered on the request form

Referrer will complete relevant clinical information and anatomical area to be viewed on the request card

Appropriate verbal and/or written information will be provided to the patient by the NP at the time of referral and this will be documented in the clinical record

3 Exclusions

X-rays will not be requested in place of an examination

Pregnancy will be excluded in female patients and LMP documented on request card

4 Referral for chest X-ray (CXR)

4.1 NPs may refer children and adults for CXR for the following indications:
Persistent unexplained cough >4/52
Haemoptysis
Unexplained SOB
Unexplained weight loss/night sweats/lymphadenopathy
Hoarseness >4/52
Severe exacerbation of COPD
Suspected heart failure
Suspected pleural effusion
Suspected TB
Suspected pneumonia
Suspected pneumothorax
Suspected inhalation of foreign body

4.2 Request for X-ray investigation should never replace admitting the patient acutely if this would be more appropriate

4.3 The following are NOT indicated:

Routine diagnosis and treatment of hypertension	Simple URTI
Routine follow-up of asthma/COPD	Uncomplicated rib fracture

5 REFERRALS (adults only)

5.1 Elbow/hand/wrist X-ray

Wrist injury, elbow trauma
X-ray may also be indicated to determine the presence of a soft tissue foreign body

5.2 Ankle/foot X-ray

Ottawa guidelines[2] apply (see reference at the end of this section)

Ankle – refer for X-ray if there is pain in the malleolar area plus:
Bone tenderness at the posterior tip of lateral malleolus, or
Bone tenderness at the medial tip of the malleous, or
Patient unable to weight-bear at time of injury and when examined

Foot – refer if there is pain in the midfoot plus:

Bone tenderness at the 5th metatarsal base, or
Bone tenderness at the navicular, or
Patient unable to weight-bear at the time of the injury and when examined
NB: if there is a history of acute injury it may be more appropriate to refer the patient
to A&E for a full assessment and management

5.3 Knee X-ray

Knee pain with locking to identify radio-opaque loose bodies

5.4 Hip X-ray

Chronic hip pain where there is a history of:

Past trauma
Full or limited range of movement with persistent symptoms
Night and/or rest pain
Associated risk factors, e.g. SLE, sickle cell, use of steroids – exclude avascular necrosis
Diagnosis in doubt

5.5 Shoulder X-ray

Persistent (6/52), severe pain unresponsive to treatment
Thoracic inlet X-ray: if suspected cervical rib (indicated by hand or forearm pain,
weakness or numbness and thenar or hypothenar wasting)

6 Ordering an X-ray investigation is equivalent to writing a prescription for radiation

7 References

1. RCR Working Party. *Making the best use of a department of clinical radiology: guidelines for doctors,* 5th edn. London: The Royal College of Radiologists, 2003.

2. Stiell I, Wells G, Laupacis A et al. Multicentre trial to introduce the Ottawa ankle rules for use of radiography in acute ankle injuries. *British Medical Journal* 1995, 311: 594–597.

8 Review

These guidelines will become effective from 1st January 2006 and will be reviewed after 12 months

Signed _____ Supporting Clinician

APPENDIX 3: PORTFOLIO DEVELOPMENT

Appendices 3–5 have been adapted with permission from the Faculty of Society and Health, Buckinghamshire New University, UK, 27 November 2006.

PORTFOLIO DEVELOPMENT

Critical reflection is central to professional growth and development and the maintenance of competent professional practice. Advanced nursing practice professionals will be required to maintain a portfolio of evidence of their competence in accordance with the Nursing and Midwifery Council (RCN 2007) Domains and Competencies. The portfolio needs to contain reflections in relation to specific activities and be formally presented. Advanced nursing practice professionals will be required to undertake critical thinking, analysis, research and technical skills through practising structured reflection which will enable them to achieve the required competencies.

A list of skills necessary to complete your portfolio is shown below.

- You should undertake a self-assessment of learning needs for discussion with your mentor/assessor.
- You should undertake a formative clinical assessment interview with mentor/assessor to determine your strengths and weaknesses in relation to the specific domains and competencies, which must then be signed and included in the portfolio.
- You should agree personal learning objectives to address the particular competence that you intend to achieve, which will be identified and achieved through the case management entries. You must demonstrate that you are working at advanced level and fulfil the criteria of the NMC domains and competencies. This should be agreed and signed by your mentor/assessor and included in your portfolio.
- You should undertake an intermediate assessment interview to assess your learning needs in relation to the domain and competencies and your overall progress with your mentor/assessor which must be signed and included in the portfolio.
- You should ensure that your mentor/assessor writes and signs a summative assessment sheet for inclusion in the portfolio at the end of your period of learning.
- You should also complete a self-assessment of your learning and discuss this with your mentor/assessor at your final assessment interview.
- You should use supportive evidence to show that you have achieved *all* the NMC domains and competencies, i.e. clinical examinations/clinical cases/critical incidences.
- You must devise a mapping grid to cross reference the evidence with the competencies.
- You should submit all work in support of your achievement in your portfolio when required by the NMC for your registration as an advanced nurse practitioner.

The learning log is also a useful tool which will help you to achieve your competencies and should be submitted as part of the marked portfolio. It should show evidence of patients through the eyes of the advancing nursing practitioner. The overall focus should be on quality not quantity and it should show the breadth and depth of patient interactions. Entries should be dated and demonstrate the learning that has taken place and should include details of both your personal and professional development.

You must ensure that you have included all the required components as listed in this document and that they have been signed and validated by your mentor/assessor. The facilitator will be a qualified nurse holding an appropriate advanced nurse practitioner qualification, or a medical practitioner with experience of working with advanced nurse practitioners.

The facilitator is responsible for promoting and developing the professional role and knowledge of the student and for assessing his/her competence in practice.

REFERENCE

Royal College Nursing (2007). *RCN Domains and Competencies for UK Advanced Nurse Practitioner Practice*. London: RCN.

APPENDIX 4: LEARNING CONTRACT EXAMPLE

CASE PRESENTATION
Name:
Mentor:
Start date: Completion date:
Discussion/description of case (practitioners should include case notes as an appendix)
Reflection on the decision-making process that was made within the consultation
My strengths and limitations (what was done well and what skills needs to be developed)
Demonstration of interprofessional collaboration and leadership skills (i.e. any involvement of the interprofessional team, referrals, etc.)
Personal action plan (learning objectives)
NMC domain and competency
Evidence produced which supports that the competence has been achieved (including policies and documents)
Signature of student   Date
Signature of facilitator   Date

Clinical Assessment – Formative

Summative Assessment by Mentor/Assessor

Observations of student learning and verification of achievement of specified competence.

Name of student: _____

EXAMPLE: STATEMENT OF PRACTICE COMPETENCE

The above-named practitioner has successfully achieved the cultural competencies relating to advanced practice and is competent in practice according to the NMC Domains and Competencies for advanced nurse practitioners.

Mentor's/Assessor's signature:

Print name:

The portfolio entries should demonstrate a mastery of the subject areas, with evidence of creative and innovative thought and encompassing various perspectives. You need to consistently apply theory and research to inform your decision-making and problem-solving in practice. A range of sources are needed to demonstrate your learning with clear articulation of progress and development.

APPENDIX 5: LEARNING CONTRACT GUIDE

Practitioners are required to set up learning contracts with your mentor/assessor within your area of clinical practice. You should select areas of practice relating to the particular competence that you wish to develop. This should be a substantial learning need that can justify a learning contract facilitated over a period of weeks. A learning contract should be developed for each competence you would like to achieve.

ORGANIZATION AND PLANNING

Select and negotiate with your mentor/assessor which competence you would like to achieve.
Agree the number of weeks for the contract.
Set time and date for the first meeting.
Agree length of first meeting.
Agree frequency of review meetings.

PROCESS

Discuss learning needs and agree objectives.
Plan a strategy for learning.
Agree assessment of learning strategy.
Discuss 'working with' activities (if any).
Discuss self-directed targets.
Discuss supervision, delegated activities, practice activities (as appropriate to the particular competence you would like to achieve).
Assess progress and provide feedback.
Time management-plot the learning process in advance and monitor progress.

OUTCOMES

Assess the level of progress made (formative).
Assess the level of achievement that is made by you (summative).
Identify strengths and areas for further development in relation to the particular cultural competence to be achieved.
Evaluate the overall effectiveness of the learning contract.

RESOURCES

Identify the literature, procedures and protocols that are needed.

Identify prescribed activities, visits, outpostings, study days and key people relevant to the learning process.
Identify the amount of contact time between mentor and learner.

PORTFOLIO

Learning contracts should be entered into the portfolio to demonstrate your progression. This will record aspects of your transition to advanced practitioner.

INDEX

Note: Appendix references are in bold.